WOMEN'S HEALTH FOR LIFE

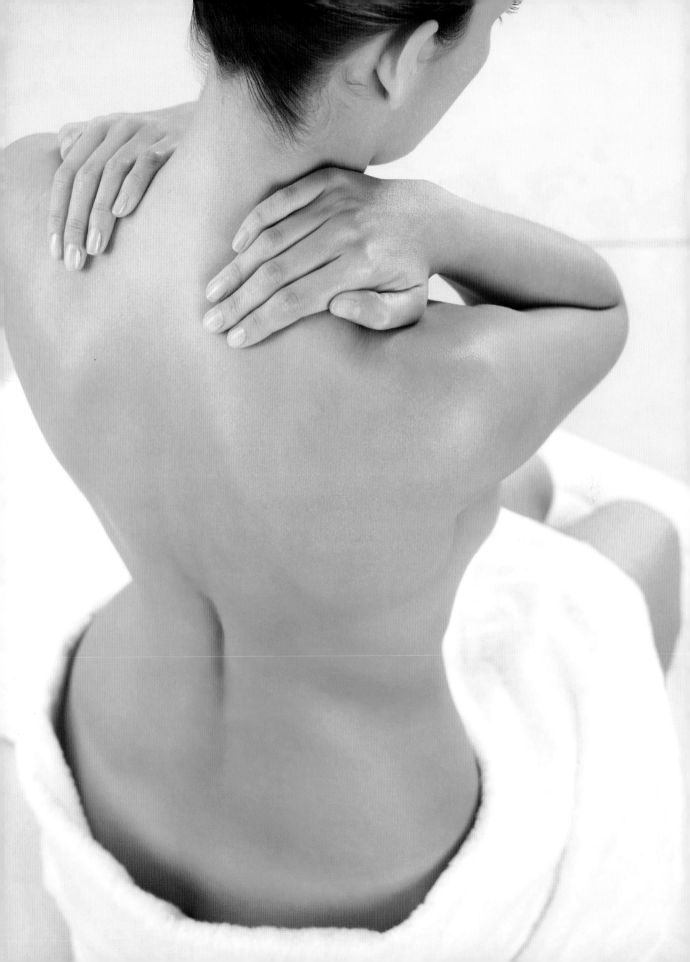

WOMEN'S HEALTH FOR LIFE

WRITTEN FOR WOMEN BY WOMEN
SYMPTOMS · TREATMENT · PREVENTION

EDITOR-IN-CHIEF **DONNICA MOORE** MD
& A TEAM OF WORLD-CLASS WOMEN DOCTORS

LONDON, NEW YORK, MELBOURNE,
MUNICH, AND DELHI

Project Editor Hilary Mandleberg
Senior Editor Jennifer Latham
Senior Art Editor Isabel de Cordova
Designers Kenny Grant, John Round
Editors Ann Baggaley, Debbie Beckerman,
Claire Cross, Jo Godfrey-Wood, Mary Lindsay,
Cathy Meeus, Pip Morgan, Martyn Page,
Nikki Sims, Susannah Steel, Kathy Steer,
Diana Vowles
Managing Editor Dawn Henderson
Managing Art Editor Christine Keilty
Senior Production Editor Jenny Woodcock
Senior Jacket Creative Nicola Powling
Picture Research Liz Moore, Jenny Baskaya
Creative Technical Support Sonia Charbonnier
Senior Production Controller Wendy Penn

First American Edition, 2009

Published in the United States by
DK Publishing, 375 Hudson Street
New York, New York 10014

09 10 11 10 9 8 7 6 5 4 3 2 1

Published in Great Britain by Dorling Kindersley Limited.

A catalog record for this book
is available from the Library of Congress

ISBN 978-0-7566-4277-8

DK books are available at special discounts when purchased
in bulk for sales promotions, premiums, fund-raising, or
educational use. For details, contact: DK Publishing Special
Markets, 375 Hudson Street, New York, New York 10014 or
SpecialSales@dk.com.

Note to readers: *Women's Health for Life* provides general
information on a wide range of health and medical topics.
The book is not a substitute for medical diagnosis, however,
and you are advised always to consult your doctor for
specific information on personal health matters. The
Publisher cannot accept any liability or responsibility for any
loss or damage allegedly arising from any information or
suggestion in this book.

Color reproduced by MDP, UK
Printed in China by Hung Hing Offset Ltd

Discover more at
www.dk.com

The Authors

EDITOR-IN-CHIEF
DONNICA L. MOORE MD is nationally regarded as a women's health expert. Known as "Dr. Donnica," she is President of the Sapphire Women's Health Group and hosts DrDonnica.com, a popular women's health information website. She has appeared on over 500 television interviews, including "The Oprah Winfrey Show," "Weekend Today," "The View," "The Rachael Ray Show," and many others. A graduate of Princeton University and SUNY Buffalo School of Medicine, Dr. Donnica has received numerous awards for her work.

JUDITH C. ANDERSON MD is Director at the Center for Bleeding Disorders and Thrombosis, Wayne State University School of Medicine, Karmanos Cancer Institute, Detroit.

CATHERINE A. BIRNDORF MD is Clinical Associate Professor of Psychiatry and Obstetrics and Gynecology at the New York Presbyterian Hospital, Weill Cornell Medical Center, New York.

ROBIN K. DORE MD, FACR is Clinical Professor of Medicine in the Division of Rheumatology at the David Geffen School of Medicine at the University of California, Los Angeles (UCLA), and a board-certified rheumatologist in private practice in Anaheim, California.

BETH B. DUPREE MD, FACS is a breast cancer surgeon in Bensalem, PA. She believes that integrating holistic therapies with state-of-the-art technology can lead to better outcomes—even in people with life-threatening disease, such as cancer.

LAUREN B. GERSON MD, MSC is Associate Professor of Medicine and Gastroenterology at Stanford University School of Medicine, Stanford, California. She is an Associate Editor for *Gastrointestinal Endoscopy* and has served as the director for multiple ASGE endoscopy courses.

ELSA-GRACE V. GIARDINA MD, FACS is trained as a cardiologist, clinical pharmacologist, and electro-pharmacologist. She is Professor of Clinical Medicine for the College of Physicians and Surgeons Columbia University, and the Director of the Center for Women's Health, Columbia-Presbyterian Medical Center.

CORDELIA GRIMM MD, MPH is Consultant to the Internal Medicine Residency Program at the Good Samaritan Hospital of Baltimore, and an Assistant

Professor of Clinical Medicine at Johns Hopkins University School of Medicine.

SUSANNA E. HORVATH MD, FAHA is an Assistant Clinical Professor of Neurology and Division Chief of Neurology at the Columbia University Medical Center, New York.

DEBRA JALIMAN MD is a board-certified dermatologist with a private practice in Manhattan. She is also an Assistant Professor at the Department of Dermatology, Mount Sinai School of Medicine, New York.

LINDSEY A. KERR MD is on the Board of Directors of the National Association for Continence and has served as their national spokesperson.

MARY JANE MINKIN MD, FACOG is Clinical Professor, Department of Obstetrics and Gynecology, Yale University School of Medicine, and she is in clinical practice in New Haven, CT. She is the women's health adviser to *Prevention Magazine*, and the medical advisor to menopause support group Prime Plus/Red Hot Mamas.

BEATRIZ R. OLSON MD, FACP is Clinical Assistant Professor of Medicine at Yale School of Medicine. She is attending physician at Waterbury Hospital and St. Mary's Hospital in Waterbury, CT. Her private clinical practice is focused on endocrinology, metabolism, and thyroid cancer. She is Endocrine consultant to Greenwich Integrative Medicine Center and founder of Lotusmedical.org.

ALEXANDRA C. SACKS MD is PGY-I Resident in Adult Psychiatry at the New York Presbyterian Hospital, Weill Cornell Medical Center, New York.

The Contributors

ANNE BALLINGER MD, FRCP is a Consultant Gastroenterologist and general physician at Queen Elizabeth the Queen Mother Hospital, Margate, Kent, UK.

TAMSIN GREENWELL MD, FRCS (UROL) is a Consultant Urological Surgeon and Honorary Senior Lecturer in Female and Reconstructive Urology at UCLH/UCL and London Bridge Hospitals, London, UK.

DAWN HARPER MBBS, MRCP, DCH, DFFP is a family practice physician in the UK. She is also a medical writer and broadcaster.

SARAH JARVIS MA, BMBCH, DRCOG, FRCGP is a family practice physician and medical writer and broadcaster in the UK.

GHADA MIKHAIL BSC, MBBS, MD, FRCP is a Consultant Cardiologist and Honorary Senior Lecturer at the Imperial College Healthcare NHS Trust, London, UK.

KAREN MORRISON MA (CANTAB), BMCHB (OXON), DPHIL, FRCP is Bloomer Professor of Neurology, and Head of the Department of Clinical Neurosciences at Birmingham University, UK.

NINA SALOOJA DM, MSC (ED), FRCP, FRCPATH is a Consultant Hematologist at the Hammersmith and Charing Cross Hospitals, London, UK.

NURHAN SUTCLIFFE MD, FRCP is a Consultant Rheumatologist at the Barts and The London NHS Trusts, London, UK.

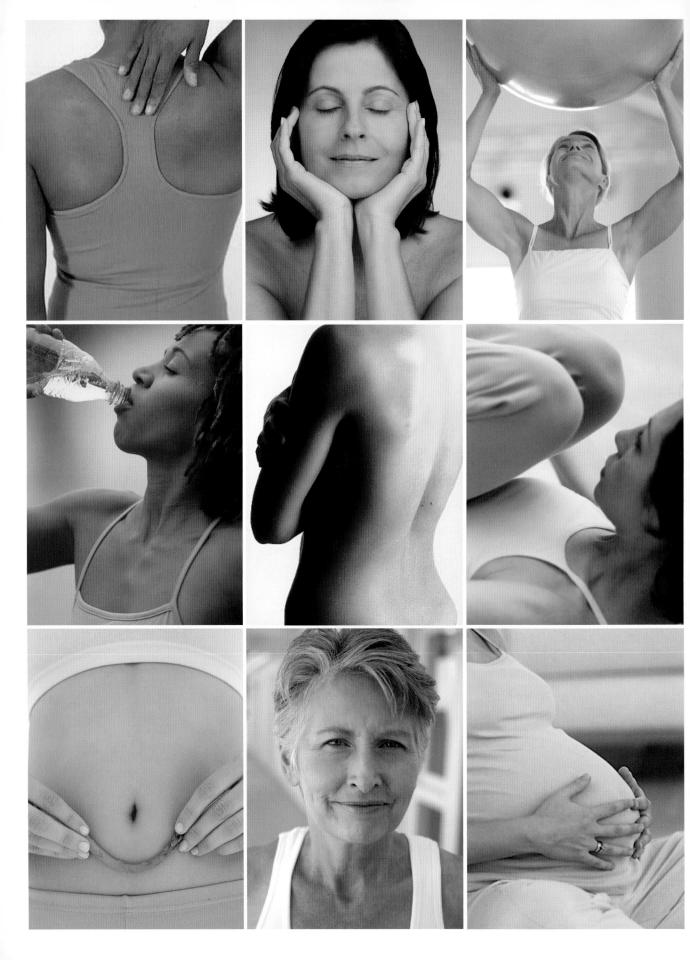

Contents

Message from the Editor-in-Chief

Women's Health for Life is a unique celebration of women's health. Designed to help you optimize your health, well-being, and quality of life, it is written for women, by women who are amongst the most credible, respected, and trusted authorities in women's health from the United States and Great Britain. Considering every woman, *Women's Health for Life* contains the most recent women's health information; provides practical advice; translates complicated data into useful tips; and offers guidance toward enhancing your health. While there are many readers who will want to read this book from start to finish, it provides easy access to the information you want when you need it most. Think of *Women's Health for Life* as a trusted reference to which you can turn—and return—any time, whether the information is for yourself or someone you care about.

Uniquely, this book provides clear illustrations, graphs, and charts to make it as easily understood as a cookbook. Unfortunately, there is no single "recipe" for health. There are many ingredients, however, and they are thoroughly discussed. While no single medical book can provide all the details about every problem, reading this book will help you to reduce your risk of infections from the flu to AIDS; prevent cervical cancer or identify an early breast cancer; identify neurologic conditions from migraines to multiple sclerosis; describe rheumatologic conditions from osteoarthritis to osteoporosis; reduce your risk of hypertension and heart disease; and how to navigate the challenges associated with contraception, menstruation, pregnancy, infertility, and menopause.

Most importantly, this book will help you protect your health, offering tips on staying fit, taking the right vitamins, and getting recommended vaccinations and tests. While this cannot be a substitute for advice from your own personal health-care provider, it may improve your interactions with health-care professionals, providing the background you need to ask informed questions. Hopefully, this will help improve your communication with your doctors and improve your health-care outcomes.

Women's Health for Life is available in a banner year for women's health: the 20th anniversary of the pivotal US Government Accountability Office report on the inclusion of women in clinical trials. This launched a groundswell of women's health advocacy in which I was thrilled to participate. The report's revelation that women were not adequately included in clinical trials stimulated changes benefiting women worldwide, including completely revising the definition of women's health itself. Before 1990, the traditional definition of women's health was linked to a reproductive orientation, focusing on organs men didn't have. Subsequently, the National Institutes of Health introduced a much broader definition of women's health: "those diseases, disorders, and conditions that are unique to, more prevalent among, or more serious in women or for which there are different risk factors or interventions for women than for men." This definition was still disease-focused and based upon the male norm. Concerns led to the current definition: any condition which affects women and their physical or mental well-being. *Women's Health for Life* presents a comprehensive view of women's health based upon this modern definition.

While the information contained throughout *Women's Health for Life* is based upon the latest women's health research, this book is not about research. The book is decidedly practical, focusing on what is available to women today. In our first four chapters, we present information useful to all women: how we differ as women from men, how we age, and how we can stay healthy. With Chapter 5, we start discussing conditions related to specific organ systems. While *Women's Health for Life* extends far beyond the reproductive system, it starts here, recognizing that's where we all come from as individuals—and that's where we've come from in the evolution of women's health. It's also the system that presents more symptoms for women throughout the lifespan and has several medicalized non-pathologic conditions. While menstruation, contraception, pregnancy, perimenopause, and menopause aren't diseases, they often require medical attention.

For the past 20 years, I've had many different roles in the modern women's health movement. My favorite is communicating useful healthcare information with the goal of improving women lives. Only you can tell me if we achieved that goal with this book.

Congratulations again for taking this important step towards improving your health. I wish you success in applying this knowledge towards a lifetime of good health.

Donnica L. Moore, MD

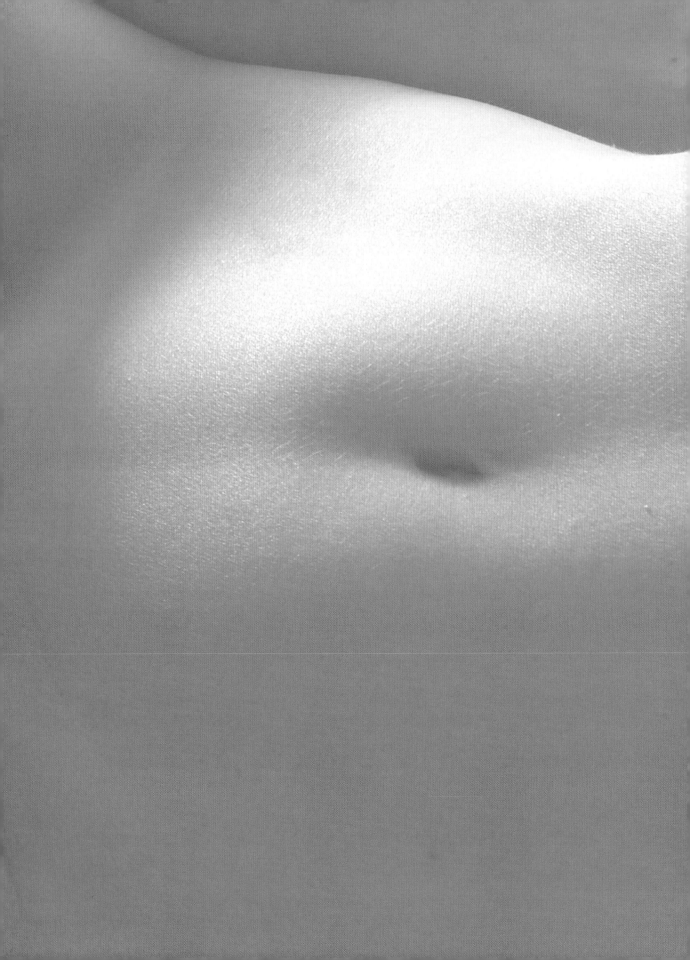

We're different

Donnica L. Moore MD
President, Sapphire Women's Health Group

Girls and boys: what are the differences?

Until puberty there are very few visible differences between boys and girls, apart from the obvious difference—the presence, or otherwise, of a penis—and the fact that boys have a slightly different build. During puberty, though, the differences—both internal and external—become much more apparent.

AN EXTRA X MAKES A BIG DIFFERENCE

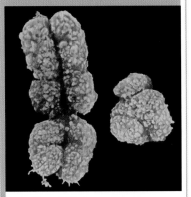

X and Y chromosomes
The X chromosome (left) is much larger than the relatively smaller Y chromosome (right).

Men have one X and one Y chromosome (XY), while women have two X chromosomes (XX). Women can pass on only an X chromosome, but a man can pass on an X or a Y. When it comes to the sex of your baby, the sperm has the final say! If a baby develops from your egg and a sperm with an X chromosome, it will be a girl (XX), but if it is fertilized by a sperm with a Y chromosome, it will turn out to be a boy (XY).

Women's bodies are designed to give birth and to nurture babies and men's are designed to father them. Puberty is when we reach sexual maturity, when, physically, we become capable of fulfilling these functions. It is, therefore, a time of enormous change, both physical and emotional.

THE START OF PUBERTY

The age at which their puberty starts is something that many children worry about. Although it varies from child to child and is influenced by a number of factors, including heredity, puberty generally begins between the ages of eight and thirteen in a girl, and between ten and fifteen in a boy.

One of the factors that influences the onset of puberty is nutrition; poor nutrition can cause a delay. As nutrition improved in the developed world between the late 19th and the mid-20th centuries, the average age when puberty started went down by well over a year. In today's developed world, malnutrition is rare and as a result, especially in the US over the last 50 years or so, there seems to be a continuing trend

toward an even lower average age of puberty. The evidence is stronger in girls than in boys, and is even more marked among African-American girls. In fact, in 1999 in the US, new guidelines were produced that suggested that puberty should only be considered abnormally early ("precocious puberty") if breast or pubic hair development starts before the age of seven in Caucasian girls and six in African-American girls.

In the UK, the changes have been less marked; there has probably only been a reduction of six months or so in the average age of puberty in the last few decades. In the UK, puberty in girls is considered to be precocious if it starts before the age of eight.

HOW GIRLS CHANGE DURING PUBERTY

The dominant female hormone is estrogen. During puberty it is produced in greater amounts and is crucial to a girl's sexual development. Its main physical effects are on:

The skeleton A girl's hips and pelvis widen, making her well suited anatomically for giving birth.

The face Girls develop jaw and facial features that are much finer and more delicate than boys'.

Body hair Girls develop pubic hair and hair under their arms.

The skin and sweat glands Girls start to experience body odor and acne.

Body fat Girls begin to get more body fat on their hips, thighs, and buttocks, as well as on their breasts. Most women are designed to have more body fat than men.

The breasts Soon after their body hair starts to appear, the breasts increase in size. Girls' nipples also change during puberty, becoming darker and more prominent and better designed for breast-feeding.

The ovaries and uterus The reproductive organs grow and mature. Girls begin their periods; the average age in the US is 12 and a half.

HOW BOYS CHANGE DURING PUBERTY

Testosterone is the main hormone that comes into play in boys during puberty. It has amazingly wide-ranging effects that last throughout life. During puberty, its main physical effects are on:

The skeleton A boy's shoulders start to widen so that by the time he is a man, he will have shoulders that are wider than his hips.

The muscles A boy's muscles become bigger and heavier. Those of his upper body in particular develop more than a girl's.

The vocal cords and the larynx (also known as the voice box) A boy's voice "breaks" and he develops a typically deeper voice.

The face Changes in a boy's bones and muscles result in the development of a heavier jaw.

Body hair Boys develop pubic and underarm hair and, depending on inherited characteristics, hair on the face, neck, chest, and back.

The skin and sweat glands, Boys start to experience body odor and acne.

The genitals A boy's penis grows, his testicles descend further and get larger, and he is able to ejaculate.

THE CHANGING BODY OF A GIRL

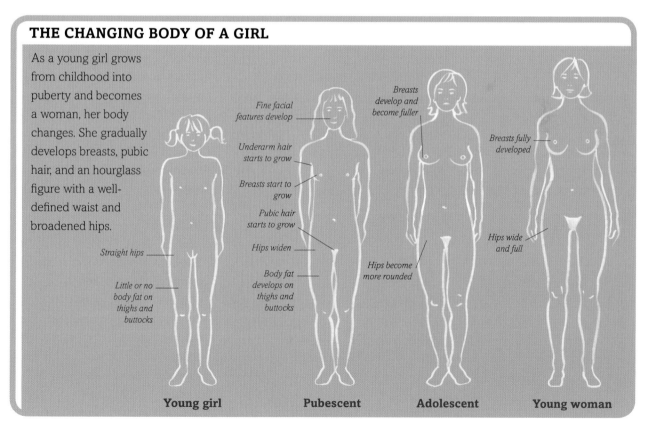

As a young girl grows from childhood into puberty and becomes a woman, her body changes. She gradually develops breasts, pubic hair, and an hourglass figure with a well-defined waist and broadened hips.

Fine facial features develop

Underarm hair starts to grow

Breasts start to grow

Pubic hair starts to grow

Hips widen

Straight hips

Little or no body fat on thighs and buttocks

Body fat develops on thighs and buttocks

Breasts develop and become fuller

Hips become more rounded

Breasts fully developed

Hips wide and full

Young girl   **Pubescent**   **Adolescent**   **Young woman**

The adult woman

By the time we reach adulthood, women are, on average, 20 percent shorter and have less upper body strength than men. There are also differences in the amount of fat and muscle on our bodies, the basic rate of our metabolism, and the structure of some of our bones and joints.

Hair Women generally have less body hair than men, although it doesn't stop many of us from feeling we have too much. Our facial hair and other body hair are usually very light, although this can become darker and coarser in later life. Our pubic hair forms a straight line at the top. Fortunately, the hair on our heads is longer lasting than the average man's. Although it becomes thinner as we age, and a little sparser, we can expect to end our lives with almost as much as we started with (unless you suffer from alopecia—see p370).

Skeleton Most women have more delicate facial features than men. Generally, we also have smaller heads, shorter necks, smaller, narrower chests, and more rounded shoulders, as well as smaller hands and feet, and shorter legs and arms.

In terms of evolution, being big was an advantage for a man if he was facing a saber-toothed tiger or another, perhaps hostile, man. Women's priorities centered around child raising, so we relied on those big burly menfolk to fend off predators while we protected our young. Women also have a broader, shallower pelvis than a man, which is essential when it comes to giving birth (see opposite).

Body fat The extra fat we gain at puberty over the hips, thighs, and buttocks, in combination with our wider hips and pelvis, gives women their traditional "hourglass" shape. Contrast this with a man's trunk, which is more like an upside-down triangle, with broader shoulders and narrower hips. Our excess body fat is probably another trick of evolution, allowing women to draw

MALE AND FEMALE BODIES

At puberty, male and female bodies become different shapes. Women have an "hourglass" shape with wider hips, while a man has broader shoulders that give his torso an inverted triangle shape.

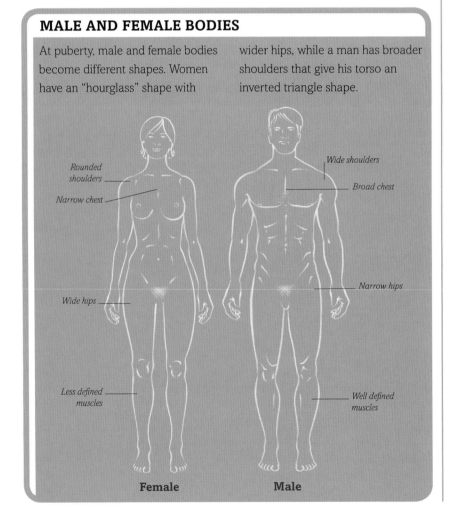

Rounded shoulders

Narrow chest

Wide hips

Less defined muscles

Wide shoulders

Broad chest

Narrow hips

Well defined muscles

Female   **Male**

on their reserves of fat to feed their young in times of famine. But the fact that we have more body fat and less body water than men is one factor that makes us more prone to the effects of alcohol (see p65).

Muscles Women naturally have smaller, less well-defined muscles than men and they are also less visible because of their covering of fat. Back in the mists of time, men needed more muscle to hunt than women did to raise young.

Breasts Our breasts usually begin to develop shortly after our body hair starts to appear. By the time puberty is complete, the breasts are sufficiently developed physically to produce milk, although this doesn't usually happen until we are well into pregnancy.

Genitals Unlike men, most of our reproductive equipment is on the inside. The only part that can be seen is the entrance to the vagina, with its two sets of lips (outer and inner labia), framing the tiny clitoris at the front where they meet.

The reproductive system

Inside her ovaries a newborn girl has many thousands of immature eggs. When her ovaries start to ovulate, they release mature eggs (the average woman produces one a month during most of the time she has periods) and she can start to reproduce.

A man can stay fertile for the rest of his life (the oldest recorded man to father a child was an Australian age 93), but a woman can't get pregnant naturally after menopause, and often not for

A WOMAN'S PELVIS COMPARED TO A MAN'S

The human pelvis consists of two large hip bones that join the sacrum at the base of the spine and meet in front at the pubic symphysis where they form the pubic arch. They create a space called the pelvic inlet that protects the bladder and, in a woman, the ovaries and womb. A woman's pelvis makes childbirth easier and is generally wider, shallower, and more delicate than a man's. Her inlet is larger and more circular, her sacrum is shorter and less curved, and the pubic arch is wider and less angular. During pregnancy the pubic symphysis joint softens and becomes more flexible, allowing the baby to pass through the birth canal during delivery. Our unique pelvis is the secret of our success in the delivery room.

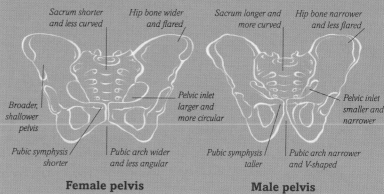

Sacrum shorter and less curved — *Hip bone wider and flared*

Broader, shallower pelvis

Pelvic inlet larger and more circular

Pubic symphysis shorter — *Pubic arch wider and less angular*

Female pelvis

Sacrum longer and more curved — *Hip bone narrower and less flared*

Pelvic inlet smaller and narrower

Pubic symphysis taller — *Pubic arch narrower and V-shaped*

Male pelvis

several years before it. What's more, we often only begin ovulating regularly a year or two after we start having periods.

Metabolism This is a term that describes how much energy the body uses. Our basal metabolic rate is equivalent to the amount of calories we burn just to stay alive without doing anything else. That includes breathing, keeping our heart, liver, and other organs going, and using our brains.

Amazingly, about 70 percent of the energy we burn is just to keep us alive. For the average woman, another 20 percent is used in physical activity and 10 percent is for digestion and creating heat to keep ourselves warm.

On average, women naturally have a lower basal metabolic rate than men, partly because we're usually smaller—and, not surprisingly, it takes more energy to keep a bigger body going.

However, even compared to a man of the same size, a woman's body has a lower metabolic rate because she naturally has a higher proportion of fat combined with a lower proportion of muscle. This also means that when the average woman eats exactly as much as the average man, she is more likely to put on weight.

Sickness and disease

Since women differ from men so much physically, it's not surprising that we differ in our susceptibility to illness, too. The good news for us is that women in the western world live, on average, five years longer than men. But that doesn't necessarily mean we have fewer diseases.

WHAT DISEASES DO WOMEN GET?

While women are slightly less likely to suffer from the biggest killers—heart disease and cancer—we're more likely to get other diseases.

Mental health problems

Women tend to have more in the way of mental health problems, such as depression (see pp210–11), anxiety (see pp204–5), and eating disorders (see pp216–17). These can seriously affect our quality of life and that of our loved ones, too.

We also suffer from Alzheimer's disease (see pp184–5) more than men, though this may be because we live longer and Alzheimer's gets more common with age. Again, this distressing condition affects our quality of life and that of our caregivers.

Bone conditions When it comes to bone conditions, we women are much more prone than men to osteoporosis, or thinning of the bones (see pp260–2).

Similarly with osteoarthritis (see pp263–5)—a joint condition that affects more women than men. Like osteoporosis and Alzheimer's, it's largely a condition that develops because of old age though it can affect young people. But the truth is that many of the conditions that women get more commonly than men are clearly debilitating but kill only slowly, if at all. Osteoarthritis and osteoporosis cause crippling pain, and can make it very difficult to live independently, but you don't die as a direct result of them.

DRUGS TESTED MAINLY ON MEN

Pharmaceutical treatments have made great strides—for example, the development of statins for reducing high serum cholesterol levels in the blood. However, most drugs were previously tested predominantly on men, leaving women wondering whether these products were as suitable for them. It is increasingly clear that women respond to some medicines differently, may need a different dose, or may experience different side effects than men. For the past decade, both government-sponsored and industry-sponsored clinical research has included women of all kinds.

Cancer Men are slightly more likely to die from cancer than we are, like smoking-related lung cancer. We, of course, are afflicted by cancers of our own, especially cervical cancer (see p107).

Heart disease and stroke More men than women die from heart disease (see pp160–75) and stroke (see p196), although, once we're past menopause, the heart-protective effect of our estrogen wanes and our risk increases sharply. Interestingly, some people who die from heart disease never even know they have it: over a third die from a heart attack without ever having had a diagnosis of heart disease.

Smoking, drinking, and taking drugs Overall, men are more likely than we are to smoke, drink too much alcohol, and take illegal drugs. This means that they're more likely to suffer (and sometimes die) from diseases linked to these unhealthy habits.

Sadly, the gap between men and women has been closing in recent years. This is because men are more health conscious, but also because women are now more likely to smoke, drink, and use drugs (see pp22–3).

PASSING ON HEMOPHILIA

We all have two of most genes—one on each of a pair of chromosomes (see p12)—inherited from our parents. A gene is a code for a particular characteristic. Some genes are "dominant," others are "recessive." If you inherit a dominant gene you will develop the characteristic associated with it. For example, the gene for brown eyes is dominant, so you will have brown eyes if you inherit a brown-eyed gene from one parent, even though you inherit a blue-eyed gene (recessive) from the other. You'll have blue eyes only if you inherit a blue-eyed gene from both parents and you'll have brown eyes if you inherit a brown-eyed gene from both.

Diseases can also be passed on through our genes. The genes for some, such as color blindness and hemophilia, are carried only on X chromosomes (see p12). These genes are recessive. Men have one X chromosome so if the one they inherit is affected, they'll get the disease. A woman has two, so if she inherits the affected X chromosome from one parent but the normal dominant gene from her other, she won't get the disease. But she will be able to pass on the affected X chromosome to a child, making her a "carrier." Very rarely—the chances are around 1 in 100,000,000—a woman can get the disease.

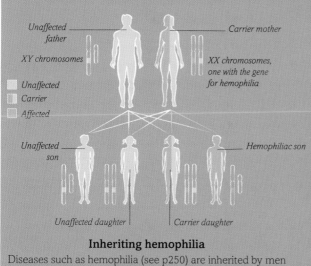

Unaffected father
XY chromosomes
Unaffected
Carrier
Affected
Unaffected son
Carrier mother
XX chromosomes, one with the gene for hemophilia
Hemophiliac son
Unaffected daughter
Carrier daughter

Inheriting hemophilia
Diseases such as hemophilia (see p250) are inherited by men on the X chromosome, which their mothers pass on to them.

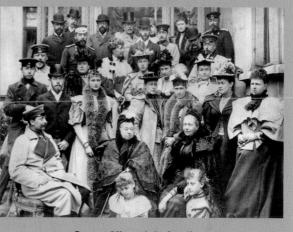

Queen Victoria's family
Many of the boys in the family of Britain's Queen Victoria inherited hemophilia, a severe blood clotting disorder.

ILLNESS AND CHANGING HORMONES

Several medical conditions tend to be more or less problematic during pregnancy or the menstrual cycle when female hormones change rapidly. They include:

Asthma During pregnancy, some women report their asthma gets better, although women with severe asthma are more likely to find their symptoms becoming worse.

Rheumatoid arthritis During pregnancy rheumatoid arthritis symptoms improve in up to three-quarters of sufferers. Unfortunately, a similar proportion experience a flare-up once pregnancy is over.

Migraine About two-thirds of sufferers have fewer episodes or less severe migraines during pregnancy, especially in the last six months. In up to 1 in 12, migraines get worse. See also menstrual migraine, p182.

Depression About 1 in 5 women get depression during pregnancy; in about 50 percent it is clinically significant. Many women with depression find their symptoms become worse in the days leading up to their period; these women are more prone to depression around menopause. Depression and mood changes are a risk of hormonal contraception and hormone infertility treatment.

Venus and Mars: the brain and intelligence

Are women better then men at multitasking but not as good at reading a map? There's no doubt that men and women have differences in behavior. Here we'll look at some of those differences and discuss the theories surrounding them. A good place to start is with the brain.

The human brain contains some 10,000–15,000 million nerve cells, called neurons, and one million billion synapses (the connections between nerve cells). But the way in which the brain functions is still, to an extent, a medical mystery, so we can't say with certainty how much the physical differences between people's brains affect or contribute to their behavior.

THE BRAIN—WHERE WOMEN ARE DIFFERENT

Women have slightly smaller brains than men (they weigh about 4oz/100g less) but, as we know, size isn't everything. Elephants, for instance, have much larger brains than humans, but nobody believes they have more intellect. And though women's brains are smaller than men's, they both have a similar ratio of brain weight to body weight. Women also have 4 percent fewer brain cells than men, but this doesn't mean they use them less! There are other male/female differences, too!

The frontal lobe of the brain plays a major part in making judgements, planning future actions, and in language. Women have far more cells here than men.

The hemispheres It is believed that these two halves of the brain probably work differently. The left side helps us think analytically, while the right side helps us look at things as a whole, involving value judgements and emotion. Men are more likely to be "left-brain dominant" while women are thought to use both hemispheres more equally.

The corpus callosum transfers information between both halves of the brain. Women have a bigger corpus callosum than men, which may account for the fact that women score better on tests of thought fluency and speech.

The limbic system affects our emotions and is, on the whole, bigger in women. Together with

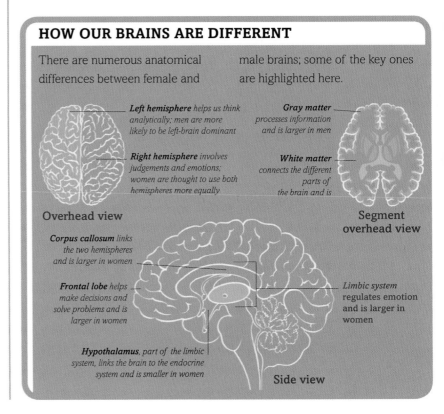

HOW OUR BRAINS ARE DIFFERENT

There are numerous anatomical differences between female and male brains; some of the key ones are highlighted here.

Left hemisphere helps us think analytically; men are more likely to be left-brain dominant

Right hemisphere involves judgements and emotions; women are thought to use both hemispheres more equally

Overhead view

Gray matter processes information and is larger in men

White matter connects the different parts of the brain and is

Segment overhead view

Corpus callosum links the two hemispheres and is larger in women

Frontal lobe helps make decisions and solve problems and is larger in women

Hypothalamus, part of the limbic system, links the brain to the endocrine system and is smaller in women

Limbic system regulates emotion and is larger in women

Side view

a female brain's greater ability to transfer information between its two sides, these facts may help account for women's greater emotional sensitivity. The bigger limbic system may also mean that women feel negative emotions more sharply, opening them up to a greater risk of depression.

Gray matter and white matter
Processing information goes on in the gray matter, while white matter connects the different parts of our brain, enabling us to carry out various tasks. Women tend to have far more white matter than men, while men are endowed with far more gray matter. Could any or all of these differences above be an explanation for the popular theory that women are generally better at "multitasking" than men?

The hypothalamus controls the endocrine system that produces many of the hormones in the body. The functions it regulates include sexual function, sleep, water content, and body temperature. In men the hypothalamus is about twice as big and contains twice as many cells as it does in women.

MEASURING INTELLIGENCE
Despite the physical differences between the male and female brain, there seems to be little, if any, difference between them as far as overall intelligence is concerned. The average IQ (intelligence quotient) score for men and for women is very similar, but that doesn't mean we're all the same. In fact, far more men than women

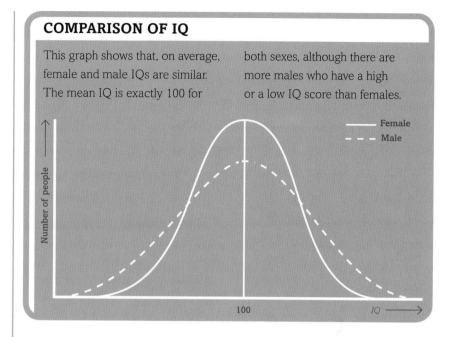

COMPARISON OF IQ

This graph shows that, on average, female and male IQs are similar. The mean IQ is exactly 100 for both sexes, although there are more males who have a high or a low IQ score than females.

Number of people

Female
Male

100   IQ

get very high or very low scores. That means that while there may be more very smart men around than there are very smart women, there may also be more men than women at the bottom of the class.

Another problem is, though, that while "average" scores tell us about the average ability of men and women in a whole population, they can't tell us how well individuals do, or the range of their results.

Nor is measuring intelligence that straightforward. The most common tests include the IQ test and the SAT test. There has been huge debate as to whether such tests disadvantage women by using situations that men (or boys) are more familiar with than women (or girls). For example, a question that asks about the relative speeds of two cars might be easier for a man or boy to answer than a woman or girl.

HORSES FOR COURSES?

Research has shown that, on the whole, men perform better than women at visual-spatial tests, so they are good at understanding the things we see and putting them in context—for instance, the way a car engine is put together. Men also tend to be better at tests involving math.

Women do better at tests involving language and words, as well as verbal reasoning. They also score better on some memory tests.

It is increasingly believed that men greatly outnumber women in top academic posts in the sciences due to institutionalized discrimination. Now that this has been recognized, greater numbers of women are rising to top posts.

Venus and Mars: personality

Do the physical differences between the male and female brain account for the personality differences between men and women? Those who believe the "nature" theory argue that they do. Others believe that "nurture," or the way we're brought up, is what makes women so different from men.

In psychology, there is reasonable consensus that personality can be described by dividing it into five broad factors or dimensions. These so-called big five are Openness, Conscientiousness, Extraversion, Agreeableness, and Neuroticism. This psychological model is often referred to as OCEAN. Each of the five factors includes several personality traits:

Openness Imagination, curiosity, a sense of adventure, and an appreciation of new ideas.

Conscientiousness A sense of duty, self-discipline, a tendency to plan ahead rather than acting on the spur of the moment, and the need for achievement.

Extraversion A tendency to seek the company of others, exuberance, energetic approach to life, looking at the positive, and assertiveness.

Agreeableness Cooperation, peacemaking, compassion, helpfulness, and a tendency to go along with the wishes of others rather than create conflict.

Neuroticism A sensitivity to anxiety, depression, or other negative emotions, moodiness, and a tendency to "blow problems out of proportion" and to see obstacles as insurmountable.

NATURE OR NURTURE?

In psychological tests, women consistently score higher in the areas of Agreeableness and Neuroticism. Perhaps surprisingly, such differences are greater in cultures where "traditional" models of the roles of the two genders have become less widespread. Thus the difference between the genders seems to be greater in Europe and the US than it is in more traditional cultures.

Nature theorists Scientists who believe in the "nature" theory argue that we're "hardwired" for either a male or female personality. They point to the differences in a woman's limbic system and the better connections between a woman's brain hemispheres (see p18) as the reason for the higher scores in the psychological tests. They also believe that the differences in the structure of a woman's brain compared to a man's account entirely for the way in which women process information. This, in turn, determines which skills in IQ tests (see p19) women will find more or less easy than men, and why women tend to look at the bigger picture when making decisions.

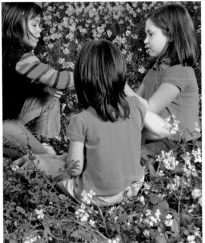 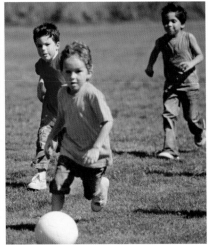

Differences between girls and boys
Stereotypically, girls are more likely to talk with each other as they sit together in the playground, whereas boys very often choose to play a physical game such as soccer.

Nurture theorists Another group of scientists argues vigorously that women are born with the capacity to have the same type of personality and intellectual skills as men. The differences are due to socialization —this is the way certain "female" personality traits are imposed on us by society and become deeply ingrained. These theorists believe that once physical strength was no longer needed for survival, men imposed other ways of subjugating women—for example, by claiming they were less intelligent or over-emotional and by relegating them to a secondary role in society.

Nature and nurture A third group argues that some innate differences exist between men and women, which society reinforces. Moreover, some think that the differences between men and women's brains are no more marked than the differences that exist between individual men or individual women. The truth is that behavior is incredibly complicated and is almost certainly influenced profoundly by both our genetic makeup and our upbringing.

PERSONALITY, GENDER, AND PROFESSION

We have looked at the differences between men and women with respect to areas of intelligence (see p19). But how much of an influence does our personality have on how we get along in our profession, and what part do gender differences in personality play? It's possible that personality may have an impact on job performance. For instance, in one study, higher job performance was linked with higher levels of Openness and Extraversion and lower performance with rising levels of Neuroticism.

However, there are many other models of personality than the five OCEAN categories, and critics of the "big five" say they do not take into account other personality traits such as Sense of Humor, Motivation, and Identity. It's possible that these characteristics may also show differences between men and women, and may have a significant effect on job performance.

Personality tests also depend on completely honest replies. Many people will be tempted to adjust their answers to give the results they think their potential employers will want. For instance, applicants for teacher training might consider exaggerating their enjoyment of being the center of attention to increase their Extraversion score.

It would therefore be unwise to come to any sweeping conclusions about likely job performance based on assessment of personality. Sadly, this means that determining your future career purely on the basis of personality testing would also be highly risky.

"Behavior is influenced profoundly by both our genetic makeup and our upbringing."

The stresses and strains of modern life

Most women have the chance to be as well educated as our male peers and we generally have similar opportunities. But the downside is that we may be juggling a career and family life. No wonder, then, that women suffer from the same ills as men, but also from the stresses of "modern life."

It was not so long ago that women were taught to aspire to nothing more in life than making a good marriage. And as recently as the late 19th century—and still true in some parts of the world—a woman was regarded as her husband's possession, to be treated entirely as he wished.

It's remarkable that many of the changes that liberated women are relatively recent. The suffragettes, for example, began their struggle in the early 20th century. Their battle was finally won in the US in 1920 when women were granted the vote on the same terms as men. Britain followed suit in 1928.

It was only as recently as World War II that women were encouraged to look for jobs outside the home, and that was to take the place of men who were enlisted in the armed forces.

But perhaps the most significant breakthrough for the liberation of women came in 1960, when the contraceptive pill was launched in the US. Within two years, more than a million American women were enjoying their sexual freedom, while controlling their fertility.

BEING ONE OF THE BOYS—AT WORK AND AT PLAY

Over many decades, women have been pushing extremely hard to be accepted as equals by their male peers. But achieving acceptance in the workplace often involves becoming "one of the boys" in the social arena—and that means drinking and smoking.

Increased drinking Women, as we will discover (see p65), aren't designed to drink as much alcohol as men. Not only are we harmed at lower levels of drinking, but we also appear to damage our bodies in a shorter space of time than men.

In the US, there has been a decrease in the average amount of alcohol consumed, with middle-aged people consuming about one-third less than 50 years ago. Though moderate drinking has seen an increase, heavy drinking is down and total alcohol consumption is down a small amount. People drank about one-third more in the 1950s and 1960s than they did in the 1970s up to 2004. But despite the decline in

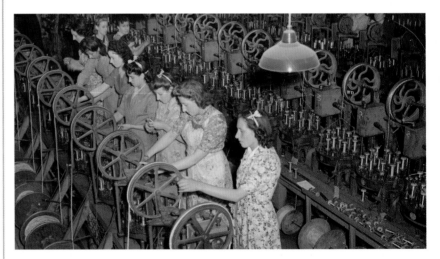

Women working in industry in World War II
These women working in a factory during World War II are typical of the thousands who started working outside the home for the first time. They were needed for the war effort.

alchohol consumption, the risk of alcohol dependence has not shown a corresponding decrease.

Nor is this change in drinking patterns confined to any particular social group of women. In fact, recent research suggests that the women in their thirties who are most likely to drink to excess are the most successful, professional women with high-pressure jobs that place them under huge stress.

Increased smoking In the past, too, women were much less likely than men to smoke. Nowadays, the gap is narrowing dramatically—possibly as young women continue to smoke or start smoking as part of a misguided attempt to keep their weight down.

EATING DISORDERS

Anorexia nervosa (sometimes referred to as "the dieter's disease") is around ten times more common among females than males. Bulimia nervosa—in which people overeat, then purge themselves by vomiting or taking laxatives—is a largely female preserve, too. These two eating disorders are psychological conditions, but they can have serious physical consequences as well as causing a great deal of family stress. For more detail, see pp216–17.

Both anorexia and bulimia have shown dramatic increases in recent decades, and it seems that the stresses and strains of modern life are mostly to blame. The "typical" woman most at risk of such eating disorders is young, attractive, and high achieving. Young women who excel at sports or occupations in which physical conditioning is paramount—ballet and athletics as well as modeling and acting—are particularly vulnerable. Often, though, these women describe their eating disorders as a kind of "coping mechanism" for the high expectations placed on them.

OUR AGING SOCIETY

Further stress on women comes from our aging society. As average life expectancy continues to rise, so does the proportion of the elderly in the population. Women are much more likely than men to act as caregivers for elderly relatives, particularly their parents. As more and more women work full time, this adds to the pressures on them.

What is more, although death rates from many serious medical conditions (such as heart disease and diabetes) are going down, the number of people debilitated by such illnesses is still going up. So as women delay having children, they are more likely to find themselves in the difficult position of having to care for both children and parents at the same time.

Women are increasingly going out to work without reducing their domestic commitments. Working women still act as the primary homemaker and caregiver for children. In a 1990s survey of doctors in their thirties, the stress of juggling domestic and professional commitments was the most common barrier to career fulfillment for women. Not one man in this survey even mentioned the problem!

Ample evidence suggests that women can't "switch off" other problems as easily as men—perhaps because of differences in their brains (see pp18–19) or social conditioning. Whatever the cause, most women juggle more tasks than men. And while this is an achievement we should all be celebrating, it can also be a recipe for stress-related illness.

"Perhaps the most significant breakthrough for the liberation of women came in 1960 with the launch of the contraceptive pill."

Understanding the changes

Donnica L. Moore MD

Through the decades

In general, women are now living longer than their mothers and much longer than their grandmothers. Our overall quality of life is better, too: we are healthier, more active, and more independent than ever before. Much of this is due to medical advances and public health measures, but we also know how to take care of ourselves more proactively. This chapter summarizes the stages we go through as our lives unfold through the decades and reminds us of the commonsense rules of health that too many of us forget to follow.

The moment you are conceived, the stage is set for a life of individuality. The genes you inherit from your parents distinguish you from everybody else on the planet, unless you're an identical twin! These genes contribute to who you are, what you look like, what your constitution is, and what diseases you may inherit.

At the same time, your changing environment—everything from your time as a developing fetus and as a newborn infant, to the hormonal merry-go-round of your adolescence—contributes not only to your health but also to the kind of illnesses from which you may suffer. These two influences—your genes and your environment—make up the two components of the "nature versus nurture" discussion. Together, they determine the essence of your mental and physical well-being. This is also the melting pot from which psychologists draw the biophysical-social model to explain the workings of mental health (p203). But while we know that genes and environment are extremely important, both can be influenced tremendously—both positively or negatively—by the lifestyle choices that we make.

TOP 10 GOOD HABITS FOR LIFE

Get into good habits when you are as young as possible, preferably in your 20s. This will help you lay the foundations for enjoying your life right through the next decades.

1 Eat a balanced diet Include five servings of fruit and vegetables a day (see pp52–5).

2 Maintain a healthy weight Calculate your Body Mass Index (BMI), see pp58–9 for how and why to do this.

3 If you smoke, stop If you need help, join a support group or talk to your doctor (see p64).

4 Moderate your drinking Limit your alcoholic intake to fewer than two units per day (see p65).

5 Drive carefully Accidents, including motor vehicle accidents, are a leading cause of death.

6 Get a good night's sleep Sleep deprivation affects your mood, productivity, relationships, and safety.

7 Practice responsible sexual behavior If you don't want to get pregnant, use contraception.

8 Brush and floss your teeth routinely Good oral hygiene protects your overall health, not just your teeth.

9 Drink 8 to 10 glasses of water per day Water is essential for many of your bodily functions.

10 Protect yourself from the sun Always wear protective clothing and sunscreen in the sun (see p66).

AS TIME GOES BY

Women differ from men in many ways but one of the most distinctive is the way we age. Women go through unique stages in life and experience particular changes, not only based upon our reproductive and hormonal status but also the kind of health problems associated with the various decades of our lives. On average, women in the US live six years longer than men. Yet, as time goes by, we also tend to suffer from more chronic illnesses and take more medication.

Usually, when we read or hear the term "the change" in conjunction with women's health, we think about menopause. Yet there are many other age-related transitions that women experience, such as reaching the "magic age" of 35 (see p32). These changes are not always dictated by age *per se*, but by when—or if—we choose to start a family. As this chapter shows, these transitions are also linked to the development of any acute or chronic medical problems we may have. These problems may affect our risks of developing other illnesses in the future, our need for additional preventive measures, or our need for further diagnostic or health screening surveillance checkups.

PREVENTION IS BETTER THAN CURE

Age inevitably causes a physical decline and our risk of developing certain diseases, such as cancer, heart disease, and osteoporosis, increases. Using a decade-by-decade approach, this chapter looks at the typical changes in women's bodies as we age, the health risk factors associated with each decade, and our changing nutritional needs. However, not all diseases have risks that depend on age, so the chapter offers many tips and tests for prevention and for taking care of our health.

Recommended checkups and screening tests begin in your 20s and should continue throughout your lives. If the list of what you need appears to mount from your 30s onward, don't be dismayed! These are just precautions. You may feel healthy now, but many medical conditions can be prevented or treated more effectively if they are caught early. There are also some suggested questions to ask your doctor as you start each decade.

Whatever your age and whatever your circumstances, the best way to minimize any health risks and prevent many problems from developing is to adopt healthy habits (see box, left). And remember two things: first, even taking small steps toward improving your health is better than doing nothing at all; and second, it's never too late to start improving your health.

FEMALE LIFE EXPECTANCY

The figures below show the estimated life expectancy at birth for females in a selection of different countries. Male life expectancy at birth in many countries is consistently five to seven years less.

Country	Life expectancy
Andorra	86.23
Japan	85.56
France	84
Canada	83.86
Switzerland	83.63
Australia	83.59
Spain	83.32
Norway	83.32
Italy	83.07
Sweden	83
Iceland	82.62
Finland	82.31
Germany	82.11
New Zealand	82.08
Greece	82.06
Netherlands	81.82
Portugal	81.36
UK	81.3
US	80.97
Ireland	80.7
Denmark	80.41
South Korea	80.10
Poland	79.44
Mexico	78.56
Saudi Arabia	78.02
Venezuela	76.48
Brazil	76.38
Turkey	75.46
China	74.82
Russia	73.03
India	71.17
Pakistan	64.83
Nigeria	48.07
South Africa	41.66

Your 20s

This decade is exciting. You are brimming with youth and vitality and unless you become a mother, you will have plenty of "me time." Use your personal time well by taking care of yourself and setting good health habits for life. It will stand you in good stead for what, hopefully, will be a long and healthy future. The earlier you start caring for yourself, the more you will benefit as you age.

FERTILITY AND SEXUAL HEALTH

Your 20s are a time when you are generally fertile and may be sexually active. The average age of a first pregnancy in the US is now 25. Since so many women become pregnant for the first time—either intentionally or unintentionally—during their 20s, family planning and preconception counseling are especially important during this decade.

We think of the importance of prenatal care as mostly benefiting the baby, but pregnancy-related complications are significant risks for the mother as well: as you can see from the figures opposite, pregnancy-related complications are the sixth leading cause of death for women in their 20s.

You may have contracted a sexually transmitted disease (STD) during your adolescence. HIV/AIDS is the most scary: it is the eighth leading cause of death for women in this age group, but there also more than 75 other STDs, and many of these can have a devastating effect on your long-term health and fertility. You need to practice safe sex religiously and have appropriate screening tests as recommended.

CANCER

It is rare for women in their 20s to be affected by cancer. However, you are never too young to be vigilant and to take precautions, especially concerning melanoma, the most aggressive form of skin cancer and, for women aged 25–29, the most common cancer of all

Make sure you protect yourself properly from the harmful effects of the sun and see your doctor if you spot that any moles have changed appearance.

ADDICTIVE BEHAVIORS

Unfortunately, for many women, the 20s may be characterized by bad habits that started with risk-taking behavior. If you do have addictive behaviors, such as smoking (see p64), alcoholism (see p220), or eating disorders (see pp216–17), try to kick them fast. You will find that there's plenty of help around if you need it.

Drive carefully, too, because accidents, including motor vehicle accidents, are the leading cause of death in women in their 20s.

MENTAL HEALTH

Mental health is important at every age, but the 20s can be a time of particular strain due to what are often major changes in your life and in your role in society. As a result, depression is common and suicide

---

QUESTIONS TO ASK YOUR DOCTOR IN YOUR 20s

The following are just some of the questions you can ask your doctor about at the start of your 20s:

- Are there any vaccines I need?
- Should I be taking any vitamins or supplements?
- Do I need to think about having any additional screening or diagnostic tests?
- Are there any behavioral or lifestyle changes I should make for optimal health?

"Take time to care for yourself and it will stand you in good stead for the future."

TESTS RECOMMENDED IN YOUR 20s

These are the tests and checkups which it is useful to have during your 20s. Some of the routine checkups, such as the breast self-exam, you can and should do yourself on a regular basis. You can ask your doctor, dentist, and optician for the others as appropriate. While different insurance plans may vary in their coverage, these are the medical recommendations.

Routine checkups

✔ Do a monthly breast self-examination (see p154)
✔ Have a Pap smear according to your doctor's recommendations: for most women, this will be every year
✔ Have your eyes tested every five years
✔ Go for a twice-yearly dental checkup and cleaning
✔ Check your skin regularly for any changes.

Additional screening tests

✔ If you are thinking of getting pregnant, see your doctor for preconception advice. You may also need screening tests and a Pap smear before you conceive.

---

is the fourth leading cause of death in this decade. The good news is that depression is treatable, both with medical therapy and "talk therapy" (see Chapter 9).

VITAMIN AND MINERAL SUPPLEMENTS IN YOUR 20s

The following vitamin and mineral supplements may help you become more healthy.

Multivitamins Most women who are menstruating benefit from a daily multivitamin with iron.

Folic acid/omega-3 fatty acids If you are breast-feeding, pregnant, or are thinking of starting a family, take a folic acid supplement (400 micrograms/day) as well as an omega-3 fatty acid supplement (200 mg/day).

Calcium and vitamin D If your diet isn't giving you 1,200 mg/day of calcium, you may need calcium and vitamin D supplements (see also p262).

VACCINES FOR YO UR 20s

Consider having the following vaccines during your 20s.

HPV This vaccine prevents two of the cancer-causing strains of human papilloma virus (HPV), which is the cause of cervical cancer. It is approved for women up to age 26. While it is ideally given before a woman becomes sexually active, ask your doctor if it is right for you.

Flu Many groups of people are on the list of who "should" receive a flu shot annually. You may think you don't need one, but if you don't want to get a bout of flu you should get the flu shot.

Tetanus You will need a tetanus booster every ten years.

Catch-up vaccines Ask your doctor if you need any vaccinations that you missed in your childhood. For example, you may have missed your rubella (German measles) vaccine (catching rubella during the first trimester of pregnancy can cause major fetal abnormalities) or your varicella (chickenpox) vaccine.

LEADING CAUSES OF DEATH FOR WOMEN IN THEIR 20s

Statistical research in the US shows that the leading causes of death among women in their 20s are:

1 Accidents	4 Suicide
2 Cancer	5 Heart disease
3 Murder	6 Pregnancy complications
	7 Birth defects
	8 HIV/AIDS
	9 Diabetes
	10 Stroke

Your 30s

The 30s are generally considered a time of robust health for most women, but this decade can also be a transitional time in terms of your physical and emotional well-being. One of the biggest physical and psychological health issues may be learning to take care of your own health needs, despite the competing demands of caring for others or focusing on your career and relationships.

35—A TRANSITIONAL AGE

Fertility is not the only physiological factor which declines in your 30s. Ironically, 35 is a "magic number" of sorts in women's health. You may notice the beginning of age-related visual changes after 35, and many women may notice changes in their hair color and in their skin. It's also a turning point because you are at increased risk of a number of medical problems and concerns, including:

- Miscarriage
- Birth defects (notably Down syndrome; see chart, opposite)
- Depression
- Breast cancer
- The beginning of bone loss
- Slower metabolism, which may make it more difficult for you to lose weight
- Fibroids
- High blood pressure
- Autoimmune diseases.

FERTILITY AND SEXUAL HEALTH

For many women, their 30s (and increasingly their 40s) are a time when they face fertility challenges and concerns.

A growing percentage of women delay pregnancy until their 30s. While this is a relatively small proportion, a woman over 35 not only has a greater risk of infertility, but is also considered to be of "advanced maternal age," which carries medical risks for the mother.

For example, if you give birth to your first child after the age of 35, you have approximately twice the risk of developing breast cancer as a woman who gave birth before the age of 20. A woman who has never given birth has a significantly increased risk of ovarian cancer.

Years ago, women over 35 weren't allowed to take the contraceptive pill. We now know that it is safe for healthy, nonsmoking women over 35 to continue taking low-dose oral contraceptives as long as they have no other contraindications.

While the average age of menopause is 51, many women enter it earlier, either naturally, surgically (by removal of the uterus or the ovaries), or as a result of chemotherapy or radiation. This may well happen during the 30s.

There is also a condition called premature ovarian failure (POF), which is estimated to affect 1 in 100 women between the ages of 30 and 39. In fact, women can be affected with POF at any age, even during their teens. Statistics show the average age of POF in the US is 27.5 years.

BONE HEALTH

The 30s are an important time for you to think about the health of your bones. While we think that our bones stop growing once we stop growing in height, they are actually continually remodeling. Women continue to build bone mass until the age of 30.

Bone mass generally remains stable until 35, after which it begins a slow but steady decline until menopause. After that, it declines relatively quickly unless you take medication to prevent it.

The most important steps that you can take in this decade to prevent bone loss include:

- Developing good exercise habits, and focusing on weight-bearing exercise. This includes walking,

TESTS RECOMMENDED IN YOUR 30s

Compared to your 20s, the number of routine checkups and screening tests that are recommended during your 30s has increased significantly. Many are precautionary while others, such as the weight/height checks and the mammogram screening, provide baseline recordings that will prove useful later on. Ask your doctor for advice about the best way to coordinate all these tests.

Routine checkups

- ✔ Do a monthly breast self-examination (see p154)
- ✔ Have a complete physical examination every year
- ✔ Have a complete gynecological examination every year
- ✔ Have a Pap smear (see p107) according to your doctor's recommendations: for most women, this will be every year
- ✔ Have your eyes tested every five years
- ✔ Go for a twice-yearly dental checkup and cleaning
- ✔ Have your weight and height measured every year: this will help measure any bone loss later on
- ✔ Have your blood pressure measured every year
- ✔ Check your lipid levels every five years
- ✔ Have a complete skin check for moles or suspicious abnormalities every one to two years (see pp358-60)
- ✔ Have an annual digital rectal exam, with fecal occult blood testing to check for colorectal cancer
- ✔ Have an annual clinical breast exam
- ✔ Have an HPV test for cervical cancer: if this is normal and you are in the same mutually monogamous relationship, this should be repeated every three years

Additional screening tests

- ✔ If you are thinking of getting pregnant, see your doctor for preconception advice. You may also need screening tests and a Pap smear before you conceive
- ✔ Have a mammogram: 35 is the age at which many doctors recommend a baseline mammogram (especially in women with a family history of early breast cancer), although the American Cancer Society recommends beginning routine mammogram screening at age 40
- ✔ Have urinalysis as recommended by your doctor
- ✔ Have your hemoglobin and hematocrit checked as recommended by your doctor
- ✔ If you are not in a mutually monogamous relationship, your doctor may recommend STD screening

running, dancing, or aerobics, and resistance exercises, such as tennis or weight training
- Ensuring that you are getting adequate amounts of calcium and vitamin D in your diet.

HEART HEALTH

It's always a good time for you to think about heart health, but your 30s are the time when risk factors for heart disease begin to increase. In this decade, it's important to

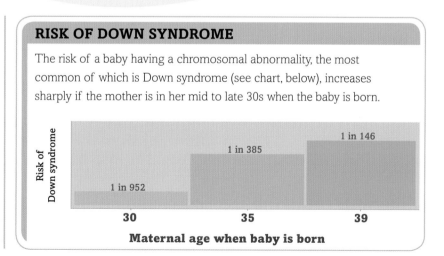

RISK OF DOWN SYNDROME

The risk of a baby having a chromosomal abnormality, the most common of which is Down syndrome (see chart, below), increases sharply if the mother is in her mid to late 30s when the baby is born.

Risk of Down syndrome

1 in 952 (30)
1 in 385 (35)
1 in 146 (39)

Maternal age when baby is born

maintain a healthy weight, address any risky habits, and correct any abnormalities in blood pressure and the levels of glucose, cholesterol, or triglycerides in your blood. Getting regular aerobic exercise is very important for maintaining a healthy heart.

WEIGHT ISSUES

Try to keep your weight under control as best you can. If you're overweight or obese, you are at increased risk of:

- Heart disease, heart attack, stroke, and type 2 diabetes
- Metabolic syndrome
- Endometrial cancer
- Gallstones
- Stress incontinence

"Between her 30s and 50s, the average woman loses 0.5 percent of bone density each year."

- Polycystic ovary syndrome
- Obstetric problems including miscarriage, preeclampsia, gestational diabetes, and needing a cesarean section
- Postmenopausal breast cancer: 30 percent of these cancers are associated with weight that has been gained after menopause.

EXERCISE

We all know that exercise is good for us and there's no such thing as being too old—especially in your 30s!—or too unwell to do some. The benefits of exercise include:

- Easier weight management
- An increase in HDL ("good") cholesterol and a decrease in triglycerides and LDL ("bad") cholesterol in the blood
- Decreased blood pressure
- Slower resting heart rate
- Increased bone density and a reduced risk of osteoporosis
- Decreased risk of colon cancer, kidney stones, breast cancer, and depression
- Decreased stress and anxiety
- Improvement in self-esteem and overall mental health
- Improvement in sleep.

VITAMIN AND MINERAL SUPPLEMENTS IN YOUR 30s

The following vitamin and mineral supplements can help you get the most out of life. However, you should note that some single-dose vitamin supplements can interact harmfully with some medications or with the absorption of other nutrients, so you

QUESTIONS TO ASK YOUR DOCTOR IN YOUR 30s

The following are just some of the questions you can ask your doctor about at the start of your 30s:

- Should I be taking any vitamins or supplements?
- Are there additional screening

or diagnostic tests that I need?
- When should I have my first/next mammogram?
- Are there any behavioral or lifestyle changes I should make for optimal health?

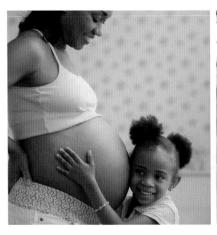
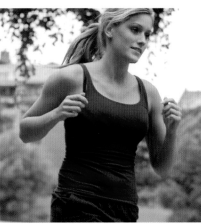
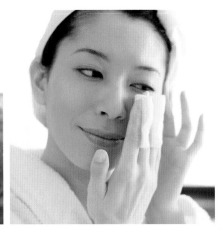

should always check with your doctor before you begin to take them.

Multivitamins Most women who are menstruating will benefit from a daily multivitamin supplement with iron; multivitamins have also been shown to reduce your risk of colds and flu.

Folic acid/omega-3 fatty acids If you are breast-feeding, pregnant, or thinking of starting a family, take a folic acid supplement (400 micrograms/day) and an omega-3 fatty acid supplement (200 mg/day). While many prenatal vitamins contain these ingredients, not all of them do—so make sure that you check the label.

Calcium If your diet is not giving you enough calcium (1,200 mg/day or the equivalent of four glasses of skim milk), you may want to take a daily calcium supplement to make up the difference. However, speak to your doctor before you do and see pp52–5 to find out more about a healthy diet.

Vitamin D This essential vitamin aids calcium absorption and bone

---

LEADING CAUSES OF DEATH FOR WOMEN IN THEIR 30s

Statistical research in the US shows that the leading causes of death among women in their 30s are:

1. Cancer (all causes)
2. Accidents
3. Heart disease
4. Suicide
5. HIV/AIDS
6. Murder
7. Stroke
8. Diabetes
9. Chronic liver disease
10. Pregnancy complications

---

health. Most multivitamins contain vitamin D, but always check the dosage. Most women need between 1,000 and 1,500 IU of vitamin D each day. While it is in many foods, vitamin D is also made in the skin in response to exposure to sunlight (even if it's not a sunny day). If you don't receive 20 minutes of daily sunlight exposure, or are diligent about using total sunscreen, you may need to consider supplements.

VACCINES FOR YOUR 30s

You may think you don't need any more vaccines, unless you're going to an exotic destination. However, you may want to consider having the following during your 30s.

Flu You may be in a high-risk group for needing a flu shot annually, but even if you aren't, you should get the flu shot if you don't want this illness.

Rubella (German measles) If there's a chance that you may become pregnant, make sure you are immune to rubella. A rubella infection during the first trimester of pregnancy can cause major fetal abnormalities.

Tetanus, diphtheria, pertussis (TDP/tDap) Ask your doctor when you had your last TDP shot. You will need a tetanus booster every 10 years.

Catch-up vaccines See p31.

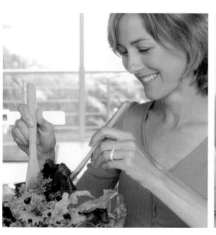
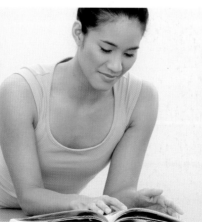
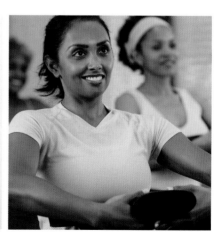

Your 40s

The 40s can be a wonderfully settling decade for women. Many describe this decade as a time when they can appreciate their accumulated life's wisdom, their professional lives have had time to develop, their family lives are often established, and, even though they are beginning to show a few more signs of aging, they are still enjoying good health.

FERTILITY AND SEXUAL HEALTH

An increasing number of women choose to become pregnant in their 40s, yet face realistic concerns about decreasing fertility. Ironically, many women in this decade are unsure about which contraceptive methods are safe for them. If they have irregular periods, they often mistakenly think that they no longer have to be concerned about getting pregnant. As a result, women in their 40s have the second highest rate of unintended pregnancy (after the teens).

If you are heterosexually active, haven't yet reached menopause, and are not using any reliable form of contraception, you can still get pregnant. The good news is that if you are a healthy, nonsmoking woman in your 40s, it is no longer considered unsafe for you to take the contraceptive pill or use the contraceptive patch, as long as you don't have any contraindications; many very low-dose alternatives are now available.

The age at which women reach menopause is, on average, 51. However, many women begin menopause earlier, either naturally or because of surgery—after they have had a hysterectomy or their ovaries removed—or as a result of chemotherapy or radiation treatment. The average age of a surgical menopause is 42.

OTHER MENSTRUAL CHANGES

Not all menstrual irregularities are due to perimenopausal changes (see box, left). Fibroids increase during the 40s and may affect up to a third of all women and up to 50 percent of African-American women. Both endometriosis and endometrial hyperplasia may become a problem, too. All these conditions may contribute to heavy menstrual cramps (dysmenorrhea; p91) and heavy menstrual bleeding (menorrhagia; p91).

PERIMENOPAUSE

The hormonal hallmark of this decade is perimenopause. This phase of hormonal flux may last up to ten years preceding your menopause (see Chapter 5). Your ovaries start to produce less estrogen and there is an inevitable reduction in your fertility.

While you may still have regular periods during this time, falling estrogen levels may cause you to notice one or more of the following symptoms:
- Changes in your menstrual flow or frequency
- Increased premenstrual symptoms
- Increased acne
- Increased moodiness or irritability
- Sleep disturbances.

You may also begin to notice menopausal symptoms such as:
- Hot flashes
- Night sweats
- Vaginal dryness
- Early bone loss (though only a test would tell you this).

If such symptoms are bothering you, there are several over-the-counter or prescription remedies available. However, you should also consult your doctor to be sure that the symptoms are due to normal, age-related hormonal changes and are not caused by another medical problem.

TESTS RECOMMENDED IN YOUR 40s

The lists of routine checkups and additional screening tests that are recommended in your 40s are almost the same as those in your 30s. A new checkup concerns talking to your doctor about bothersome perimenopausal symptoms, while extra screening tests include measuring your blood glucose and having a baseline check on your heart and lungs if you are or were a smoker.

Routine checkups

- ✔ Do a monthly breast self-examination (see p154)
- ✔ Have a mammogram every other year
- ✔ Have a complete physical examination every year
- ✔ Have a complete gynecological examination every year
- ✔ Have a Pap smear (see p107) according to your doctor's recommendations: for most women, this will be every year
- ✔ Have your eyes tested every two years
- ✔ Go for a twice-yearly dental checkup and cleaning
- ✔ Have your weight and height measured every year
- ✔ Have your blood pressure measured every year
- ✔ See your doctor if you are experiencing any perimenopausal symptoms that bother you
- ✔ Check your lipid levels every five years
- ✔ Have a complete skin check for moles or suspicious abnormalities every one to two years (see pp358-60)
- ✔ Have an annual digital rectal exam, with fecal occult blood testing to check for colorectal cancer
- ✔ Have an annual clinical breast exam

Additional screening tests

- ✔ If you are thinking of getting pregnant, see your doctor for preconception advice. You may also need screening tests and a Pap smear before you conceive.
- ✔ If you are not in a mutually monogamous relationship, your doctor may recommend STD screening, including the HPV test for cervical cancer
- ✔ Have urinalysis as recommended by your doctor
- ✔ Have your hemoglobin and hematocrit checked (anemia is very common in menstruating women and fibroids are now an increased risk) as recommended by your doctor
- ✔ Have blood glucose testing (a screen for diabetes) every five years until 65
- ✔ Have a baseline electrocardiogram (EKG) and a chest X-ray or CT scan if you are/were a smoker.
  Have an HPV test for cervical cancer: if this is normal and you are in the same mutually monogamous relationship, this should be repeated every three years

MAMMOGRAMS

The optimal number of times to have mammography screening during your 40s is still debated. While lung cancer is the leading cause of cancer death among American women overall, breast cancer is the leading cause among Hispanic-American women. Added to this, African-American women are at greater risk of a more aggressive breast cancer at a younger age. Some specialists recommend annual mammograms for women over 40, though many feel that changes in the breast tissue make it harder to spot abnormalities in the under 50s.

The question about how often you need to have a mammogram relates only to women who don't have any symptoms at all. If you discover a new, abnormal, or changing breast lump, discuss this immediately with your doctor.

LIBIDO

Many women have reported that they experience a decreased libido during their 40s, even before they reach menopause. It is unclear whether this is driven by hormones, psychology, or social forces, but it is probably a combination of all three. If you are feeling that your libido has decreased, the best thing to do would be to discuss it with both your partner and your doctor.

Many women are not aware, for example, that decreased libido is a potential side effect of many medications, including birth control pills and some antidepressants (which are increasingly prescribed to women in this age group).

> **"Women in their 40s have the second highest percentage of unplanned pregnancies."**

MENTAL HEALTH

While the overwhelming majority of women in their 40s enjoy good mental health, up to 10 percent of them (twice as many as men) may experience significant clinical depression. A common myth about aging is that depression increases after menopause and continues to increase with age. This is not true; the average age of depression in women is 44 and it appears to decrease afterwards.

Obvious risk factors for depression include separation, divorce, loss, and chronic illness. But there are other, hormonally related causes, as well as smoking, having had PMS, having started menstruating at a young age, and never having been pregnant.

OTHER PHYSICAL CHANGES

"Female, fertile, fat, and 40" is an old medical expression describing the classic risk factors for a number of medical problems, from type 2 diabetes to gallstones. Changes in your metabolism seem to make it suddenly more difficult to lose weight and much easier to put it on, especially around the abdomen.

Perhaps the condition of greatest concern is one that is only just being understood: during this decade, you are at a much greater risk of developing metabolic syndrome. While the definition of this syndrome varies, the consensus is that it includes a constellation of conditions that create a high risk for coronary artery disease. These conditions include type 2 diabetes, obesity, increased LDL ("bad" cholesterol), low HDL ("good" cholesterol), high blood pressure, elevated triglycerides, and insulin resistance.

Other changes you are likely to experience during your 40s include:

- Visual changes (especially the need for reading glasses)
- Hair becoming grayer
- Some hair loss (or growth in the wrong places)
- Urinary incontinence (may begin or get worse)
- Early bone loss. You may not notice it, but it may start, especially if you are at greater risk for osteoporosis.

QUESTIONS TO ASK YOUR DOCTOR IN YOUR 40s

The following are questions you should ask during your 40s:

- Should I be taking any vitamins or supplements?
- Are there additional screening or diagnostic tests that I need?
- When should I have my first/next mammogram?
- Are there any lifestyle changes I should make for optimal health?
- If I am at risk for heart disease, should I take a daily baby aspirin?

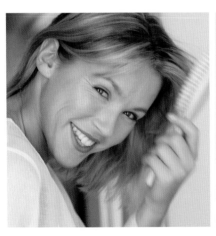
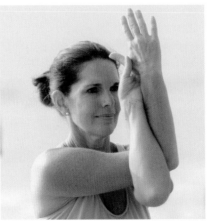
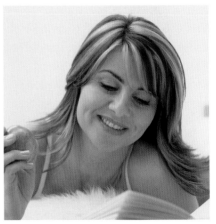

VITAMIN AND MINERAL SUPPLEMENTS IN YOUR 40s

The following supplements can help you get the most out of life. Some single-dose vitamin supplements can interact harmfully with some medications or with the absorption of other nutrients, so check with your doctor before taking them.

Multivitamins Most women who are menstruating will benefit from a daily multivitamin with iron.

Folic acid/omega-3 fatty acids If you're breast-feeding, pregnant, or thinking of getting pregnant, take folic acid (400 micrograms/day) and omega-3 (200 mg/day). Not all prenatal vitamins have these ingredients, so check the label.

Calcium If your diet is not giving you enough calcium (1,200 mg/day), you may need to take a daily calcium supplement to make up the difference. Speak to your doctor first and see pp52–5 to find out more about a healthy diet.

Vitamin D This essential vitamin aids calcium absorption and bone health. Most multivitamins contain vitamin D, but always check the dosage. Most women need between 1,000 to 1,500 IU of vitamin D each day. While it is in many foods, vitamin D is also made in the skin in response to exposure to sunlight (even if it's not a sunny day). If you don't receive 20 minutes of daily sunlight exposure, or are diligent about using total sunscreen, you may need to consider supplements.

VACCINES FOR YOUR 40s

You might need one or two vaccines during your 40s, such as:

Flu You may not be in a high risk group, but if you don't want the flu, be sure to get a flu shot.

Rubella (German measles) In case you become pregnant, make sure you're rubella immune. If you catch rubella in the first trimester of pregnancy, your baby can develop major abnormalities.

Tetanus, diphtheria, pertussis (TDP/tDap) Ask your doctor when you had your last TDP/tDap shot (see p33).

Catch-up vaccines See p29.

LEADING CAUSES OF DEATH FOR WOMEN IN THEIR 40s

Statistical research in the US shows that the leading causes of death among women in their 40s are:

1 Cancer (all types)
2 Heart disease
3 Accidents
4 Suicide
5 Stroke
6 Chronic liver disease
7 HIV/AIDS
8 Diabetes
9 Chronic lower respiratory diseases
10 Murder

"Vitamin and mineral supplements can help you get the most out of life."

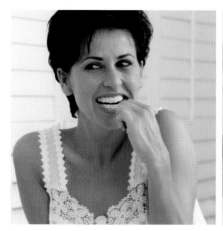
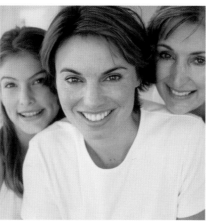
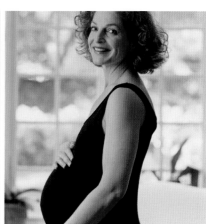

Your 50s

Most women go through menopause in their 50s. For many, the years following menopause are a cause for celebration, leading to renewed energy as they embrace the "third act" of their lives. Women no longer have to worry about contraception or unplanned pregnancies, and they can now enjoy the increased independence that comes with their children leaving the nest.

MENTAL HEALTH

More good news: myths about "the empty nest syndrome" leading to depression have been proven to be unfounded for the majority of menopausal women.

Depression is not associated with menopause except for women with specific risk factors. These include women who:
- Have previously suffered from major depression
- Experienced moderate premenstrual syndrome (PMS)
- Experienced postpartum depression
- Have experienced a major loss, such as the death of a spouse or a child
- Smoke
- Have a young child still at home.

SEXUAL HEALTH

For many women, one advantage of menopause is that they no longer have to worry about contraception. Consequently, women in this age group often forego condom usage with a new partner. This means that the incidence of sexually transmitted diseases (STDs) in women in their 50s has been increasing. In fact, Centers for Disease Control and Prevention (CDC) data show that, in 2005, 15 percent of new HIV diagnoses were among men and women over the age of 50. If you are sexually active and are not in a mutually monogamous relationship, you are at the same risk of getting STDs as younger women unless you practice safe sex.

BONE HEALTH

Many other subtle changes within the body result from the decline of estrogen production. Bone loss is the most dramatic: 20 percent of your lifetime expected bone loss will occur during the first five years of menopause, after which it will continue to decrease more slowly. For this reason, the National Osteoporosis Foundation (NOF) recommends that women with risk factors other than being female, menopausal, and Caucasian have a bone density test in their 50s (see p261 for risk factors).

OTHER CHANGES

The following changes may also occur during this decade:
- You'll probably need glasses for some tasks
- Your hearing starts to fade
- A continued decrease in your metabolism accounts for persistent weight gain, even though you may have the same calorie intake as before and get the same amount of exercise. It seems that the weight is simply harder to lose
- Fat deposits around your middle are more likely to occur and be

---

LEADING CAUSES OF DEATH FOR WOMEN IN THEIR 50s

Statistical research in the US shows that the leading causes of death among women in their 50s are:

1 Cancer (all types)
2 Heart disease
3 Accidents
4 Chronic lower respiratory diseases
5 Stroke
6 Diabetes
7 Chronic liver disease
8 Septicemia
9 Kidney diseases
10 HIV/AIDS

TESTS RECOMMENDED IN YOUR 50s

The tests and checkups that you began in your 30s and 40s continue into your 50s, with the exception of preconception advice, which you are no longer likely to need. Now is the time to discuss menopausal concerns with your gynecologist and bone density tests with your doctor. Perhaps the most important new addition is to have a colonoscopy to screen for colon cancer.

Routine checkups

✔ Do a monthly breast self-examination (see p154)

✔ Have an annual mammogram (see p155)

✔ Have a complete physical examination every year

✔ Have a complete gynecological examination every year and discuss any menopausal concerns and treatments

✔ Have a Pap smear according to your doctor's recommendations: for most women, this will be every year

✔ Have your eyes tested now every two years

✔ Go for a twice-yearly dental checkup and cleaning

✔ Have your weight and height measured every year

✔ Have your blood pressure measured every year

✔ Check your lipid levels every five years

✔ Have a complete skin check for moles or suspicious abnormalities every one to two years (see pp358-60)

✔ Ask when you should have your first bone density test (see p260)

Additional screening tests

✔ Have an annual digital rectal exam, with fecal occult blood testing for colorectal cancer

✔ Have an annual clinical breast exam

✔ Have a colonoscopy once every ten years

✔ If you are not in a mutually monogamous relationship, your doctor may recommend STD screening, including the HPV test for cervical cancer

✔ Have urinalysis as recommended by your doctor

✔ Have your hemoglobin and hematocrit checked (anemia is common in menstruating women and fibroids are an increased risk)

✔ Have blood glucose testing (a screen for diabetes) every five years until age 65

✔ Have an electrocardiogram (EKG) or other cardiac testing as indicated

---

more persistent. This is an increased risk factor for heart disease and leads to an increase in blood triglyceride levels

- Skin changes become more obvious with increased facial wrinkles, liver spots, skin tags, and overall dryness
- While increased forgetfulness is common during this decade, you should discuss any significant

change in memory with your doctor so it can be evaluated.

SLEEP

Some experts attribute forgetfulness to sleep disturbances associated with menopause. Many surveys of menopausal women report that women find sleep disturbances to be the most disruptive menopausal symptom of all.

In addition to these hormonally mediated sleep disturbances, a snoring disorder in a bed partner can also disrupt a woman's sleep! Whatever the reason for the sleep deprivation, it can be very upsetting, cause excessive daytime drowsiness, and interfere with cognitive or skilled functions.

EARLY-ONSET ALZHEIMER'S

You may worry that increased forgetfulness is a sign of early Alzheimer's, the most common form of dementia, which is believed to affect five million Americans.

"Approximately 30 percent of American women will not experience any disruptive menopausal symptoms."

Of those, more than 4.5 million are over 65 years of age (and half of these are over 85 years of age).

However, there is a condition called "early-onset Alzheimer's," which can affect anyone under 65. It is very difficult to calculate how many people are actually affected: estimates range from 200,000 to 500,000 Americans, most of whom are in their 50s.

Early-onset Alzheimer's often results from a genetic defect that is inherited on the chromosomes. So, if you know you have a family history of early-onset Alzheimer's, make sure you discuss this with your doctor. While any truly impaired cognitive function must be seriously evaluated at any age, experts are currently concerned that early-onset Alzheimer's is grossly underreported.

BOWEL HEALTH

Turning 50 is a major birthday, but your most valuable gift is one you should get for yourself: a screening colonoscopy. The good news is that if the results are normal, you don't have

---

QUESTIONS TO ASK YOUR DOCTOR IN YOUR 50s

The following are just some of the questions you can ask your doctor about at the start of your 50s:

- Should I be taking any vitamins or supplements?
- Are there additional screening or diagnostic tests that I need?
- Do I need a bone density test?
- When should I have my next mammogram?
- Are there any lifestyle changes I should make for optimal health?
- Do I need to make any changes in any of my medicines?
- If I'm at risk of heart disease, should I take a daily baby aspirin?

---

to repeat it for another 10 years. Colon cancer is the second most common cancer killer of women. Women who have had endometrial or ovarian cancer are at greater risk of developing colon cancer, as are women with a family history of colon cancer.

The American College of Obstetricians and Gynecologists has stated that colonoscopy is the preferred colon cancer screening test for women because it gives the doctor better access to the right side of the colon—this is more often the site of a type of advanced cancer that is more likely to develop in women. See Chapter 13 for more information.

VITAMIN AND MINERAL SUPPLEMENTS IN YOUR 50s

The following vitamin and mineral supplements can help you get the most out of life. However, some single-dose vitamin supplements can interact harmfully with some medications or with the absorption of other nutrients, so check with your doctor before taking them.

Multivitamins Unless your doctor tells you otherwise, you probably no longer need iron in your multivitamin supplements.

Calcium If your diet is not giving you enough calcium (1,500 mg/day) after menopause, you may want to take a daily calcium supplement to make up

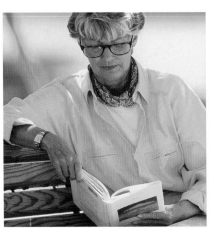
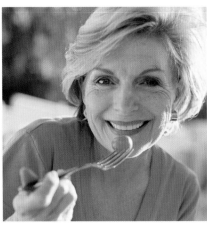
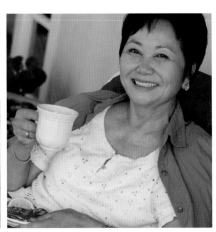

the difference. Be sure to speak to your doctor before you do and see pp52–5 to find out more about a healthy diet.

Vitamin D This vitamin helps to absorb calcium and is good for your bones. Most multivitamins contain vitamin D, but check the dosage—most women need between 1,000 to 1,500 IU a day. Vitamin D is contained in many foods, but your skin also makes it in response to sunlight. If your skin doesn't receive approximately 20 minutes of daily sunlight exposure, you may need to consider supplements.

VACCINES FOR YOUR 50s

Unless you are traveling outside the country or your doctor tells you otherwise, these are probably the only vaccines you might need:

Flu There are many qualifiers on the list of who "should" get a flu shot annually; it can be summed up as being recommended for anyone who doesn't want to get the flu.

Tetanus, diphtheria, pertussis (TDP or tDap) Ask your doctor when you had your last TDP shot. You will need a tetanus booster every 10 years.

MENOPAUSE

The average age of menopause among women in the US and Canada is 51. For most women, menopause not only signifies the end of menstruation; when it's over, it also brings about a feeling that has been described as "postmenopausal zest" (see p137)

It is a myth that all women experience menopausal symptoms. In fact, approximately 30 percent of American women will not experience any disruptive menopausal symptoms. However, that means that approximately 70 percent will. While menopausal symptoms vary significantly in terms of the age of onset, severity, frequency, and duration, classic menopausal symptoms include hot flashes, night sweats, vaginal dryness (leading to irritation and painful sexual intercourse), mood swings, irritability, and sleep disturbances (see Menopause, pp136-41).

HORMONE REPLACEMENT THERAPY

One of the biggest health questions for menopausal women who have moderate to severe menopausal symptoms is whether or not to use hormone replacement therapy (see p137-8). One major concern is whether this therapy may or may not increase a woman's risk of serious health consequences, notably breast or endometrial cancer.

Among the huge amount of information available is a confusing study from the Women's Health Initiative (WHI), the largest ever study of menopausal women. This study confirms only one thing: that each woman must consider her own individual circumstances, symptoms, risks, and benefits in consultation with her doctor. Women in their 50s should be reassured by the 2006 reanalysis of the WHI data, which showed that there was no increase in the risk of heart disease among those women aged 50 to 59 who were taking estrogen.

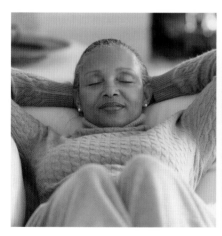

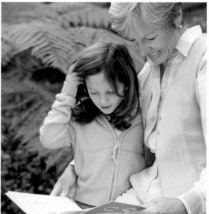

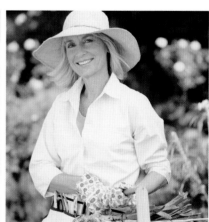

Your 60s

Women in their 60s are more active than ever before. Many continue to work beyond the usual retirement age, take up new activities, and embark on new relationships. In fact, the average, healthy, 60-year-old woman can expect to live another 24 years and for 18 of those, she should be in good, very good, or excellent perceived health—and she won't have given up on her sex life, either.

EXERCISE

Try to keep active: if you enjoy a specific activity, continue with it, but if you're not active it's never too late to start. Consider the following physical activities:

- Walking, swimming, and low-impact aerobics reduce cardiac risk and maintain endurance and overall fitness
- Weight-bearing exercises, such as tennis, are particularly good for preventing osteoporosis
- Weight-building exercises, such as light weight training, build and maintain muscle mass and bone strength
- Exercises, such as yoga and Pilates, maintain flexibility and help prevent falls.

"Walking, swimming, and low-impact aerobics reduce cardiac risk and maintain overall fitness and endurance."

MENTAL HEALTH

The impression that women in this age group suffer from increasing depression and isolation has largely been shown to be inaccurate, but women with difficult physical changes to contend with (see below) need to take special care of their mental health.

PHYSICAL CHANGES

Physical signs of aging are now more apparent. Sight and hearing continue to decline, with 30 percent of all people over 65 having significantly impaired hearing. Urinary incontinence is an increasing problem in the mid-60s, when 10 percent of women are affected (see Incontinence, p339-42). Bladder, vision, and hearing problems, as well as decreased physical activity, may contribute to social isolation.

BONE HEALTH

Women with osteoporosis may start to develop a slight hunch and lose a little height. Arthritis may disfigure your fingers and make some other joints less flexible.

DISEASES OF THE 60s

Heart disease is a close second to cancer as the main killer of women in their 60s. There is an increased incidence of other diseases, such as Parkinson's disease and brain tumors. On average, Parkinson's starts at about 60 years of age.

VITAMIN AND MINERAL SUPPLEMENTS IN YOUR 60s

Check with your doctor before taking supplements since some single-dose vitamins can interact harmfully with

QUESTIONS TO ASK YOUR DOCTOR IN YOUR 60s

The following are just some of the questions you can ask your doctor about at the start of your 60s:

- Should I be taking any vitamins or supplements?
- Are there additional screening or diagnostic tests that I need?

- Are there any lifestyle changes I should make for optimal health?
- If I am at risk for heart disease, should I take a baby aspirin once every day?
- When should I have a bone density test?

TESTS RECOMMENDED IN YOUR 60s

In your 60s, you need to continue with a number of recommended checkups and tests, many of which you should have already had previously. The annual mammogram continues as an important routine test. You now also need a baseline bone density test, too, to monitor osteoporosis. The only new blood test is one that assesses the health of your thyroid gland.

Routine checkups

✔ Do a monthly breast self-examination (see p154)
✔ Have an annual mammogram (see p155)
✔ Have a complete physical examination every year
✔ Have a complete gynecological examination every year
✔ Have a Pap smear (see p107) according to your doctor's recommendations: for most women, this is every year
✔ Have your eyes tested annually for glaucoma, cataracts, and macular degeneration
✔ Have your hearing tested every year
✔ Go for a twice-yearly dental checkup and cleaning
✔ Have your weight and height measured every year
✔ Have your blood pressure measured every year
✔ Check your lipid levels every five years
✔ Have a complete skin check for moles or suspicious abnormalities every year (see pp358-60)
✔ Have a baseline bone density test (see p260) by the time you are 65
✔ Have an annual clinical breast exam
✔ Have an annual digital rectal exam, with fecal occult blood testing for colorectal cancer

Additional screening tests

✔ Have a colonoscopy once every ten years
✔ Have an electrocardiogram (EKG) or other cardiac testing as indicated
✔ Have blood glucose testing (a screen for diabetes) every five years until 65, then annually
✔ Have a thyroid screening test, known as the TSH test, to check your thyroid gland once you reach 60
✔ Your doctor may recommend STD screening, depending on your risk factors.
✔ Have urinalysis as recommended by your doctor
✔ Have your hemoglobin and hematocrit checked as recommended by your doctor

medications or with the absorption of other nutrients.

Multivitamins Unless your doctor tells you otherwise you probably no longer need iron in your multivitamin.

Calcium and vitamin D If your diet does not give you the calcium you need (1,500 mg/day), you may need to take calcium and vitamin D supplements.

VACCINES FOR YOUR 60s

Make sure you receive vaccines for the following diseases:
Pneumonia (see p234)

Flu Have an annual flu vaccination.
Tetanus You should have a tetanus booster every 10 years.

Zoster Since 2005 there has been a vaccine to prevent shingles. It reduces your risk by 50 percent.

LEADING CAUSES OF DEATH FOR WOMEN IN THEIR 60s

Statistical research in the US shows that the leading causes of death among women in their 60s are:

1 Cancer (all types)
2 Heart disease
3 Stroke
4 Chronic lower respiratory diseases
5 Diabetes
6 Accidents
7 Alzheimer's disease
8 Pneumonia/influenza
9 Kidney diseases
10 Septicemia

Your 70s

An increasing number of women live active, healthy lives well into their 70s and beyond. In fact, a 75-year-old woman in the US has, on average, an additional 12.8 years to enjoy. The challenge is to do all you can to make those years as healthy and as mobile as possible, remembering that it's never too late to take steps to improve your health.

MENTAL AND PHYSICAL WELL-BEING

Mental and social health are just as important as physical health for women in their 70s. Because of longer life expectancies for women than men, and the tendency for many women to marry men who are older, most women can expect to spend some of their later years as singles. However, "single" should not mean "alone."

To prevent this isolation, many women in their 70s work part-time (paid or voluntary), join clubs, take classes, form exercise groups, or pursue other interests. Pets can also be great companions.

Studies have shown that women who become socially isolated are three times more likely to die from cancer. Although depression does not increase in this decade, it does raise the mortality rates of other medical problems if left untreated.

While most women over 70 are able to maintain a healthy quality of life, the Women's Health and Aging study found that 32 percent of American women over 70 had difficulty performing—or were unable to perform—basic self-care activities. The most common

causes of this kind of disability were musculoskeletal pain, general weakness, and balance problems.

EXERCISE

Staying physically active is one of the most important ways of staying well. Running after your grandchildren is a great form of exercise, but a recent study found that women aged 72–79 who did some form of moderate physical activity for at least one hour per week were far less likely to have symptoms of arthritis.

It is a myth that older people should avoid doing exercise. On the contrary, it would be harmful to your health if you didn't! You simply need to find a physical

activity that suits you. Regular flexibility exercises such as yoga or stretching are good for you, as are swimming and supervised strength training. Unless your doctor has told you otherwise, age itself is no reason to discontinue any activity that you have previously enjoyed. If in doubt, check with your doctor.

LIBIDO

Another common myth about people in their 70s and beyond is that their sex lives are over. Yet, many of them are still sexually active. However, one large-scale study revealed that about half of the men and women surveyed reported at least one sexual problem. Among women in the

---

QUESTIONS TO ASK YOUR DOCTOR IN YOUR 70s

The following are just some of the questions you can ask your doctor about at the start of your 70s:

- Should I be taking any vitamins or supplements?
- Are there additional screening or diagnostic tests that I need?
- Should I still have an annual mammogram and Pap smear?
- Have I been tested recently for diabetes or thyroid problems?
- Are there any lifestyle changes I should make for optimal health?
- If I am at risk for heart disease, should I take a baby aspirin once every day?
- Would I benefit from some form of physical therapy?

TESTS RECOMMENDED IN YOUR 70s

The lists of checkups and tests that are recommended for you in your 70s remain similar to those in your 60s. Make sure you keep your appointments for the routine checkups, especially the mammograms and the tests for glaucoma, cataracts, and macular degeneration of the eyes. Tests for blood pressure, bone density, and colon cancer are important, too.

Routine checkups

✔ Do a monthly breast self-examination (see p154)
✔ Have an annual mammogram (see p155)
✔ Have a complete physical examination every year
✔ Have a complete gynecological examination every year
✔ Go for a twice-yearly dental checkup and cleaning
✔ Have a baseline bone density test (see p260) if you did not have it at 65
✔ Have your eyes tested annually for glaucoma, cataracts, and macular degeneration
✔ Have your weight, height, blood pressure, and hearing checked every year
✔ Have a complete skin check for moles or suspicious abnormalities every year (see pp358-60)

✔ Have blood glucose testing (a screen for diabetes) every year
✔ Have another thyroid screening test, known as the TSH test, to check the health of your thyroid gland
✔ Have an annual clinical breast exam
✔ Have urinalysis as recommended by your doctor
✔ Have your hemoglobin and hematocrit checked
✔ Have an annual digital rectal exam, with fecal occult blood testing for colorectal cancer

Additional screening tests

✔ Check your lipid levels every five years
✔ Have a colonoscopy once every ten years five years
✔ Have an electrocardiogram (EKG) or other cardiac testing as indicated

---

study, the most common problems were low desire (43 percent), vaginal dryness (39 percent), and an inability to climax (34 percent).

Decreased libido and an inability to achieve orgasm are complex sexual issues. However, vaginal dryness can be easily treated, either with an over-the-counter, water-based lubricant or with a prescription estrogen cream.

Most seniors with treatable sexual problems have not discussed their symptoms with a doctor. There are various reasons for this: they think, mistakenly, that nothing can be done or that their problem is just a part of aging; or else they are too embarrassed to talk about it.

DIGESTIVE HEALTH

Digestion slows down after the age of 70 due to dental problems, a fall in gastric acid production, and the decreased movement of food through the gut. The result may be constipation and indigestion.

Decreased appetite can become a problem, too. It is often caused by a reduced sense of taste and smell, or by illness or muscle wasting. If you have decreased energy, you may think that it is a "normal" sign of aging, but it may be that you are

LEADING CAUSES OF DEATH FOR WOMEN IN THEIR 70s

Statistical research in the US shows that the leading causes of death among women in their 70s are:

1 Heart disease
2 Cancer (all types)
3 Stroke
4 Chronic lower respiratory diseases
5 Diabetes
6 Alzheimer's
7 Pneumonia/influenza
8 Kidney diseases
9 Accidents
10 Septicemia

deficient in protein, calories, iron, vitamin B12, or vitamin D. Ask your doctor about taking a daily multivitamin or if you should consult a qualified nutritionist.

Various preventive measures can help improve the health of your digestive system. These include:

- Eating small meals frequently
- Increasing your dietary fiber (or take a supplement)
- Taking digestive supplements since some women benefit
- Drinking eight glasses of water per day
- Walking for about 20 to 30 minutes each day.

BONE AND TEETH HEALTH

Tooth loss is increasingly common in this decade, due to poor dental hygiene, osteoporosis of the jaw, and gum disease.

Increasingly fragile bones in women over 70 make it vital that they do not fall. Bone density testing, osteoporosis treatment, and taking calcium and vitamin D supplements are important, too. In women over 75, the most common

"Various preventive measures can help improve the health of your digestive system."

surgery is hip fracture repair—but 20 percent die within one year of surgery and 25 percent need long-term care in a nursing home.

EYE AND EAR HEALTH

Poor vision can contribute to falls as well as make daily living more challenging. Similarly, hearing may become increasingly impaired in your 70s and beyond.

Don't be shy or embarrassed about telling your doctor your hearing needs help: there are many types of hearing aids that are neither obvious nor intrusive.

SKIN HEALTH

In your 70s and beyond, the skin continues to become increasingly thin, dry, itchy, and fragile, making bruises, cuts, and infections more common. While most of the skin problems are benign, you should still be alert to changes that are potentially cancerous. People over

70 may also experience decreased sensitivity to temperature changes. Hypothermia, in particular, can be serious, so make sure your home is adequately heated when the weather is cold outside.

VITAMIN AND MINERAL SUPPLEMENTS IN YOUR 70s

The following vitamin and mineral supplements can help you get the most out of life. However, some single-dose vitamin supplements can interact harmfully with some medications or with the absorption of other nutrients, so check with your doctor before taking them.

Multivitamins Unless your doctor tells you otherwise, you probably no longer need iron in your multivitamin.

Calcium If your diet is not providing you with an adequate amount of calcium (1,500 mg/day or the equivalent of four glasses of skim milk), you could take

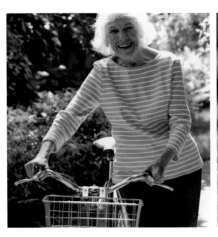

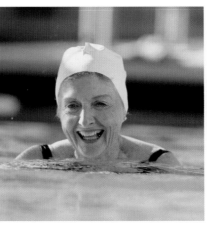

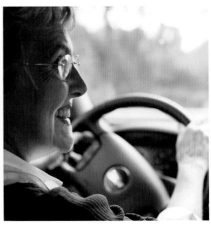

a calcium supplement every day to make up the difference. However, be sure to speak to your doctor before doing so and see pp52-5 and p262) for more about a healthy diet.

Vitamin D This essential vitamin aids calcium absorption and bone health. Most multivitamins contain vitamin D, but always check the dosage. Most women need between 1,000 to 1,500 IU of vitamin D each day. While it is in many foods, vitamin D is also made in the skin in response to exposure to sunlight (even if it's not a sunny day). If you don't receive 20 minutes of daily sunlight exposure, you may need to consider supplements.

VACCINES FOR YOUR 70s

As in your 60s, make sure you receive vaccines for the following:

Flu Have a flu shot every year.

Pneumonia All adults over 65 should receive this vaccine to lower the risk of pneumonia.

Tetanus You should have a tetanus booster every 10 years.

Zoster Have this vaccine against shingles if you missed it in your 60s.

DEMENTIA AND ALZHEIMER'S DISEASE

Memory problems and dementia are increasingly a cause for concern for women in their 70s. Alzheimer's (see pp184-5) is one of the most common forms of dementia, and the average age at which it starts is 72. A significant number of people with Alzheimer's also develop signs of Parkinson's disease, such as rigidity of the body and walking abnormalities. Certain factors increase the risk of Alzheimer's:

- Smokers can develop it 2.3 years earlier than nonsmokers. Other studies estimate the increased risk of Alzheimer's and other forms of dementia with smoking is 50 percent
- This "smoking" effect is even greater in individuals who have a genetic predisposition to develop Alzheimer's
- Those who consume two or more alcoholic drinks per day can develop Alzheimer's 4.8 years earlier than nondrinkers

- People with all three of the above risk factors can develop Alzheimer's disease an average of 8.5 years earlier than their risk-free counterparts.

We now know that you can reduce your risk of Alzheimer's by:

- Stopping smoking and reducing alcohol intake
- Getting regular exercise (see p197). The greatest benefit of this simple habit may be in reducing the risk, or delaying the onset, of Alzheimer's. This is because neurons in the brain (particularly in the hippocampus, the area most affected by Alzheimer's) continue to regenerate throughout life. The process is fueled by cerebral blood flow in the brain, which can be increased by aerobic exercise
- Taking vitamin E and omega-3 fatty acid supplements. However, their benefits have not yet been proved, nor have their effective doses been established.

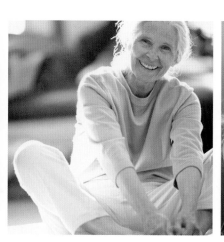

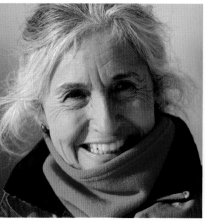

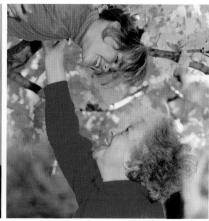

Staying well

Beatriz Rodriguez Olson MD FACP
Clinical Assistant Professor
Yale University School of Medicine

Staying well

Obesity, diabetes, and heart disease seem to be the curse of the Western world today. Doctors refer to these conditions as "multifactorial," which simply means that lots of different things can put us at risk of developing them. Some, like our genetics, we can't do much about, but most of the risk factors for these and lots of other conditions are entirely in our own hands. How we live our lives, what we eat and drink, and how we handle stress all play a part in how healthy we are, and even how long we will live.

We all lead increasingly busy lives, and perhaps women more so than men: more women work today than ever before, but many are still trying to juggle jobs with running the home. It is not unusual for women to start doing at 7 pm what their mothers and grandmothers spent all day doing. This leaves precious little time to be proactive about health, and too many women put their own needs at the bottom of the list, which is a false economy for all concerned.

It is easy to take good health for granted, but if you don't take care of yourself you won't be able to take care of anyone else. If you are lucky, your warning call will be a gentle nudge, like one too many colds this winter because your immune system just isn't strong enough to

OUR PSYCHOLOGICAL WELL-BEING

It's not just our physical health that we need to maintain if we want to enjoy good health in the fullest sense—living a longer, more purposeful, and happier life is in part due to the relationships that we cultivate and enjoy.

The meaningful relationships that we have with a partner, family, friends, and wider community can help to nourish us emotionally and benefit our psychological well-being, as can spirituality in whatever form we best relate to it. Our sense of identity and our self-worth is inevitably grounded in these significant relationships, and being able to share our hopes, dreams, goals, and successes within a loving, intimate relationship or with a good friend is as important as being there to support each other through the conflicts, challenges, anxieties, and disappointments that we all encounter in life. Relaxing with friends and enjoying people's company can also help us unwind, which decreases our stress levels (see pp62–3) so that we feel revived and revitalized once again.

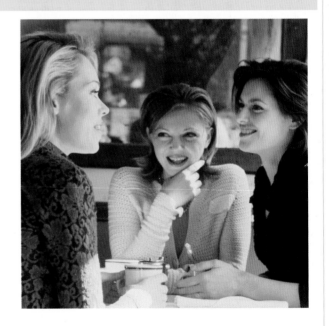

fight off infection. However, ignoring your own needs can have much more serious consequences. Most women don't expect to have a heart attack, but the fact is that heart disease is the number one killer of women in the US, followed by cancers of the lung, breast, and colon. Inquiring about your blood pressure and cholesterol levels, finding ways to stop smoking if you do, and following through with monthly breast exams, screening mammograms and colonoscopy when appropriate, can improve your chances of being healthy and enjoying long-term health.

It is no surprise that thousands of women spend a great deal of time and money on looking good on the outside. Whether it is hairdressing, cosmetics, or freshening up our wardrobes, we are more likely to take care of our external appearance than men but, frighteningly, few of us take our internal health seriously enough.

Just a few simple changes to your lifestyle could keep you feeling well longer. Eating well, exercising regularly, and keeping stress under control will boost your immune system and keep you healthy longer. There is nothing in this chapter that will require superhuman willpower. In fact, the exact opposite is true. Most of us can stick to a restrictive diet for a week or two or cut out alcohol for short periods. Once these become habits, it is not very difficult to maintain that lifestyle for as long as our health goals require.

ACHIEVABLE GOALS

If positive lifestyle changes are to have any effect on your health and longevity, they have to be achievable and sustainable, so there is no need to worry about having to begin training for a marathon. The goal of this chapter is simply to point you in the right direction to help you make relatively minor changes to your lifestyle that could make a significant impact on your health and well-being, leaving you and your family to enjoy your good health longer.

"It's easy to take good health for granted, but if you don't take care of yourself you won't be able to take care of anyone else."

PROTECT YOUR IMMUNE SYSTEM

Every day our bodies are exposed to literally thousands of bacteria and viruses, which could potentially cause infection. Our immune system protects us from succumbing to the vast majority of them. It is easy to take our immune system for granted, but if you get more than your fair share of the coughs and colds that go around, you probably need to be more proactive about taking care of yourself:

Eat a balanced diet Healthy eating habits can boost your immune system (see pp52–5). The nutrients zinc, vitamin C, and selenium are particularly important for a healthy immune system (see pp54–5).

Deal with your stress A little bit of stress can be good for you, making you feel more alert, but chronic stress will depress your immune system. (See pp62–3 for ways to deal with stress.)

Take time out to relax A yoga or Pilates class is a great way to unwind and exercise your body.

Don't rely on excess caffeine or alcohol to get you through the day—it will depress your immune system. Drink lots of water instead, and try swapping caffeine and alcohol for herbal teas and fruit juices.

Stop smoking—smokers absorb 30 percent less vitamin C from their diet. They also get more chest infections and upper respiratory tract infections than nonsmokers, and are at increased risk of many diseases (for information on giving up smoking, see p64).

Get enough rest How much sleep you need varies from person to person, but not getting enough sleep undoubtedly suppresses your immune system, and chronic sleep deprivation will play havoc with your immune system. For more information on getting a good night's sleep, see pp60–1.

Keep smiling According to research from the American Psychological Association, a positive attitude really can help protect against illness.

Wash your hands regularly Colds are passed mainly by hand to hand contact, and from there to the eyes and nose—and not via droplets in the air from other peoples' coughs and sneezes.

Eat a healthy diet

Eating healthily is all about ensuring that you eat a balanced diet of beneficial foods, and in the western world we are fortunate enough to have easy access to a whole variety of different foods all year round. So there really is no excuse to let your health suffer as a result of a poor diet.

A good diet increases your chances of living a longer, healthier life by reducing the risk of diseases such as heart disease, stroke, and diabetes. It may even help to reduce the risk of developing some cancers.

Eating healthily doesn't mean cutting out all your favorite foods and treats, but you do need to eat more of certain types of fresh foods. Eating the occasional bar of chocolate or a fast food meal is fine, but making these foods part of your staple diet is not.

CARBS AND FIBER

Around half of our daily calories should come from the complex carbohydrates found in all fruit, vegetables, and grains and cereals such as rice, pasta, and potatoes. Try to eat at least five portions of fruit and vegetables a day. Frozen, canned, and dried fruit and vegetables are just as nutritious as fresh. Don't fall into the trap of thinking of "carbs" as the enemy: complex carbohydrates are an excellent and filling energy source and used in correct portions, will not make you fat. With processed carbohydrates such as breads, pastas, grains, and cereals, try to choose the whole-grain, unrefined options, such as whole-wheat bread and brown rice. These foods are high in fiber and help to fill you up without being high in calories. It's also important to remember what you eat with these foods. Use olive oil instead of butter or margarine on bread for fewer calories.

FOOD ALLERGIES AND INTOLERANCES

While food allergies have doubled in the US in the past decade, many people who think they are "allergic" to a food may be intolerant of it, rather than allergic.

An allergy occurs if the body's immune system reacts to a food in a dramatic way. Symptoms include itchy skin and a rash that looks like hives (urticaria). In severe cases, the lips, tongue, and throat swell, the heart rate increases, blood pressure drops, and wheezing may occur due to the narrowing of the airways. Known as anaphylaxis, this reaction is life-threatening if the obstructed airways and extreme low blood pressure are not treated quickly. An allergic reaction will often occur within an hour of contact with the allergen, and gets worse with repeated exposure. Common food allergens include:

● Peanuts and tree nuts
● Cow's milk
● Eggs
● Fish and shellfish
● Soy
● Wheat (gluten, Celiac disease). Possible triggers, identified from a patient's story, can be confirmed with blood tests or skin prick tests.

Food intolerance affects as many as 1 in 5 of us. The symptoms can be vague and include abdominal pain and bloating, nausea, constipation, or diarrhea. The key difference is the timescale and the variability—people who are intolerant to a food develop symptoms several hours, or even days, after exposure to it, and may go through phases when they are able to tolerate it again—unlike allergy sufferers. Keep a food and symptom diary for a few weeks if you think you have an intolerance, and talk to your doctor.

The right food combinations

For a well-balanced diet, eat a range of healthy foods in the correct portions. Complex carbohydrates, whole-grain starchy foods, and proteins release energy gradually, preventing the body from rapid swings in sugar levels, thus helping you feel satiated for longer. Vegetables and fruits are important sources of fiber, vitamins, minerals, and antioxidants. Protein-rich foods are also vital for building and repairing your body cells. To gauge the correct size of each food portion, use the palm of your hand as a guide.

Complex starchy carbohydrates

One third of your daily energy intake should be complex carbs. Include 1 portion per meal.

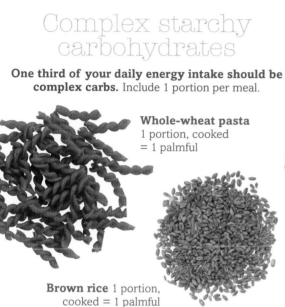

Whole-wheat pasta
1 portion, cooked
= 1 palmful

Brown rice 1 portion, cooked = 1 palmful

Protein

Choose 2 portions a day. Include at least 2 portions of fish a week, 1 portion of which should be oily fish.

Salmon steak
1 portion = 1 palmful

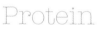

Lentils 1 portion, cooked = 1 palmful

Chicken 1 portion = 1 palmful

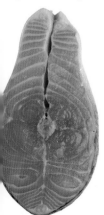
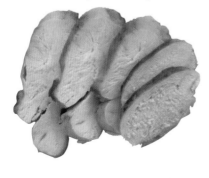

Vegetables and fruit

Eat at least 5 portions of fruit and vegetables a day. Try to choose from a wide range of different colored fruit and vegetables.

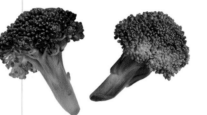

Red pepper
1 portion = ½ a pepper

Broccoli 1 portion = 1 palmful (e.g. 2 large spears or 4 small ones)

Apricots
1 portion = 1 palmful
(e.g. 2 small apricots)

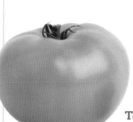

Tomato 1 portion = 1 medium-sized tomato

Dairy

Choose 2–3 portions a day. Select from cheese, milk, and yogurt, and choose low- or reduced-fat options.

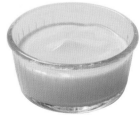

Milk
1 portion = 1 small glass (7 fl oz/ 200 ml)

Low-fat yogurt 1 portion = 1 small container (5 fl oz/150 ml)

Refined grains are known as simple carbohydrates, and the processed products made from these refined grains, such as white bread, cakes, and pastries, should be eaten sparingly.

Fruits, vegetables, whole grains, beans, lentils, and other legumes are rich in fiber, which keeps your digestive system healthy, lowers cholesterol, and may decrease the risk of cancer. If you eat a more processed diet, you do not get the fiber you need and you get more partly hydrogenated and saturated fats, which are detrimental to your body's metabolism.

MILK AND DAIRY PRODUCTS

These foods are high in calcium, protein, and vitamins, but they can be high in fat; opt for low- or reduced-fat dairy products, such as low-fat or skim milk. Check the labels: some low-fat foods have added sugar to mask loss of flavor..

MEAT AND FISH

Lean meat, such as poultry, and fish, are rich in protein, vitamins, and minerals. Try to eat at least two portions of fish a week, at least one of which should be an oily fish such as salmon, mackerel, or fresh tuna, which are rich in omega-3 oils. Otherwise, take an omega-3 fatty acid supplement.

FATS AND SUGARS

The fats found in nuts, seeds, and oily fish provide vitamins A, D, E, and K, and essential fatty acids—which help

HOW MUCH SALT CAN I HAVE?

The high salt diet that we eat in the west works against how we were ancestrally developed, and so predisposes us to salt-sensitive problems. Adults should eat no more than 6 g (about 1 teaspoon) of salt a day; given that three quarters of our salt quota is included in the food we buy, it is easy to see how we exceed that amount. Check prepared food labels for salt content, try swapping salt for herbs when you cook, and avoid adding salt to your food. Your food may taste bland at first, but in time your taste buds will get used to it.

FIVE ESSENTIAL MINERALS

Minerals promote muscle activity, keep cells and nerves healthy, and help the body repair itself. The recommended daily allowance (RDA) of five key minerals are given below, together with the average mineral content per 4 oz (100 g) of the foods listed.

ZINC
RDA: 15 mg

Helps maintain a healthy immune system. Good sources include shrimp (2.2 mg), oysters (59 mg), cow's liver (15.9 mg), and whole-wheat bread (1.6 mg).

CALCIUM
RDA: 800 mg

Crucial for strong bones and teeth. Good sources include cheddar cheese (739 mg), low-fat yogurt (162 mg), low-fat milk (120 mg), tofu (510 mg), and broccoli (40 mg).

POTASSIUM
RDA: 3,500 mg

Promotes muscle activity and nerve function, and prevents cramps. Found in most foods; good sources include bananas (400 mg), avocados (450 mg), and red kidney beans (420 mg).

IRON
RDA: 14 mg

Important for the manufacture of red blood cells. Lack of iron can lead to fatigue, anemia, and hair loss. Good sources include red kidney beans (2 mg), cow's liver (12.2 mg), and dried apricots (3.4 mg).

MAGNESIUM
RDA: 300 mg

Necessary for a healthy nervous system. Good sources include nuts, such as almonds (270 mg), steamed spinach (34 mg), and whole-wheat bread (66 mg).

make healthy cell membranes. Limit these foods to a third of your daily caloric intake, since fat contains more calories per gram than any other foods. Fats can be divided into three types:

- Monounsaturated—found in olive oil, nuts, and avocados
- Polyunsaturated—found in oily fish, sunflower oil, and spreads
- Saturated—found in sweet and savory snacks, processed meat products, prepared meals, cookies, cakes, pastries, and some dairy. Limit these foods to a third of your daily caloric intake.

Unsaturated fats increase "good cholesterol," while saturated fats increase "bad cholesterol" (see p163). If you see the word "hydrogenated" on a food label, it means that some of the unsaturated fats in a food have been converted to saturated fats.

Like fat, sugar is high in calories, and provides no nutritional benefit, so limit sugary foods in your diet.

NINE ESSENTIAL VITAMINS

Small quantities of vitamins are needed by our bodies in order for them to work efficiently and resist illnesses. The recommended dietary allowance (RDA) of nine key vitamins are given below, together with the average vitamin content per 4 oz (100 g) of the foods listed.

VITAMIN A
RDA: 700 mcg

Strengthens the immune system. Good sources include dairy foods. Beta-carotene, found in yellow and orange foods such as carrots, turns into Vitamin A in the body.

VITAMIN B1
RDA: 1.4 mg
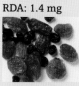
Necessary for converting carbohydrates into energy. Good sources include raisins (0.12 mg), eggs (0.09 mg), whole-wheat bread (0.25 mg), and bran flakes (0.8 mg).

VITAMIN B2
RDA: 1.6 mg

Helps keep the eyes, skin, and nervous system healthy. Good sources include rice (0.02 mg, cooked), mushrooms (0.31 mg), low-fat milk (0.24 mg), and eggs (0.45 mg).

VITAMIN B6
RDA: 2 mg

Allows the body to use and store energy from the food we eat. Good sources include chicken (0.36 mg), turkey (0.49 mg), cod (0.21 mg), and peanuts (0.59 mg).

VITAMIN B12
RDA: 1 mcg
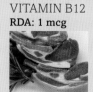
Prevents anemia, helps maintain a healthy nervous system, and relieves irritability. Good sources include lamb (3 mcg), salmon (5 mcg), cheddar cheese (2.4 mcg), and eggs (2.7 mcg).

VITAMIN C
RDA: 60 mg

Increases the body's resistance to infection and free radicals. Good sources include oranges (54 mg), red pepper (140 mg), and steamed broccoli (44 mg).

VITAMIN D
RDA: 5 mcg

Vital for strong bones and crucial for calcium absorption, immune function, vascular health, and metabolism. Good sources include sardines (8.8 mcg) and salmon (7.10 mcg).

VITAMIN E
RDA: 10 mg
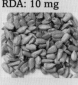
Protects from free-radical damage and keeps skin, nerves, and muscles healthy. Good sources include sunflower seeds (37.7 mg), peanuts (10 mg), and almonds (23.9 mg).

FOLATE
RDA: 200 mcg

Breaks down protein in the body and helps prevent birth defects in newborn babies. Good sources include steamed broccoli (64 mcg), peas (33 mcg), and chickpeas (66 mcg).

Exercise to stay healthy

We are leading increasingly sedentary lives and unless we make some fundamental changes, our children are likely to do even less exercise than we do. Exercising regularly will boost your energy levels, help combat stress, improve your sleep, keep you slim, and protect against weight-related illnesses.

TOP TIPS TO WALK 10,000 STEPS A DAY

Walking the equivalent of 3–4½ miles (5–7.5 km) every day is easier to achieve if you try these options:

- Wear a pedometer (see below) on your waistband and measure the number of steps you take. An average pace is 20–30 in (50–75 cm). If you have an office-based job, you may walk as little as 2,000 paces a day, so throughout the day check your pedometer to motivate you to reach your target
- Get off the bus or subway a stop early each morning
- Never use the elevator or escalator when alone
- Park your car as far away from the entrances as possible
- Don't use a phone for internal calls—walk over instead.

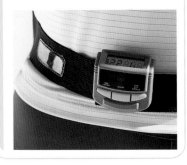

Lifestyles of women have changed changed dramatically in the past century. One hundred years ago, we didn't have convenience stores or Internet shopping, washing machines or vacuum cleaners, and most people didn't have cars. Women used around 4,000 calories a day simply doing the chores, so they had no need for a personal trainer or gym membership. Today, we typically use a little over half of those daily calories and almost certainly take in a lot more, so it should come as no surprise that we are getting fatter. With this worrying trend comes an increased risk of a multitude of diseases, including heart disease (see pp158–75), diabetes (see pp320–5), and even depression (see pp210–11).

Women often give up formal exercise at a younger age than men. In the US women are, on average, less physically active than men with about 53 percent of women, compared to 60 percent of men, engaging in moderate to vigorous activity three or more days per week.

HOW MUCH EXERCISE IS ENOUGH?

As a minimum, you should walk at least 10,000 steps a day (see box, left). In addition, you should try to exercise moderately for 30 minutes five times a week, or aerobically three times a week. It doesn't matter what you do as long as it gets your heart pumping. Choose something you enjoy, such as a dance class or swimming, and if you exercise with a friend you will be more likely to stick to a routine, especially as women often put themselves at the bottom of a long list of family and work commitments. Be realistic about your day—it may be better to get up early and fit in your exercise at the start of the day, or follow an exercise DVD at home

CALCULATE YOUR MAXIMUM HEART RATE (MHR)

To calculate how hard you should work your heart, subtract your age from 220. Your training range (beats per minute) is 70–85% of your MHR.

For example: if you are 40 years old, your MHR should be:

220	—	40 Your age	=	180 MHR	70–85% of 180	=	126–153 pulse rate Training range

while the children are at school. While personal trainers are wonderful helpers, there are many other ways to stick to your plan. Set yourself targets—whether it is fitting into that little black dress for a special occasion or joining a fun run—so that you have something to help you keep motivated.

ARE YOU EXERCISING HARD ENOUGH?

If you can talk easily as you exercise, you aren't pushing yourself hard enough, but if you are gasping for breath, you are overdoing it. Somewhere in the middle is just right. To begin with, you may find just walking briskly is all you need to do push yourself, but as you get more fit you'll have to work harder to achieve the same result. It's not necessary to invest in a heart rate monitor if you take your pulse regularly and aim for a pulse rate of 70–85 percent of your maximum heart rate (see box, opposite) as you exercise.

EXERCISE AND WEIGHT LOSS

You need to expend 3,500 calories to lose one pound of fat. It is difficult to be too dogmatic about how many calories we burn doing different activities, since the amount depends on how energetically you take part in that activity and how much you weigh: heavier women use more calories doing exactly the same activity as their slimmer counterparts. As a rough guide, a 125 lb (57 kg) woman will use up the following calories with each half hour of exercise:

Three ways to stay strong

Strength-training exercises are an important part of any fitness routine, helping to keep muscles toned and bones healthy. The exercises below work many of the major muscle groups—and they are quick and easy to do anywhere.

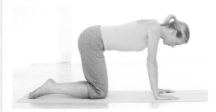

Upper body 1
A great exercise that will tone your arms, chest, and belly. Kneel on all fours, back straight, belly pulled in.

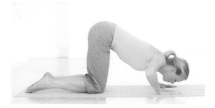

Upper body 2
Bend your elbows out the sides and slowly lower your chest to the floor. Slowly push back up; repeat 8 times.

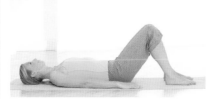

Lower body 1
This exercise will keep your spine strong, and your bottom and thighs toned. Lie with your knees raised, feet hip-width apart.

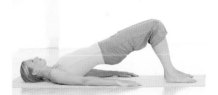

Lower body 2
Pull your belly in, squeeze your bottom, and slowly lift your hips into the raised position. Lower gently; repeat 25 times.

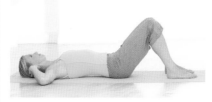

Strong core 1
For strong abdominal muscles, lie on your back, knees bent, feet hip-width apart. Rest your fingertips at the side of your head.

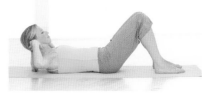

Strong core 2
Pull your belly in and curl up slowly until your shoulders are off the floor. Don't tuck your chin in. Curl down; repeat 8 times.

- Playing golf—110 calories
- Horseback riding—120 calories
- Dog walking—125 calories
- Housework—135 calories
- Gardening—160 calories
- Gym workout—160 calories
- Dancing—170 calories
- Aerobics—170 calories
- Cycling—240 calories
- Swimming—250 calories
- Jogging—280 calories
- Tennis—300 calories.

Weight issues

Obesity is a major growing health problem in the United States. Nearly 60 percent of Americans are considered either obese or overweight. While 35 percent of women are considered obese compared to 33 percent of men, obesity rates in women vary with race.

AM I OVERWEIGHT?

You are considered overweight if you carry too much fat for your height. Doctors use a calculation called a Body Mass Index (BMI) to assess your weight in relation to your height (see box, below), although if you are an athlete or very muscular—muscle weighs more than fat—you can have a higher BMI even though you may have a healthy level of body fat and be at the peak of fitness.

Waist and hip measurements For this reason, many doctors rely more on waist measurement as an indicator of risk for weight-related diseases, in particular diabetes and heart disease. If your waist measures more than 31 in (79 cm), you are at increased risk of these diseases, and the risks are very high if your waist measures more than 34 in (86 cm). To calculate your waist-hip ratio and measure the proportion of fat stored around your waist in comparison to your hips, measure your waist at its narrowest point, then your hips at their widest point. Divide the waist by the hip measurement to calculate your waist-hip ratio. A ratio of more than 0.8 defines you as an apple shape (see box opposite), which means that you are at risk of serious health problems.

THE RISKS OF BEING OVERWEIGHT

Being overweight will make you look and feel older, but it is how it ages you on the inside that is most important. If being overweight doesn't bother you from a cosmetic point of view, it is easier to accept your weight as normal and ignore the health warnings. But being obese can knock as many as ten years off your life. The health risks make sobering reading:

Diabetes Being overweight is the main cause of Type 2 diabetes (see pp322–5), which predisposes you to a range of serious illnesses including heart disease, stroke, kidney disease, and blindness.

High blood pressure The heavier you are, the higher your blood pressure is likely to be (see p161), which increases your risk of heart disease and stroke.

Heart disease and stroke Obese women are 3.2 times more likely to have a heart attack (see p166), and 1.3 times more at risk of stroke (see p196).

CALCULATE YOUR BMI

To calculate your own BMI, divide your weight* by the square of your height in meters. If your BMI is:

Below 18.5 you are underweight
18.5–25 you have a healthy BMI
25–30 you are overweight

Over 30 you are clinically obese
Over 40 you are morbidly obese.
*weight in kg = pounds ÷ 2.2

For example: if you are 5 ft 3 in (1.6 m) and weigh 143 lb (65 kg), your calculation would be:

1.6 m (5 ft 3 in)		1.6 m (5 ft 3 in)		2.56		65 kg (143 lb)		2.56		25.39
Height in meters	**✕**	Height in meters	**=**	Height (squared)		Weight in kilograms	**÷**	Height (squared)	**=**	**Your BMI**

CALCULATE YOUR DAILY CALORIE REQUIREMENT

If you have a healthy BMI, you can calculate your daily calorie requirement for a healthy weight: [(0.062 x your weight in kilograms) + 2.036] x 239.

If you are between ages 35–55, deduct 200–300 calories from this total. If you are 55 or over, deduct 400–600 calories.

Then multiply the number of calories by your activity level to reach your correct daily intake:
- no formal exercise: multiply by 1.4
- 30 minutes of moderate exercise a day: multiply by 1.5
- three or more sessions of intense aerobic activity a week: multiply by 1.6

For example: if you weigh 143 lb (65 kg), are 41 years old, and exercise aerobically three times a week, the calculation would be:

$$\left[\; (0.062 \times 65 = 4.03) + 2.036 = 8.205 \; \right] \times 239 = 1,449$$
Your weight (143 lb/65 kg)   Basic calories

$$- \; 200 = 1,249 \times 1.6 = 1,998$$
For ages 35–55   Activity level   **Total calories per day**

High cholesterol The heavier you are, particularly if the weight is in the belly, the higher your cholesterol and triglycerides, increasing your risk of heart disease, stroke, and diabetes.

Cancer The heavier you are, the higher the risk and recurrence of breast, uterus, ovary, and kidney cancers.

Infertility Overweight women are more likely to have irregular periods, PCOS, difficulty in getting pregnant, and are at increased risk of complications in pregnancy (see pp124–31).

Osteoarthritis Obese women are three times more likely to suffer from arthritic knees (see pp263–5).

Depression Overweight women are more likely to suffer from depression (see pp210–11).

THE RISKS OF BEING UNDERWEIGHT

If your BMI calculation is below 18.5, your body has fallen below a critical weight and you are at risk of infertility and osteoporosis. Low weight can occur with eating disorders or too much exercise. If this is the problem, psychiatric counseling can help.

ACHIEVING A BALANCE

If you're overweight or underweight, first figure out how many calories your body needs to stay healthy (see box above), and follow the advice on healthy eating (see pp52–5). If you need to lose weight, reduce your weekly allowance by 3,500 calories to lose a steady 1 lb (0.5 kg) a week.

APPLE SHAPED

If you are overweight and "apple shaped" (a healthy apple shape is shown below), you are more at risk of developing diabetes or heart disease than if you store fat on your thighs and bottom (pear shaped). This may be because apple shapes store fat around their internal organs, making them resistant to the effects of the hormone insulin (see p324).

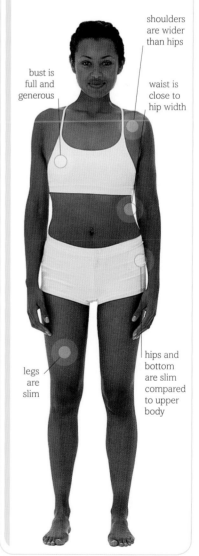

shoulders are wider than hips

bust is full and generous

waist is close to hip width

legs are slim

hips and bottom are slim compared to upper body

Sleep well

A good night's sleep is essential to our physical and emotional well-being. Most of us can deal with the occasional bad night, but disturbed sleep on successive nights can weaken your immune system, leave you feeling irritable and less able to concentrate or make decisions, and make you prone to stress.

Although we all vary in our need for sleep—our requirements change according to our activity levels during the day, and throughout our lives—experts believe that between seven and nine hours of sleep a night is probably the optimum amount. Of course, there is more to sleep than the number of hours we actually spend in bed.

NORMAL SLEEP PATTERNS

At night we oscillate between two types of sleep pattern—rapid eye movement (REM) sleep, and non-rapid eye movement (NREM) sleep. We probably spend about a quarter of the time in the lighter REM sleep (when most of our dreaming is thought to occur) and the rest in the deep, more refreshing NREM sleep, which is divided into four stages, each stage being a little bit deeper than the last.

If we are constantly disturbed during the night, we are deprived of the NREM sleep—what could also be called "battery recharge sleep"—that we need, and we therefore wake up tired and not feeling refreshed.

YOGA FOR RELAXING

To help you unwind at the end of the day, try this simple yoga sequence known as the hare pose. It will help you relax your body and calm your mind ready for bed. Hold each posture for 10 seconds, turning your attention inward. Feel a great stretch in your back, hips, and knees as you repeat the pose three times.

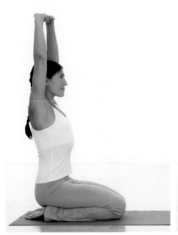

Step 1
Kneeling on a soft surface, stretch your hands toward the ceiling, fingers interlocked, palms facing upward.

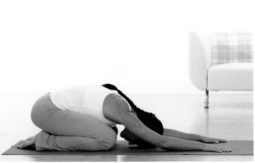

Step 2
Bend forward and stretch your arms out in front of you. Open your knees if you need to. Rest your forehead on the floor.

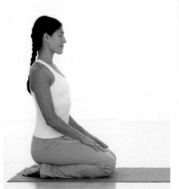

Step 3
Return to a seated position, palms on thighs. Close your eyes and breathe deeply and slowly.

PROBLEMS WITH SLEEP

Persistent sleep problems are very common; your sleep pattern can easily be affected by how you are feeling. Women are twice as likely as men to suffer from insomnia, and social factors such as being unemployed or divorced seem to increase the risk of developing it. The incidence of insomnia also seems to increase the older we get, because we tend to need less sleep and sleep less deeply.

Listed here are some of the factors that may influence the quantity and quality of sleep that you get, and some suggestions as to how to resolve them so that you sleep more easily.

Stress Try to resolve any stressful problems you encounter before you go to bed. However, if your mind is still preoccupied, take a pen and paper to bed with you so that you can jot down any thoughts as you think of them. This should help you switch off properly and get to sleep knowing that you will have an memory aid when you wake. For more information on dealing with stress, see pp62–3.

Anger There is a lot to be said for not letting the sun go down on an argument. Try to resolve all disputes outside the bedroom.

Depression Sufferers of depression may find that they can get to sleep quite easily, but wake in the early hours and are unable to get to sleep again. If you suffer from low moods or depression and you repeatedly wake too early, talk to your doctor.

Hormones The hot flashes and night sweats that occur around menopause are a common cause of sleep problems. If you are struggling to sleep, don't rule out a short course of HRT. Your doctor will explain the risks and benefits to you, but if you decide that HRT isn't for you, there are nonhormonal alternatives that may prove helpful.

Pain Few of us can get to sleep, let alone stay asleep, when we are in pain, so if you are struggling with pain, talk to your doctor about fine tuning your treatment.

Noise Whether you have a noisy neighbor or a snoring partner, use a pair of good-quality earplugs to block out the noise.

Room temperature and light Being too hot or cold in bed can affect your ability to get to sleep, as can too much light in the room. Adjust the conditions to suit you better and help you settle quickly.

Caffeine Avoid drinks that contain caffeine—including coffee, tea, and cola—after 6 pm.

Alcohol Don't rely on alcohol—it may help you get to sleep by making you feel tired, but it interferes with your normal sleep rhythms and you won't get a proper night's sleep.

Smoking Nicotine is a stimulant. If you have to smoke, at least avoid smoking after 6 pm.

Drugs If you notice a change in your sleep pattern after you have started taking medication, talk to your doctor. The new drug could be to blame, and there may be a more suitable alternative.

TOP TIPS FOR A GOOD NIGHT'S SLEEP

There are several golden rules to follow if you want to be assured of a restful night.

- **Stop working** at least an hour before you go to bed to allow yourself enough time to unwind and relax
- **Make your bedroom as calm** and as comfortable as possible so that going to bed is a peaceful experience
- **Go to bed at the same time** each night and avoid catnaps during the day at all costs. A good night's sleep is all about routine
- **Be active during the day**, but avoid exercising late at night—it may boost your energy levels, which can make it harder for you to wind down in order to get to bed at your usual time
- **Don't read or watch TV in bed.** Your bedroom should be for sleeping and sex, and your brain needs to know that!
- **Once you are in bed**, don't toss and turn and worry about whether you can get to sleep. If you are not asleep within 20 minutes of going to bed, get up again, go to another room, and read until you are tired enough to try to get to sleep again. However, choose your reading matter carefully—a thriller could leave you feeling even more awake.

Managing stress

Most of us find it impossible to live a totally stress-free life, and it's probably unlikely that we would want to; a little bit of stress can be exhilarating, and enables us to get things done. If we have too much stress to deal with, however, something has to give—and it shouldn't be our health.

When we experience stress or feel anxious, the stress hormones that our bodies release in response to the situation cause our heart rate and blood pressure to increase and put us in what is known as "fight or flight" mode. For our ancestors, that meant being able to react quickly enough to flee from an approaching mammoth, but today's "mammoths" don't come and go in an instant; they can hang around for days, weeks, or even months.

These days it is common for most women to find themselves multitasking as they handle busy work and home lives. Many of us have become accustomed to our pressured lifestyles and are able to cope well in crises, but sometimes these chronic demands not only increase adrenaline, but also the cortisol production by our adrenals, thus causing metabolic stress. This chronic stress then increases our risk of anxiety and depression, decreases

our creativity, and alters our immune system so that we are more prone to infections from viruses and other illnesses, more likely to consume more calories than we need, and neglect to exercise.

RESPONDING TO STRESS

While it is difficult to measure how much stress we actually experience, our ability to handle stress is affected by the amount of rest we get, prior experiences with stress, and genetics.

DEEP-BREATHING MEDITATION

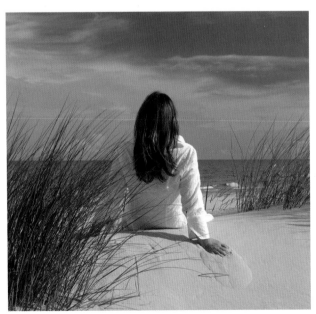

Use this simple meditation to relax and re-energize your body and mind:

1 Sit in a comfortable position, or lie flat on a bed or on the floor with your knees bent. Place one hand on your abdomen and the other on your chest. Close your eyes if you want.

2 Quiet your body and mind. To help you relax, imagine you are on the beach or some other favorite location; savor the sights, sounds, and smells.

3 Now slow your breathing: breathe in for a count of 5, pause for 1–2 seconds, then breathe out for a count of 5.

4 Consciously release all your tension with each out breath. Feel your abdominal muscles push out the last of each breath, and your diaphragm expand as you inhale. Repeat as many times as you'd like; even 5–10 minutes will help to you to feel calmer and centered.

What might wind one person up into a frenzy can pass straight over another's head. If your stress level is under control, you should feel mentally alert and vibrant, able to concentrate, make decisions, eat well, and then switch off and relax at the end of the day. If you feel anxious or tense, however, perhaps with a thumping heart or a knot in your stomach, or if you have any physical symptoms related to stress (see right), you need to do something about the stress levels in your life, and sooner rather than later.

WHEN STRESS AFFECTS YOUR HEALTH

Recognizing the signs of stress in yourself can go a long way to helping you know when to slow down. Common signs of stress building up include:

- Disturbed sleep and feeling tired all the time
- Depression, anxiety, panic attacks
- Frequent minor infections from a weakened immune system
- Migraine and tension headaches
- Flare-ups of skin problems, such as eczema and psoriasis
- Indigestion or symptoms of irritable bowel syndrome.

If you recognize any symptoms, the chances are that ongoing stress in your life is adversely affecting your health and you need to deal with it (see box, below). It's also important to re-learn how to relax, so practice some simple relaxation techniques or meditation (see box, opposite). If you feel overwhelmed or do not know where to start, speaking with a doctor or counselor may help. See below for further tips on managing stress.

TOP TIPS ON MANAGING STRESS

Women can get caught in the trap of wanting to be everything to everyone and then take on too much, which can put huge pressure on your time and dramatically increase your stress levels. Try these solutions:

Make lists Write down everything that you have to do in the week ahead, and then prioritize. It will help you to plan your time carefully so that the really important things get done first. If anything at the bottom of the list gets missed or time runs out on you, the chances are that it won't really matter.

Delegate No one can, or should, expect you to do everything on your own; your partner or children may not tidy up the house as well as you, but they can certainly try!

Communicate There is nothing wrong with admitting that you aren't coping with all the pressures on your time, and even the people you live with won't necessarily know how much you are juggling if you don't say. You may find that simply talking to a close family member or friend about how stressed you feel, and the reasons why, will help hugely.

Accept offers of help Whether you have a neighbor who can help with taking the kids to school, or a colleague at the office who offers to help with your workload, the probability is that they can see that you are under pressure and want to help.

Learn to say "no" Women are slow learners here, and it is often not until we are in our mid- to late forties that most of us finally learn how to say "no." If you haven't got time to do something, say so. There are only 24 hours in a day and, try as you might, you won't find any more.

Find some "me time" It doesn't matter if it's a session at the gym or having lunch with a friend, taking some time out of your routine will help you switch off and then be more efficient the next day, not to mention being a better mom and partner. Women are notorious for feeling guilty about doing anything for themselves, but remind yourself that there are no winners if you are stressed and short-tempered.

Exercise regularly Regular exercise reduces stress levels and wards off depression. If you are feeling tired all the time, forcing yourself to exercise may seem like a ludicrous suggestion, but it really does work, because it leaves you feeling energized and refreshed.

Most of us can manage our stress levels by making just a few of these simple adjustments, but if you are still overwhelmed by stress and feel swamped, or if stress is making you physically unwell, you must seek help from your doctor.

Kicking bad habits

Giving up bad habits is never easy, and it requires a lot of willpower, but one thing is certain—you really need to want to give up. It doesn't help for your partner or children to urge you to quit smoking or cut out alcohol if you're ambivalent about it, but once you have made the decision, their support will be invaluable.

SMOKING

When it comes to living a long and healthy life, smoking is not an option. The truth is that half of all smokers will die from smoking-related diseases, and women are more susceptible to these diseases than men—diseases such as chronic obstructive pulmonary disease (see pp240–1), heart disease (see pp158–74), and cancers. Overall, smoking carries almost twice the risk of developing heart disease in women as it does in men, and you don't have to be a heavy smoker to be susceptible. One study of Danish women showed that those who smoked just three cigarettes a day were at almost double the risk of having a heart attack. The risk of developing other, non life-threatening, conditions, such as osteoporosis (see pp260–2), cataracts (see pp190), psoriasis (see pp356–7), gum disease, and tooth loss, are also higher if you are a smoker. Stopping smoking can make a big difference to your health: if you quit smoking before the age of 35, your life expectancy is only slightly less than those who have never smoked; if you quit smoking by the time you reach 50, your chances of dying from a smoking-related disease decrease by about 50 percent.

TOP TIPS FOR QUITTING SMOKING

Giving up smoking isn't easy, but there are several steps you can take to help give you the determination you will need to stop:

Think of the cost Smoking 20 cigarettes a day for a year can cost approximately the same as a family vacation. Stop for a moment and think what else you could spend that money on.

Write down the pros and cons of smoking Which is the longer list? Keep the list of reasons why you want to stop in your pocket so that you can read it again if your resolve begins to weaken.

Keep a diary of when you smoke Recognizing when you have your weakest moments will give you a better chance of avoiding temptation when you decide to quit.

Set a date to quit You will need all your willpower if you are going to be successful, so if you are under a lot of pressure, now may not be the best time. However, don't fall into the trap of finding endless excuses.

Make a plan of what you will do instead Giving up smoking is a life-changing event, and taking up a new hobby may help take your mind off things.

Be ready for weak moments You will have them. Ask your family and friends to help you through by focusing your attention on something else.

Think about your children If you smoke, your children will be exposed to the dangers of secondhand smoke, and are three times more likely to smoke themselves.

Stop completely You may prefer the idea of cutting back gradually, but even if you smoke fewer cigarettes, your nicotine desire will remain the same.

Get professional help Research shows that the chances of quitting permanently are greatly improved if you have the backup of a smoking support group or organization. Your doctor will be able to advise you on this and on the various medicines, such as gums, sprays, pills, and patches, that are available.

TOP TIPS FOR KEEPING TO RECOMMENDED ALCOHOL LIMITS

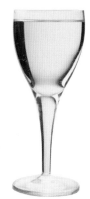

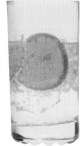

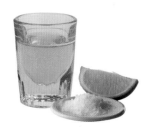

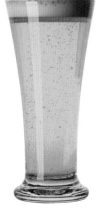

Red or white wine
small glass, 4 fl oz (125 ml)
12% ABV
Units: 1.5

Gin and tonic
large single measure,
1 fl oz (35 ml)
Units: 1.4

Tequila shot
large shot, 1 fl oz (35 ml)
Units: 1.3

Beer
10 fl oz (284 ml)
5% ABV
Units: 1.4

Admitting that you have a problem with alcohol is the first step toward getting better. The second is to find practical ways to cut back on the amount you drink, or quit drinking entirely. Try these tips:

Keep a journal Make a note of every alcoholic drink you have for a week and calculate your units using the formula above. It may shock you, but don't cheat.

Only drink while you are eating.

Have at least two alcohol-free days a week.

Offer to drive if you go out, and stick to soft drinks.

Find a soft drink you like If you are serious about cutting back on the amount you drink, or stopping entirely, you need to find a substitute. If you want to have a drink or two, alternate each glass of alcohol with a soft drink—it will help hydrate you and slow the rate at which you drink.

Think of the calories Alcoholic drinks may vary in their caloric value, but they are all fattening—and that doesn't include the increase of food intake and snacking that occurs as your willpower gradually fades.

ALCOHOL

In recent years there has been a marked increase in the number of women who regularly drink more than the recommended 14 units of alcohol per week. Forget the old guidelines of a glass of wine being a unit of alcohol—our glasses are getting bigger, and our wine stronger. A more accurate calculation is to look at the percentage of alcohol in your drink. That indicates the number of units in a liter of that drink. The standard size of a glass

of wine is now 6 fl oz (175 ml), and if the wine you are drinking is 13 percent alcohol by volume (ABV), your drink is equivalent to 2.3 units. Suddenly, exceeding the recommended limits is easy to do.

Women are more susceptible to the harmful effects of alcohol than men, and alcohol now kills more women than cervical cancer. It seems that too many of us are choosing to put our health at risk by exceeding this recommended weekly limit of alcohol.

Do you have an alcohol problem?
If you answer "yes" to two or more of these questions, you have an alcohol problem. Have you ever:

- Felt you should cut down on your drinking?
- Been annoyed by others criticizing your drinking?
- Felt guilty about your drinking?
- Had an alcoholic drink to help you start the day?

 Had a black-out episode?
Your doctor will be able to advise you on where to get the help you need.

Top-to-toe health care

Taking care of your body and cultivating a positive self-image is all about making the most of what you have. Contrary to the media's preoccupation with surgical enhancement, there is little that the majority of us need to, or should want to, change if we are taking good care of ourselves inside and out.

Hair care

Creating a healthy head of hair is a multibillion dollar industry, but how we take care of our hair on a day-to-day basis is just as important as having a haircut every few weeks.

MAINTAINING HEALTHY HAIR
Try these simple suggestions to keep your hair in optimum condition:
Wash your hair regularly Regular shampooing and conditioning will keep your hair looking and feeling healthy. Dirt accumulates in your hair as much as it does on your skin, so wash your hair as often as you want. However, avoid using hair products containing chemical preservatives, such as parabens and sodium lauryl sulphate, since they act like detergents and strip your hair of its natural oils.

Detangle your hair first using a wide-toothed comb. Soak your hair thoroughly with warm water before shampooing it, pour the shampoo onto your hands, and rub them together before applying it to your scalp. Take at least 30 seconds to massage the shampoo into your hair. If you wash your hair every day, you should only need one application. Rinse your hair for twice as long as you think you should—dull hair is often a result of inadequate rinsing.
If you have dandruff, regular use of a dandruff shampoo should keep it under control. Dandruff is not due to a dry scalp; in fact, it is more likely due to an oily scalp.
Condition your hair after every wash Apply conditioner to the ends of your hair, not on the scalp.
Use the products designed for your hair type If you are not sure whether your hair is fine, medium, or coarse, ask your hairdresser.
Beware of overheating your hair Ration the use of hair dryers and straighteners. Towel your hair dry by gently patting it, and use a wide-toothed comb to comb it. If you use a hair dryer, choose one with a wide nozzle and use it about 6 in (15 cm) from your hair. Blow-drying already dried hair will cause hair damage, as will the overuse of hair straighteners.
Eat healthily Eating foods rich in vitamins, minerals, and iron help keep your hair healthy too.
Don't smoke Gray hair is largely determined by our genes, but smoking will make you prone to premature graying.

HOW MUCH SUNSCREEN DO I APPLY?

We often apply too little sunscreen when we are outside in strong sunlight. It is thought that the average adult needs about 2 mg of sunscreen to protect each square centimeter of skin, which means that you need approximately 1 fl oz (35 ml)—about a sixth of a bottle, or a shot glass-full—to cover your body. Reapply more sunscreen at least every two hours, since sweating and being active can easily remove it.

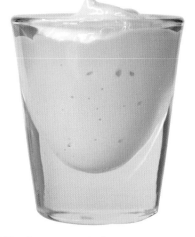

Life-size amount of sunscreen

Posture

Good posture is essential for the proper functioning of your muscles and joints; poor postural habits can lead to neck pain, shoulder tension, headaches, and back pain. In addition to the "Ws" exercise shown below, the exercises on p57 will also help improve posture.

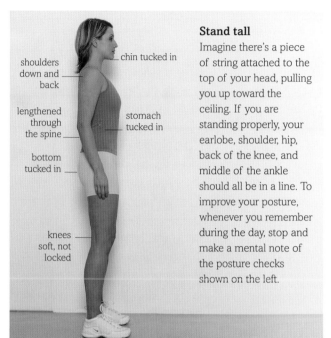

shoulders down and back

chin tucked in

lengthened through the spine

stomach tucked in

bottom tucked in

knees soft, not locked

Stand tall
Imagine there's a piece of string attached to the top of your head, pulling you up toward the ceiling. If you are standing properly, your earlobe, shoulder, hip, back of the knee, and middle of the ankle should all be in a line. To improve your posture, whenever you remember during the day, stop and make a mental note of the posture checks shown on the left.

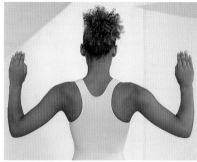

"Ws" Step 1
You can do this exercise anywhere to strengthen the muscles in your mid-back. Put your arms out to your sides as shown, elbows bent.

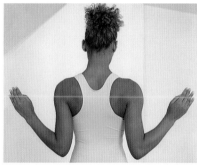

"Ws" Step 2
Draw your shoulder blades down and together as you move your elbows slowly and smoothly to your sides. Repeat 10 times.

Skin care

Develop good skin-care habits now so your skin is radiant for years to come.

CARING FOR YOUR SKIN
Avoid stressed, dehydrated skin by following these simple steps:
Protect yourself from excessive sun exposure Some sun exposure is important for our skin to make Vitamin D, which is vital to the health of our bones, metabolism, and immune system. The lighter your skin, the less exposure it needs. After a daily minimal dose of sun (5–15 minutes depending on your skin color), cover up with sunblock to prevent further exposure to UV rays. Tanning is not recommended as it ages the skin and can increase the risk of skin cancer.

Don't smoke Smoking causes the skin to age prematurely, since it reduces the blood flow to the skin, depleting it of vital oxygen and nutrients. This damages the elastin and collagen fibers in skin. What's more, repetitive facial movements when you inhale smoke from a cigarette cause deep facial lines, especially on the upper lip and around the eyes. Tobacco smoke also contains many toxins that wreak havoc on your skin and affect its ability to repair itself.

Treat your skin gently Hot water from long showers or baths can strip the natural oils from your skin, so limit your bathing time and turn the water temperature down. Strong soaps and certain product ingredients (see below) leave skin dry or irritated. Pat your skin dry rather than rubbing and then use moisturizer.

Moisturize regularly Trap moisture in your skin by slathering on a moisturizer, which forms a seal over your skin and prevents water loss. Ideally, your moisturizer should contain SPF 15 or higher. Avoid any products with artificial colors, fragrances, and preservatives (parfum, parabens, and sodium lauryl sulphate).

Ears

Unlike eye tests, there is no need to have routine hearing tests unless you think you have a particular problem. However, if your family complains that you are not answering them, or that you have the TV on too loud, you need to get your ears checked.

EAR MAINTENANCE
Like eyes, our ears are largely self-maintaining, but you may sometimes have an occasional problem:
Deafness from ear wax The most common cause of deafness is earwax, which affects one in three people over the age of 50. Ear wax is made up of dead cells and a substance called cerumen produced by the gland in the lining of the ear canal. Don't be tempted to use cotton swabs to try to remove the wax, since this causes irritation to the delicate lining of the ear canal, and results in further inflammation and more wax production. A five-day course of eardrops, available from pharmacies, will soften the wax and deal with the problem, but if the wax is still impacted see your doctor to ask about syringing.

Eyes

Good eyesight is crucial to our quality of life, yet many of us take it for granted. In fact, 85 percent of what we learn is through the eyes and brain, so you should look after your eyes properly.

Eye care
Our eyes do most of their own minor maintenance work, but there are important precautions we need to take to ensure good eyesight:
Have regular eye tests
Even if you think that your vision is fine, make an eye test appointment every couple of years, and more often if you have visual problems (see pp189–91).
Don't smoke Tobacco smoke contains 4,000 chemicals, many of them toxic to the eyes. Smoking can cause or worsen several eye conditions, including cataracts (see p190) and age-related macular degeneration (see p191).
Protect your eyes from the sun
Ultraviolet light can cause cataracts (see p190), corneal damage, and macular degeneration (see p191), one of the most common causes of blindness in the US. Wear a wide-brimmed hat to reduce UV rays by 50 percent and choose your sunglasses carefully. Price is no guarantee of quality—if they don't carry a label confirming that they conform to UV safety standards, don't buy them.
Eat healthily Vitamins A, C, and E are all important for healthy eyes, and a diet rich in the antioxidants lutein and zeaxanthin—found in dark-colored fruits and vegetables—may help safeguard your vision (see p55).

Teeth, gums, and mouth

Poor dental hygiene will leave you with discolored teeth, plaque, inflamed gums, cavities, and bad breath, but may also increase your riks of heart disease. With regular brushing and flossing, you may enjoy healthy teeth well into old age.

GOOD ORAL HYGIENE
There are several simple, but vital, routines to follow if you want healthy teeth, gums, and mouth:
Get regular checkups Unless they suggest otherwise, most dentists recommend checkups every six months and a regular visit to the hygienist.
Brush your teeth well with a pea-sized blob of toothpaste containing fluoride. Brush your teeth with short, gentle strokes at least twice a day after meals for 2 to 3 minutes. Replace your toothbrush every three months with a toothbrush that has soft, rounded bristles; hard bristles can hurt or damage your gums.
Floss regularly Use a piece of floss about 16 in (40 cm) long and wind it around the middle finger of each hand. Grip the floss between your thumb and forefinger and gently place the floss between each tooth in turn, curving it around the tooth and bringing it up the side of the

"Gum disease may be linked to other diseases in the body, so taking care of your teeth and gums has many health benefits."

tooth away from the gum. Repeat the process twice on each side of every tooth.

Watch your diet Sugar causes the bacteria that live naturally in your mouth to produce acid, which attacks tooth enamel and causes dental decay. Cut down on sugar in your diet and, if you have to give yourself a sweet treat, eat it at one sitting to reduce the number of times your teeth are under attack. Chewing sugar-free gum after meals will stimulate saliva production and will help neutralize the acid.

Don't smoke Smokers are at increased risk of stained teeth and gum disease (which results in the loosening, and then loss, of teeth).

Hands and feet

Don't forget your hands and feet in your health-care regimen—apart from your face, they are usually the most frequently exposed parts of your body, and can be a real giveaway to your age and health.

HAND AND FOOT CARE

Adopt a regular routine to care for your hands and feet:

Use a good moisturizer or emollient cream on your hands, especially in winter or after doing dishes. Moisturize your feet in summer to prevent the skin around your heels from becoming too dry.

Remove hard skin around the soles of your feet to keep them smooth.

Use a pumice stone or special foot file after a bath or shower to remove the softened skin.

Check your nails for changes in your health. Look out for spoon-shaped nails called koilonychias (a sign of low iron levels), or nails that lift off and flake, or have ridges, which can be linked to thyroid disorders (see p326), psoriasis (see p356), or due to a fungal infection. A horizontal ridge in the nail is often caused by a past illness: normal healthy nails grow at about 0.1 mm a day, but they stop growing when we are seriously ill.

Always cut your toenails straight across and don't be tempted to shape them as you would your fingernails, since this can leave you prone to ingrown toenails.

RESTORATIVE FOOT MASSAGE

Our feet are amazing structures, yet we rarely think about them until something goes wrong. Reduce the likelihood of problems by wearing well-fitting shoes (feet get wider as we age, so get them remeasured from time to time), and if you love high heels, wear them only for special occasions—your feet will thank you! This quick 5-minute foot massage is wonderfully relaxing, and can help relieve mild aches and pains.

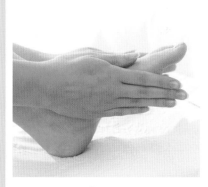

Step 1

Apply a little massage oil to one foot and use both hands slowly and firmly to stroke from toes to ankle 3–4 times.

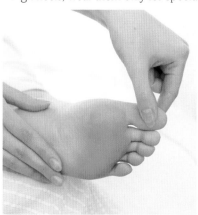

Step 2

Gently circle the ankle one way and then the other 3–4 times, then rotate and massage each toe in turn.

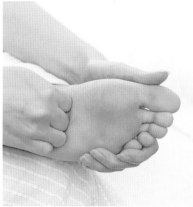

Step 3

Knead the sole of the foot with your knuckles, focusing on any tender areas, then repeat Step 1 to finish.

Knowing the signs

Donnica L. Moore MD
President, Sapphire Women's Health Group

Introduction

Your body is a miraculous, highly tuned collection of muscles, nerves, blood vessels, and organs, connected by an intricate network of pathways that carry messages from one part to another. It is exquisitely adapted to your needs—but it is constantly exposed to the stresses and strains of daily life, and all too often the delicate balance is disrupted. Because some of our organs have an impact on the functioning of other, often distant parts of your body, a problem in one area can produce symptoms in an unconnected part.

In this section, we give you some pointers about what symptoms in any one part of your body might mean. Sometimes the connection is clear—a burning pain in your stomach, made worse by eating, is likely to be related to your stomach. But often, the signals your body sends out don't make sense if you're not versed in the mysteries of medical science. For instance:

- Swollen ankles could mean your heart isn't pumping properly (in which case you may also find that you are breathless unless you sleep propped up on several pillows)
- Pitting of your nails could mean that you're suffering from a condition associated with skin problems
- If your doctor wants to rule out a clot in your lung, she will check you out for a painful red calf, which could be the underlying cause
- A butterfly rash on your skin could mean that you have an autoimmune condition (in which your body's defense systems turn on your own body), which can make you prone to heart and kidney problems.

IF YOU HAVE SKIN PROBLEMS

Other symptoms are found in widespread parts of the body. The skin is a particularly good example because it is often an excellent barometer of what is going on in the rest of your body. For instance:

- Dull, lifeless skin can be an indication of being run down (see Chapter 3, Staying well, pp48–69)
- Dry skin can be an indication of an underlying thyroid hormone problem

- Developing acne again later in life have can be a symptom of polycystic ovary syndrome (see p95)
- Lemon-yellow tinge to the skin can be a pointer to kidney disease
- Yellow skin (and yellowing of the whites of the eyes) can be a sign of liver damage or inflammation
- Excessive bruising can suggest a problem with the blood clotting system
- Finding very mild signs of the skin condition psoriasis can indicate joint disease in some cases
- Blotchy purple bruises that don't blanche when you press on them can be a sign of meningitis or blood poisoning—get help urgently!

IF YOUR LYMPH NODES ARE SWOLLEN

The lymphatic system runs throughout your body in a complex series of interconnecting channels, which meet at junctions. Here, the lymph cells created by your body to fight off infection are stored and congregate if there is a threat such as an infection. Sometimes a single lymph node or group of nodes becomes enlarged because of a local infection—such as tonsillitis, which can cause swollen glands in your neck. But in other conditions large numbers of lymph nodes spread all over your body can become swollen.

Many apparently innocuous signs could mean that there is a more serious underlying condition, but on the other hand, many signs that may, at first sight, seem worrying can have an innocent cause that requires nothing more than time for a full recovery.

SYMPTOM GUIDES

The symptom guides on the following pages will give you a general idea of what signs and symptoms in one part of your body may mean, and they will also point you to the relevant sections where you can find out more. These guides are, however, not a replacement for medical advice, and if you are at all worried or concerned about anything, you should see or call your doctor who will be able to advise you.

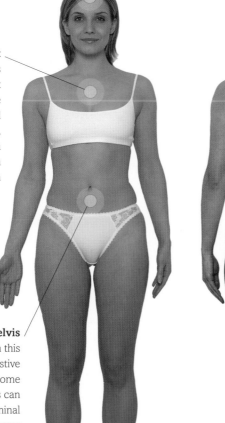

Head and face
This section covers not only pains in your head, neck, and face, but conditions affecting your balance. It also offers a brief pointer to what might be at the root of changes in mood

Neck and back
The spine, stretching from the neck to the coccyx, is held in place by innumerable joints, muscles and pieces of connective tissue

Upper chest
The upper chest includes some of your most crucial organs—the lungs and heart, essential for life; and the breasts, which play such a fundamental part in marking us as women

Pelvis
As the site of the female reproductive organs, the focus in this section is firmly on the woman. But as you can find out in the more detailed sections, there may be a more general underlying cause

Abdomen to pelvis
Most of the headings in this section relate to the digestive system. But some gynecologic problems can also cause abdominal symptoms

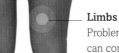

Limbs
Problems in an individual limb can come from joints, muscles, blood vessels, or nerves. More generalized limb problems can stem from conditions of the immune system or the central nervous system

Head and face

You may have experienced a headache, but could you tell the difference between a migraine and meningitis? The brain has a widespread impact on your body. But some parts of the nervous system can cause local symptoms affecting your eyes or ears.

Head

Headaches:

- Moderate pain worsening as the day progresses: p180
- Nausea, dislike of bright lights, with severe throbbing pain: see migraines p182
- With rash, nausea, fever, and dislike of bright lights: exclude meningitis p181
- Worse on waking, nausea, impaired vision/balance: exclude brain tumors p181

Unusual changes in mood:

- With changes in menstrual pattern and libido: see menopause pp136–41
- With undue worry or panic, fatigue: see generalized anxiety disorder p204, panic disorder p205; if related to social situations: see social anxiety disorder p206
- With compulsions/obsessions: see obsessive compulsive disorder p207
- With persistent sadness, weight loss/gain: see depression pp210–11; if seasonal: see SAD p213
- With emotional numbness, irritability, insomnia: see post-traumatic stress disorder pp208–9
- With racing thoughts, poor concentration, distractability, inflated self-esteem: see bipolar disorder p212
- During pregnancy: see prenatal depression p214

- Soon after giving birth: see postpartum depression p215
- Fear of losing or gaining weight: see anorexia nervosa p216, bulimia nervosa p217
- Personality disorders: see pp218–19
- Related to substance abuse, alcohol, and prescription drugs: see addictions pp220–1
- Lack of desire for sex: see hypoactive sexual desire disorder p222
- Lack of arousal during sex: see female arousal disorder p222, female orgasmic disorder p223
- With declining memory: exclude Alzheimer's disease p184–5

Dizziness:

- Lightheaded, sweaty, and pale: see dizzy spells and falls p192
- Sudden onset, nausea, vomiting: see vertigo/Meniere's disease p192
- With nausea, vomiting, impaired vision: see vestibular neuritis, pp193, labyrinthitis pp193
- Partial or total loss of consciousness with jerking or twitching limbs, abnormal sensations, detachment from reality: see epilepsy pp194–5

Skin

Rash:

- Intermittent flushed hot skin, associated with sweating: see menopause pp136–41
- Dark irregular patches: see melasma p361
- In butterfly pattern across nose and cheeks: see lupus p269

Lips:

- Tingling, blisters: see cold sores p367

Pimples:

- With greasy skin and blackheads: see acne vulgaris pp362–4
- With redness and thread veins: see rosacea p364
  Sore with blisters and honey-colored crusts: see impetigo p367

Hair

Hair loss:

- Thinning most at temples: see female pattern baldness p371
- Small round bald patches: see alopecia areata p370
- Major hair loss: see telogen effluvium p369
- Generally thinned hair with weight gain: see thyroid disorders p326

Eyes

Painful eyes:

- With redness, discharge, itching: see conjunctivitis p190
- With reduced vision, aversion to light: see glaucoma p191
- Dry, with dry mouth: see Sjögren's syndrome p271

Yellow eyes:

- See liver disorders pp296–9, gallstones pp294–5

Low vision:

- Near- or farsighted: see eye conditions p189; macular degeneration p191
- Aversion to light, pain in the eyes: see glaucoma p191; with tingling in the face, numbness in limbs, unsteadiness: exclude multiple sclerosis p198

Blurred vision:

- With yellow or reddish tinged vision, distortion: see cataracts p190

Ears, nose, and throat

Earache:

- With itchiness, pus: see otitis externa p186
- Sudden ache, reduced hearing: see otitis media p187
- Recurrent pain: see "glue ear" p187
- Ringing or buzzing noises: see tinnitus p188
- Hearing loss: see p188

Blocked nose:

- With pain over forehead/cheek bones: see sinusitis p235

Neck swelling:

- Moves with swallowing: see thyroid disorders p326, goiter p329, Grave's disease p329

Sore throat:

- With sneezing and cough: see colds p232
- With fever: see flu p232
- With hoarse voice: see laryngitis p236
- With a runny nose and fever: see pharyngitis p237
- Chronic hoarseness: see vocal cord nodules p237

Mouth

Dry mouth:

- Intense thirst, frequent urination, fatigue, blurry vision: see Type 1 diabetes pp320–1
- With dry eyes: see Sjögren's syndrome p271

Difficulty swallowing:

- With chest pain: see esophageal disorders p293

Slurred speech:

- With facial drooping, weakness, tingling in limbs, clumsiness, impaired vision: see stroke p196

Tongue

- Inflamed: see glossitis p288
- Irregular patches, smooth, red: geographical tongue p288; if black and "hairy": see tongue disorders p288
- White patches, sore, inflamed: see oral thrush p288

Upper chest

As you'll discover in chapter 7 (heart and circulation),
women are not immune from heart disease. The chest
also houses the lungs, which can be affected by long-
term conditions (such as asthma) and acute ones (such
as pneumonia). The heart and lungs are housed in the
rib cage, with bones, joints, and muscles
which can also cause symptoms.

Chest

Sharp chest pain:
- Worse on breathing with coughing up of blood and
  shortness of breath: see pulmonary embolism pp252

Central chest pain:
- With belching, acidic taste in mouth, and
  often related to eating: see gastroesophageal reflux
  pp290–1
- With difficulty swallowing: see esophageal disorders
  p293
- Traveling to neck, jaw, or left arm, brought on by
  cold temperature, exercise, or stress, and relieved
  by rest: see angina p164
- Heavy or squeezing, may radiate to arms, jaw, neck, back,
  or stomach, with sweating and nausea; shortness of
  breath; increasing fatigue, feeling dizzy, light-headed:
  exclude heart attack pp165, 166
- With breathlessness, dizzy spells, swollen ankes: see
  valvular heart disease p174

Palpitations:
- Heart beating too fast, too slowly, or irregularly: see
  palpitations, p167

Cough:
- With nasal congestion and fever: see bronchitis, p232
- Persistent cough: see chronic cough p233
- With blood in phlegm, with fever and malaise: see
  pneumonia p234
  And wheeze: see asthma p238
- Longstanding with gradually increasing breathlessness:
  see COPD p240; also with rapid weight loss, exclude lung
  cancer p242

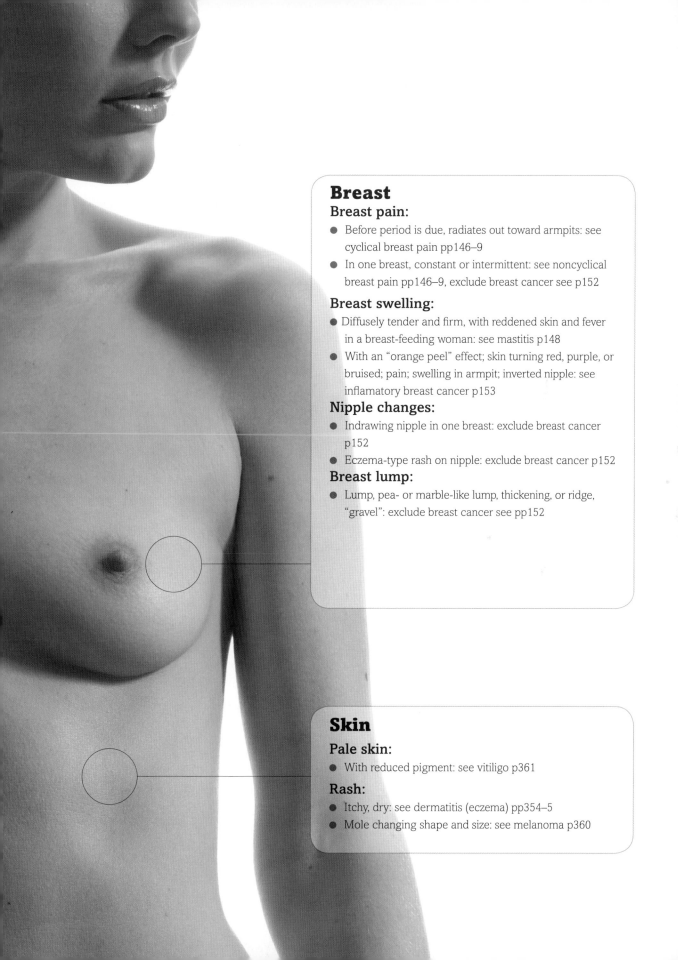

Breast

Breast pain:
- Before period is due, radiates out toward armpits: see cyclical breast pain pp146–9
- In one breast, constant or intermittent: see noncyclical breast pain pp146–9, exclude breast cancer see p152

Breast swelling:
- Diffusely tender and firm, with reddened skin and fever in a breast-feeding woman: see mastitis p148
- With an "orange peel" effect; skin turning red, purple, or bruised; pain; swelling in armpit; inverted nipple: see inflamatory breast cancer p153

Nipple changes:
- Indrawing nipple in one breast: exclude breast cancer p152
- Eczema-type rash on nipple: exclude breast cancer p152

Breast lump:
- Lump, pea- or marble-like lump, thickening, or ridge, "gravel": exclude breast cancer see pp152

Skin

Pale skin:
- With reduced pigment: see vitiligo p361

Rash:
- Itchy, dry: see dermatitis (eczema) pp354–5
- Mole changing shape and size: see melanoma p360

Abdomen to pelvis

Many people refer to their "stomachs" when what they're talking about is their abdomen. The stomach actually occupies only a small portion of your abdominal cavity. Most of the rest is taken up with your large and small bowel, with your liver at the top right hand side.

Stomach

Diarrhea:
- Chronic: see diarrhea p302
- With abdominal pain and fever: see gastroenteritis p300
- With blood and mucus: see inflammatory bowel disease p310
- Alternating with constipation, rectal bleeding, and weight loss: exclude colorectal cancer pp307–9

Constipation:
- Chronic: see constipation p303, diverticular disease p312
- Recent, with cramping abdominal pain: see diverticular disease p312, exclude colorectal cancer pp307–9
- With pain and bleeding when moving bowels: see hemorrhoids p314
- Tearing on opening of bowels, rectal bleeding, itching around the anus: see anal fissure p315
- With unexplained weight gain: see underactive thyroid p327; plus a loss of appetite, weight loss, muscle spasms, minor depression: see parathyroid gland disorders p330

Abdominal pain in pregnancy

- To one side, and less than 3 months pregnant: see ectopic pregnancy p125
- More than 3 months pregnant: see abruption p128
- With lots of morning sickness, sleeplessness, rapidly gaining weight in first trimester: see multiple births p131
- With high blood pressure, swollen feet, headaches, occasional nausea, vomiting: see preeclampsia p128
- Regular contractions, breaking of water before week 37: see premature delivery p129
- Vaginal bleeding, cramping pains in lower abdomen, nausea/sore breasts: see miscarriage p124
- Vaginal bleeding, shoulder pain: see ectopic pregnancy p125

Upper abdomen

Upper abdominal pain:

- Nausea, bloating, belching, heartburn: see Indigestion and ulcers p292
- On the right side, traveling to the right upper back, pale stools, nausea, yellowing eyes and skin: see gallstones p294
- Aches and pains around liver, mild fever, fatigue, nausea: see hepatitis B p118; with pale stools and dark urine: see hepatitis p296
- Weight loss, fever, jaundice: see alcoholic liver disease p297
- Easy bruising, jaundice, mild confusion, swollen abdomen: see cirrhosis pp298–9
- With jaundice, difficulty swallowing: exclude esophageal cancer p306

Lower abdomen

Lower abdominal pain:

- Before menstruation: see PMS pp92–3
- Severe on one side, pressure on rectum: see ovarian cyst p94, exclude urinary tract cancer p348
- Fever, pungent vaginal discharge, severe pain: see pelvic inflammatory disease p98
- With swelling in the groin: see hernia p291
- In waves with diarrhea: see gastroenteritis p300
- Loose, bulky, greasy feces, bloating, itchy rash: see celiac disease p301
- Associated with alternating diarrhea and constipation, and relieved by passing gas: see irritable bowel syndrome pp304–5
- Irregular periods, headaches, blurry vision: see pituitary gland disorders p330
- Weight gain around the abdomen, reddening in the face, increased hairiness: see adrenal gland disorders p331
- With urinary frequency: see urinary incontinence p339
- With painful urination: see urinary tract infection p336, bladder pain syndrome pp343–5
- Radiating to pain in the back: see kidney stones pp346–7

Pelvis, genitals, and bladder

Only women can have children, and only women have the reproductive organs that give them that ability. From puberty through the reproductive years to menopause, these reproductive organs go through constant change every month.

Genitals

Vaginal discharge:

- Premenopause and postmenopause: increasingly heavy periods, and between periods and after sex, heavy, foul-smelling discharge: see cervical dysplasia p106 (exclude cancer of the uterus p104)
- Unpleasant, often fishy odor: see vaginitis p108
- "Cottage cheese" appearance, vaginal/vulval irritation: see yeast infections p109
- Blood-stained, rectal pain, postcoital bleeding: exclude cancer of the vagina p111
- With burning feeling in vagina and urethra, anal irritation, bleeding in between periods: see gonorrhea p114
- With lower abdomen pain, burning while urination: see chlamydia p115
- Green/yellowish, itchy or sore, and smells: see trichomoniasis p119

Painful vagina:

- During sex: see dyspareunia p109; with unusual bleeding and heavy, watery discharge: exclude cervical cancer p107
- With discharge: see vaginitis p108 and vulvitis p113
- Burning pain: see vulvodynia p112
- With ulcers: see genital herpes p116

Vaginal bleeding:

- Heavy periods: see menorrhagia p91
- Absent periods: see irregular periods p90
- Irregular: see irregular periods p90
- Irregular with hot flashes: see menopause pp136–41
- With pain: see dysmenorrhea p91
- Irregular, noticable facial hair and oily skin: see polycystic ovary syndrome p95
- With bleeding between periods: see endometrial polyps p100
- Heavy periods, pelvic pressure, pain, frequent urination, constipation: see fibroids p99
- With constipation, infertility: see endometriosis p101, endometrial hyperplasia p103
- With vaginal discharge, lower abdominal pain, fever: see endometritis p102
- Between periods, piercing pelvic pain: see adenomyosis p102
- Ranging from spotting to heavy bleeding, no abdominal pain, during pregnancy: see placenta previa p130

Lumps around the vagina:

- Heaviness, protruding into the vagina: see uterine prolapse p105
- Spasms, fear of penetration, pain, loss of desire: see vaginismus p110
- With pain and swelling: see Bartholin's gland cyst p113
- With roughened surface: see genital warts p117

Skin

Rash:

- With painless sores on vulva, anus, tongue, or lips: see syphilis p115

Swollen nodes:

- Blisters, headaches, fever, burning sensation when urinating: see genital herpes p116

Bladder

Painful urination:

- With increased frequency of urination: see urinary tract infection p336
- With fever and backache: see pyelonephritis 338
- With increased frequency, lower abdominal pain, blood in urine: see bladder pain syndrome pp343–5
- Urinating very frequently, intense thirst, blurry vision, lack of energy: see type 1 diabetes 321; with recurrent skin infections: see type 2 diabetes p322; during pregnancy: see gestational diabetes p127
- Blood in urine, frequent urination and urgency; also pain in side that won't go away: exclude urinary tract cancer pp348–9

Change in urination:

- Involuntary leakage of urine: see urinary incontinence pp339–42
- Frequent, sudden urge to pass urine: see urinary incontinence pp339–42

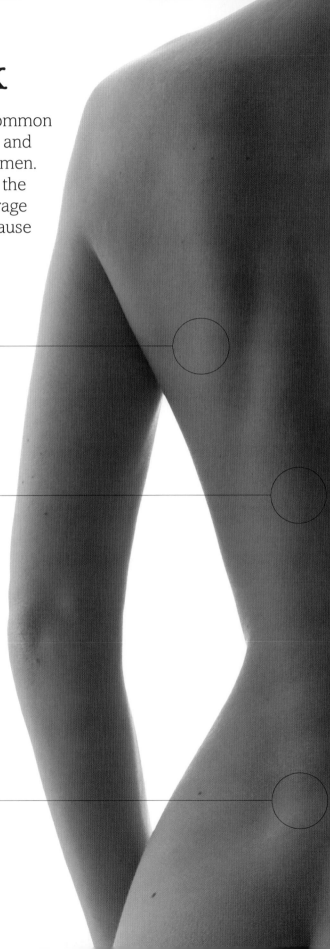

Neck and back

Lower back pain is the single most common cause of missed work in this country, and neck pain is also very common in women. Not only the physical daily strains on the body, but also the stresses of the average woman's constant juggling act, can cause symptoms in the muscles and bones of the back.

Shoulder

- Pain, tenderness, loss of range of movement in joint: see painful shoulder p282

Upper back

Back pain:

- Central and associated with loss of height: see osteoporosis pp260–2

Mid back pain:

- On one side, with fever over 100°F (38°C): see pyelonephritis p338
- Pain in waves, traveling to the groin: see urinary tract stones pp346–7

Lower back

Lower back pain:

- Before menstruation: see PMS pp92–3
- Traveling to buttock or thigh: see back and neck pain pp272–5
- Gradual or sudden pain, with stiffness, often recurrent: see mechanical low back pain p272

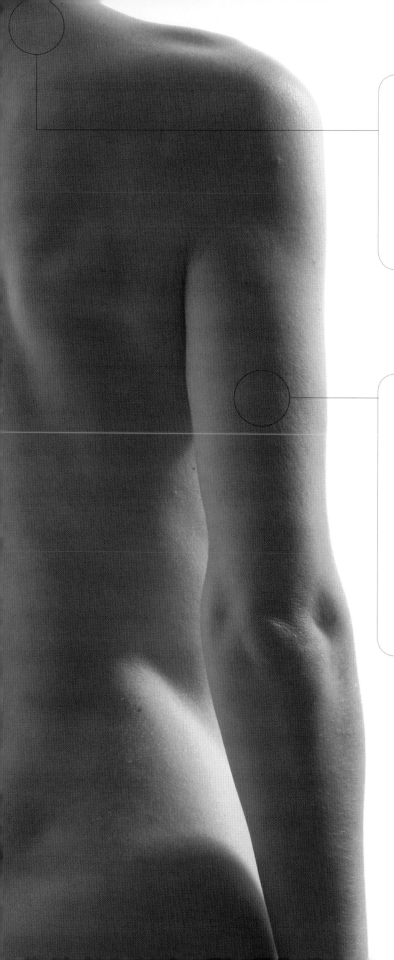

Neck

Neck pain:

- Traveling into shoulders and arms: see cervical spondylosis p272
- Associated with generalized muscle pains, swollen joints, tingling, headaches: see fibromyalgia pp276–7
- Pain, stiffness, tenderness, swelling: see repetitive strain injury p280

Skin

Rash:

- Itchy, dry; with scaling and blistering: see dermatitis pp354–5
- Scaly, raised, salmon-pink color: see psoriasis pp356–7
- Nonhealing, scaly and rough: see squamous cell carcinoma p359; with weeping scabs: see basal cell carcinoma p359
- With reduced pigment: see vitiligo p361
- Easy, spontaneous bruising, prolonged/major bleeding: see bleeding disorders p250

Limbs

The joints and muscles of the limbs are vulnerable to sprains, strains, and wear and tear. Some symptoms, however, can point to an underlying problem with the heart or circulatory system, which may need urgent medical attention.

Hands

- Pain, aching, numbness, and tingling in the hands: see carpal tunnel syndrome p283
- **Tremors:**
- Often on the same side initially, stiff limbs, slow movements: exclude Parkinson's disease p197

Joints

Joint pain:

- Painful joints, but no redness, getting gradually worse: see osteoarthritis p263
- Pain and swelling, morning stiffness: see rheumatoid arthritis p266
- Several painful, hot, red joints after recent infection: see reactive arthritis p267 With swelling in big toe joint: see bunion p265
- Pain moves from joint to joint, weakness, persistent sore throat, chills: see chronic fatigue syndrome pp278–9
- With dislike of heat, thinning of hair, diarrhea: see overactive thyroid p328

Skin

Pale skin:

- Pale skin, easy bruising, enlarged lymph glands in neck/groin: anemia pp248–9, exclude blood cancers pp254–5

Rash:

- With reduced pigment: see vitiligo p361
- Multiple purple colored, like bruises, not blanching with pressure: exclude meningitis p181, clotting disorders pp250–1
- Small, yellow pimples with pus, itching: see folliculitis p366

Arms

Arm pain:

- With shoulder pain and stiffness and restricted movement: see painful shoulder p282
- Around elbow, pain and bony lump on joint: see tennis elbow p281, golfer's elbow p281
- Associated with central, heavy chest pain: see heart attack pp165–7
- Shooting pain in arm: see cervical spondylosis p272
- Worse after repetitive movements: see repetitive strain injury pp280–1
- With weakness, numbness, tingling, slurred speech, impaired vision: see stroke p196

Legs

- Shooting pain in leg going to ankle: see back and neck pain pp272–5
- Aching legs with swollen veins: see varicose veins p175
- Swollen ankles with breathlessness: see heart failure p166
- Hot, red, swollen calf, pain, feeling of a cramp: see deep vein thrombosis p252
- Weakness and clumsiness in the legs, with numbness or tingling: see multiple sclerosis p198
- Stiffness in the legs, with slurred speech, muscle twitching: exclude motor neurone disease p199

Feet

Toes:

- Pain, numbness, changes in skin color: see Raynaud's phenomenon p270

Nails:

- Brittle, tingling in toes/fingers, swollen ankles: see blood deficiency problems pp248–9

Warts:

- With black spots, painful: see warts p366

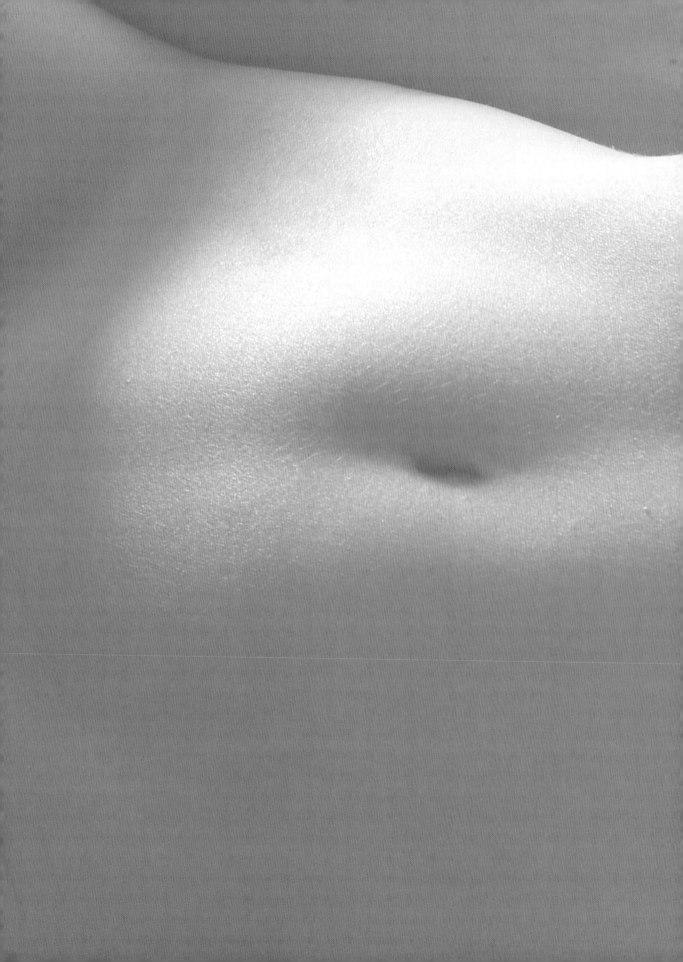

Hormones, fertility, and menopause

Mary Jane Minkin MD
Clinical Professor of General Obstetrics and Gynecology
Yale University School of Medicine

Reproductive system

The central role of your reproductive system is carried out by the ovaries. Even before you are born, your ovaries contain hundreds of thousands of eggs that will be released—usually one a month throughout your reproductive years—ready to be fertilized by male sperm. Unfertilized eggs are shed with the lining of the uterus during menstruation. This process is controlled by a finely balanced hormonal system, which starts to function at puberty and continues for about 40 years until your fertile phase ends at menopause.

THE FEMALE REPRODUCTIVE SYSTEM

These diagrams show the main female reproductive organs, which are positioned low down in your abdomen, between your pelvic (hip) bones. The uterus (womb) lies just above the bladder and in front of the rectum. On either side of the uterus are the egg-bearing glands, or ovaries, which also produce the female sex hormones. Close to each ovary is a fallopian tube, a duct that carries eggs to the uterus.

The muscular walls of the uterus are capable of expanding dramatically during pregnancy to hold a developing baby. In childbirth, the cervix (the neck of the uterus) and the vagina both open out to allow the baby to pass through into the world.

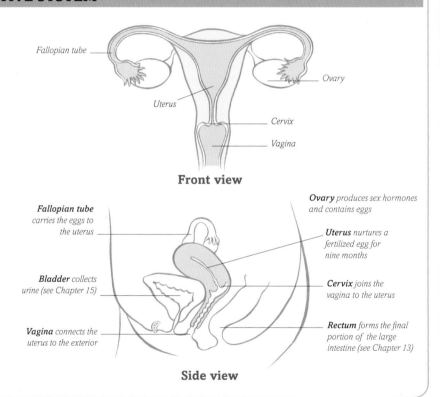

Front view

Fallopian tube

Ovary

Uterus

Cervix

Vagina

Fallopian tube carries the eggs to the uterus

Bladder collects urine (see Chapter 15)

Vagina connects the uterus to the exterior

Ovary *produces sex hormones and contains eggs*

Uterus *nurtures a fertilized egg for nine months*

Cervix *joins the vagina to the uterus*

Rectum *forms the final portion of the large intestine (see Chapter 13)*

Side view

Most of your reproductive organs are hidden deep within your pelvis. The visible parts of the system at the entrance to the vagina are known together as the vulva. These are the clitoris and the soft flaps of skin called the labia. The vagina is a flattened tube that connects with the cervix, or neck of the uterus. The uterus is a thick-walled chamber where a developing baby is nurtured during the nine months of pregnancy. A pair of ovaries (the female sex glands) lie to either side of the uterus. The fallopian tubes, which open at one end into the uterus, reach out toward the ovaries with fingerlike projections. These "fingers" gather up the eggs as they are released from the ovaries (see opposite) and guide them into the tube.

Jointly, the ovaries contain about 400,000 eggs, one or more of which may be released every month. The ovaries also make the female sex hormones—estrogen and progesterone—that are vital for sexual development, the menstrual cycle, and fertility, as well as the male hormone, testosterone, in much smaller quanitites.

YOUR MENSTRUAL CYCLE

Each month a woman's body goes through a cycle in preparation for conception and pregnancy. In the ovary an egg ripens inside a fluid-filled sac called a follicle (see right). At the same time, the lining of the uterus starts to thicken. When the fully mature egg is released from the ovary, it is delivered into the fallopian tube. If it meets a male sperm in the fallopian tube, fertilization may take place. The egg takes several days to complete its journey to the uterus. If it is fertilized, it may embed in the thickened lining of the uterus to start a pregnancy. If the egg is not fertilized, both it and the lining of the uterus are shed in menstrual bleeding. The cycle continues as another egg comes to maturity in the ovary.

HOW THE HORMONES ARE INVOLVED

As we have seen, the female sex hormones estrogen and progesterone are secreted by the ovaries. The time this takes place and how much is secreted are controlled by the follicle-stimulating hormone (FSH) and the luteinizing hormone (LH), which are produced by the pituitary gland in the brain. Release of these hormones occurs in peaks and troughs during your menstrual cycle, with estrogen and LH reaching highs just before you ovulate.

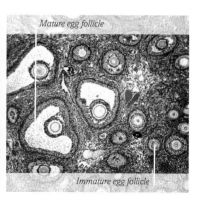

Developing egg follicles

Eggs within the ovary are in various stages of development, as seen in this magnified image. Usually only one egg matures and is released during each monthly cycle of ovulation.

SECTION THROUGH AN OVARY

In each of your ovaries, there are many thousands of immature eggs in their follicles; other eggs are just beginning to ripen, while some are reaching full maturity. When ovulation occurs, the egg follicle ruptures to release the mature egg. The empty follicle produces the hormone progesterone, which triggers thickening of the lining of the uterus.

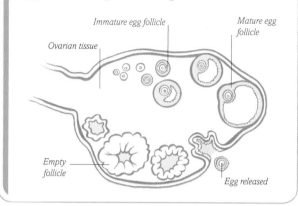

LIFE AFTER CHILDBEARING

In the past, because of poorer health and nutrition—and because many women were exhausted after spending most of their fertile lives either pregnant or breast-feeding—the end of the childbearing years was often closely followed by the end of life. These days, fortunately, the situation is very different and women can expect to live upwards of 30 years after menopause. For some women, the lack of estrogen can have profound effects on well-being, both mental and physical. On the downside, at this time some of us may have "empty nest" syndrome when children leave home, problems with a partner, and frail elderly parents to care for. However, this can be a joyful time; you've got your life back after years of nurturing a family, accidental pregnancy is no longer a worry, and the stresses of your younger years have blown away.

> "Women can now expect to live upwards of 30 years after menopause."

Menstrual problems

Menstruation is a highly complex cycle governed by your hormones. Your menstrual cycle is unique: what is regular for you might be abnormal for someone else, just as light or heavy periods vary from woman to woman. Fortunately, most menstrual problems are minor and easily treatable.

Irregular periods (oligomenorrhea)

Your first periods are likely to be unpredictable in timing and length. After a year or so, most women settle into a regular cycle, but erratic periods often become the norm again before menopause.

WHAT IS IT?
Many women have a menstrual cycle that varies from the 28-day average. A cycle that is routinely shorter or longer is not seen as a problem. However, irregularity may be caused by a hormone imbalance or a disorder, such as PCOS (see p95).

WHAT NEXT?
If irregularities persist, or if you develop other problems, consult your doctor.

MY TREATMENT OPTIONS
You may be prescribed an oral contraceptive, or if you are approaching menopause, you may be offered hormone replacement therapy (HRT).

HOW CAN I HELP MYSELF?
For two or three months, note down the dates of your periods, to see if irregularity is normal for you.

DO I HAVE THE SYMPTOMS?

Your menstrual cycle will be considered irregular if you experience:
- Periods occurring more frequently, with fewer than 23 days between them
- Periods occurring less frequently, with more than 35 days between them.

See your doctor if you are concerned by any irregularities in your menstrual cycle, or if your periods are very frequent or very infrequent.

Absence of periods (amenorrhea)

The most common cause of absent periods is pregnancy. Amenorrhea can also be a side effect of illness or stress, over-exercising, or extreme weight loss.

WHAT IS IT?
Amenorrhea is lack of menstrual periods (or absence of menses).

WHAT NEXT?
Visit your doctor to discuss the problem. Once pregnancy or menopause have been ruled out, your doctor may want to check for hormonal disorders. This may include a blood test and an ultrasound or CT scan.

MY TREATMENT OPTIONS
If the cause of your amenorrhea cannot be identified, you may be given hormonal treatment to restart your periods; ask your doctor about any side effects.

HOW CAN I HELP MYSELF?
Keep a check on your lifestyle. Avoid excessive exercise or dieting.

DO I HAVE THE SYMPTOMS?

You should talk to a doctor if:
- You haven't started having periods by the age of 16.
- You have missed 3 periods.

Heavy periods (menorrhagia)

Some women have heavier menstrual flows than others; it isn't necessarily a problem. However, leakage may be annoying and loss of iron through excessive bleeding can cause anemia (see pp248–9).

WHAT IS IT?

Heavy periods may be due to disorders of the uterus (see pp98-9) or hormonal imbalances, but the cause is not always obvious.

WHAT NEXT?

Consult your doctor. He or she will examine you and may do blood tests to measure your iron and hormone levels. Your doctor may also take a sample of tissue from your uterus, using a speculum placed in your vagina. Other tests may include an ultrasound scan or a transvaginal scan (taken through the vagina).

MY TREATMENT OPTIONS

Treatments could include the following. Ask your doctor to explain any possible side effects.

- Oral contraceptive pill (see p134).
- Progesterone-coated IUD (see p132).
- Iron medication (for anemia)
- Thyroxine (for an underactive thyroid gland)
- Laser surgery (for endometriosis, see p101)
- Surgery (for fibroids, see p99).

DO I HAVE THE SYMPTOMS?

Heavy flow (with or without pain) is usually defined by one or more of the following:

- Bleeding that lasts for seven days or more
- Bleeding that cannot be controlled by sanitary napkins or tampons
- Large blood clots being passed.

See your doctor if your flow fits these descriptions.

HOW CAN I HELP MYSELF?

If you are anemic, try to eat plenty of iron-rich foods. These include lean meat, liver, leafy green vegetables, whole grains, and nuts.

Painful periods (dysmenorrhea)

There are two types of painful periods: primary dysmenorrhea, which occurs once ovulation is established; and secondary dysmenorrhea, which affects women who have not had period pain before.

WHAT IS IT?

Primary dysmenorrhea is linked to a rise of natural chemicals in the body at ovulation, which can cause pain. Secondary dysmenorrhea is a sign of an underlying disorder.

WHAT NEXT?

If you develop painful periods, see your doctor to make sure you have no reproductive disorder. You may have an internal examination, cervical swabs taken, and possibly an ultrasound scan. In addition, you may have an examination by laparoscopy (see p98).

MY TREATMENT OPTIONS

Drug treatment often relieves the pain. Ask your doctor about any possible side effects. He or she may suggest the following:

- Anti-inflammatory drugs such as ibuprofen (which block the action of the pain-causing chemical prostaglandin).
- Antispasmodic drugs
- Combined oral contraceptive.

DO I HAVE THE SYMPTOMS?

Pain begins just before or just after bleeding starts and may be:

- Wavelike cramps in the lower abdomen
- Aches in the lower back and in the legs
- A dragging sensation in the pelvic area.

See your doctor if period pain becomes too uncomfortable.

HOW CAN I HELP MYSELF?

Taking over-the-counter analgesics may be enough. If not, try placing a covered hot-water bottle on your pelvis for extra relief.

Premenstrual syndrome

In the week or so before their periods start, many women experience a collection of uncomfortable symptoms known as premenstrual syndrome. Bloating, migraines, and moodiness are just a few of the things that can make life difficult. But there are various ways in which you can ease the symptoms.

WHAT IS IT?

PMS is a chronic, cyclic mood disorder distinguished by a set of physical, psychological, and emotional symptoms that affects approximately 4 out of 10 women of childbearing age in the second half of their menstrual cycle. The symptoms of premenstrual syndrome (PMS)—once known as premenstrual tension (PMT)—are thought to be caused by hormonal changes just before menstruation. While up to 85 percent of American women experience some premenstrual discomfort, only 5 to 10 percent experience symptoms severe enough to interfere with their daily lives. The symptoms of PMS usually disappear after the first day of menses.

A more severe version of PMS, called premenstrual dysphoric disorder (PMDD, see opposite), can seriously impair a woman's ability to function normally. Some types of depression are also affected by PMS. If you suffer from depression (see pp210–11) most days of the month, you may find that you feel worse in the lead-up to your period.

DO I HAVE THE SYMPTOMS?

Over 150 symptoms of PMS have been identified. They may vary from month to month but you're likely to have at least some of the following:

- Breast tenderness or lumpiness
- Feeling bloated
- Feeling moody or irritable
- Depression and/or anxiety
- Fatigue
- Trouble concentrating or decision making
- Headaches or migraines, if you're a sufferer
- Back and muscle stiffness
- Disrupted sleep
- Food cravings
- Reduced libido.

Some women may also suffer from nausea, vomiting, cold sweats, hot flashes, and dizziness.

See your doctor if you have any of these symptoms and they are causing you distress.

WHAT NEXT?

If PMS is affecting your lifestyle, talk to your doctor. You may be asked to make a symptom chart over several menstrual cycles to confirm the diagnosis.

MY TREATMENT OPTIONS

The past 15 years have seen some developments in treating PMS but success isn't always consistent. Your best option is to try different things over several months. Ask your doctor about any potential side effects when discussing your treatment options.

Antidepressants SSRI antidepressants (see p227), such as fluoxetine and paroxetine, may be prescribed if your symptoms include fatigue, food cravings, mood swings, and sleeping problems. If your symptoms are approaching PMDD levels, you may be on a daily dose, but for more manageable symptoms you need to take the drugs only for the two weeks before menstruation.

Diuretics If you can't control your weight gain, bloating, and fluid retention by diet and exercise alone, diuretics can help your kidneys secrete excess water and make you feel less bloated.

Combined oral contraceptives The older oral contraceptives, which regulate hormone production, are surprisingly ineffective for dealing with PMS—in fact, some women actually have worse symptoms on the "pill." However, a newly developed progestin—drospirenone—has helped some women. Because this drug is present in some of the newer oral contraceptives, it can be used for contraception at the same time as treating your PMS.

Synthetic steroid hormone

Danazol is occasionally prescribed for PMS. It decreases production of the hormones estrogen and progesterone, which relieves the symptoms of PMS.

HOW CAN I HELP MYSELF?

There are many self-help remedies for PMS, although they may not all work for you.

Aerobic exercise This has been the mainstay of PMS therapy for years. Aerobic exercise for at least 30–45 minutes three to four times a week, will help increase endorphins (the "feel good" hormones) in your brain, which are powerful natural pain relievers. (See pp56–7 for advice on exercise.)

(See pp56–7 for advice on exercise.)

PMDD—SEVERE PMS, OR SOMETHING ELSE?

Doctors are divided in their opinions about PMDD. Is it a variant of PMS or a type of depression? Though some doctors don't believe in PMDD, it is a documented disorder. PMDD symptoms are severe manifestations of PMS. There are interesting differences in how SSRI antidepressants affect sufferers. Women with PMDD note improvement within a day of starting an SSRI, whereas a depressed woman may not notice improvement for 3–4 weeks. Women with PMDD need to take SSRIs only for the 10 days when they have symptoms, whereas a depressed woman needs medication daily. Women with PMDD are at higher risk of postpartum depression (see p215), so if you've recently given birth and are feeling depressed, talk to your doctor.

Change your eating Many experts recommend a low-salt, low concentrated-carbohydrate, and high complex-carbohydrate diet before your period.

Calcium A few studies have shown that 1200 mg calcium per day, in three doses, can be helpful.

Vitamins E and B6 Vitamin E, in doses of 200–400 units per day and vitamin B6, in doses of 100–200 mg per day, may reduce breast discomfort.

Herbal remedies Some women swear by herbal remedies (see below), but there are not sufficient scientific data to substantiate their effectiveness. One of the most popular is evening primrose oil, which is reported to improve breast pain; the usual dosage is 1000 units (2 standard capsules) per day. Herbal remedies aren't regulated in the same way as drugs, so make sure you buy them from a reputable supplier and always follow the manufacturer's advice on dosage.

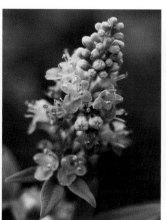 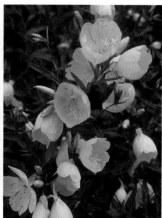 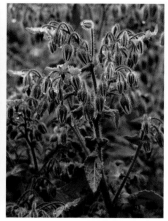

Herbal remedies to keep PMS at bay
Vitus agnus-castus (far left), usually taken as a tincture, is thought to help balance hormones; the seed oil from evening primrose (center) and borage (left) contain omega-6 fatty acids that have anti-inflammatory properties, which may ease breast pain.

Ovarian disorders

The ovaries store all the eggs you will ever have, and are undoubtedly the key to reproduction. They also secrete female sex hormones that regulate your menstrual cycle and affect your physical and emotional well-being. Because the ovaries lie deep in your pelvis, problems are not always immediately obvious.

Ovarian cyst

This disorder is very common and nearly always harmless. Unless you have a very large cyst that presses on nearby organs such as the bladder, or a smaller one that causes pain, you may not know you have one. It is comparatively rare for an ovarian cyst to become cancerous, and this is more likely to occur in women over 40.

WHAT IS IT?

Ovarian cysts are swellings, usually filled with fluid, that are found inside or on the ovaries. The most common type occurs in one of the follicles, or sacs, where eggs develop. Another type, known as dermoid cysts, are formed from body cells and can contain tissues that are normally found in such parts as teeth and hair.

Cysts range in size from tiny to so large that they can make your abdomen look swollen. Most cysts occur singly; multiple cysts are caused by a hormonal disorder called polycystic ovary syndrome (see opposite).

WHAT NEXT?

If your doctor suspects you have an ovarian cyst, you'll probably have an ultrasound scan, which is taken through your abdomen, or a transvaginal scan (taken through your vagina). These scans can confirm the presence of a cyst, reveal its size, and, importantly, look at the blood flow to the cyst. Massive blood flow could indicate that a cyst is cancerous (new blood vessels often develop around cancer cells). However, in the vast majority of cases, ovarian cysts are not malignant.

MY TREATMENT OPTIONS

Ovarian cysts often disappear of their own accord, and no treatment is needed. However, you are likely to need regular checkups to make sure that a cyst isn't growing larger.

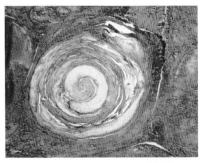

Dermoid cyst
This ovarian cyst arose from various body cells. It contains tissues usually found in parts such as bone and teeth.

Drainage If a fluid-filled cyst continues to grow, your gynecologist may drain it.

Surgery Sometimes it is necessary to remove a cyst surgically, especially if it is large. Occasionally, it is not possible to take out just the cyst and the ovary must be removed as well.

HOW CAN I HELP MYSELF?

Don't ignore any pelvic symptoms (see above). Talk to your doctor.

Polycystic ovary syndrome

Polycystic ovary syndrome (PCOS) affects about 5–10 percent of premenopausal women in the US. It produces a variety of symptoms that may be difficult to diagnose.

WHAT IS IT?

In PCOS, a hormone imbalance results in lack of ovulation and overproduction of the male hormone testosterone, which is normally produced in minute amounts by the ovaries. Often, many small, fluid-filled cysts develop in the ovaries and the menstrual cycle is seriously disrupted or stops entirely. PCOS is a major cause of infertility and may also increase the risk of other diseases, including diabetes (see pp320–5) and cancer of the uterus (see p104). Because of the testosterone, male characteristics, such as excess facial and chest hair, are common symptoms of PCOS.

WHAT NEXT?

If PCOS is suspected, your doctor will take some blood samples to test your hormone levels. You will probably also have an ultrasound scan to look for ovarian cysts.

MY TREATMENT OPTIONS

Treatment of PCOS will depend on how severe your symptoms are and whether you are planning to have a baby. Ask your doctor about the side effects of any drugs.
Hormone therapy If you're not trying to get pregnant, you'll probably be prescribed an oral contraceptive to regulate your periods and suppress the growth of ovarian cysts. The "pill" will also help control excess hair growth.
Infertility treatment If you are not ovulating and you want to have a baby, you'll need to be treated with fertility drugs, such as clomiphene. Many women with PCOS have successful pregnancies following infertility treatment.
Drugs to reduce the risk of diabetes Because PCOS can cause raised glucose levels, and possibly diabetes, your doctor may prescribe metformin, a drug used to lower glucose levels.

HOW CAN I HELP MYSELF?

Trying to keep your life on an even keel can help PCOS symptoms.
Watch your weight You are likely to have higher than normal levels of glucose in your blood as a side effect of PCOS, so you should be extra vigilant about weight gain.

DO I HAVE THE SYMPTOMS?

You may not have any symptoms and the disease may only be diagnosed if you are being assessed for infertility. Possible symptoms include:
- Irregular periods, or even absence of periods
- Noticeable facial hair
- Very oily skin and acne
- Being overweight.
PCOS also puts you at a greater than average risk of developing diabetes.
See your doctor if you notice any of the above symptoms.

Eating healthily and getting plenty of exercise will help adjust your glucose levels and lessen your risk of developing diabetes.
Take control of stress Your hormone levels can be upset by stress. Try relaxation techniques to keep the stress in your life at a manageable level.

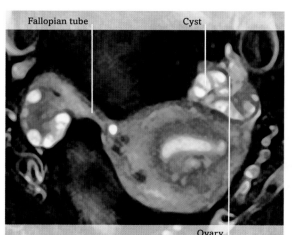

Fallopian tube | Cyst | Ovary

Multiple cysts
This MRI scan shows a large number of cysts (white spheres) affecting both ovaries (green) in a woman with PCOS. The condition is a major cause of infertility. The cysts are not cancerous.

Ovarian cancer

Around 7,000 women are diagnosed with ovarian cancer every year, most of whom are past menopause. Doctors don't know what causes ovarian cancer, but there are various factors that may marginally increase your risk.

WHAT IS IT?

Occasionally, a cancerous tumor develops from an ovarian cyst (see p94) but more often the disease occurs without any early warning signs. There are several types of ovarian cancer. The majority of these cancers form from the cells that cover the surface of the ovary. Less commonly, cancers develop from the cells that make eggs in the ovary. There are also other,

rarer, cancers of the ovary that cannot be linked with any certainty to particular cell types.

A woman with ovarian cancer may not realize that anything is wrong in the initial stages. Often, symptoms arise only after the cancer has spread from the original site in the ovary (a process known as metastasis), when there may be pain and swelling in other organs.

WHAT NEXT?

If your doctor suspects you have ovarian cancer, he or she will probably refer you to a specialist for tests. You will have an ultrasound scan (taken through your abdomen) of your pelvic region or a transvaginal scan (taken through your vagina), and possibly some blood tests. There is one blood test that detects what is known as a "tumor marker"—in this case a protein, CA-125, which is produced by certain cancerous tumors. However, the test is by no means foolproof and is therefore not used routinely. Research is being done on other blood tests, but so far none is currently available for widespread screening.

If the results from the first round of tests are inconclusive, you will have more detailed investigations such as a CT or MRI scan, or laparoscopy (see p98). At the same

time, your doctor may remove a small sample of tissue from one or more areas to test for cancerous cells.

If you have relatives with ovarian or breast cancer (see Am I at risk?, opposite), your doctor will discuss genetic testing with you. The breast cancer gene test can detect if you are carrying the BRCA gene, which is associated with a very high risk of ovarian cancer. If you do carry this gene, your gynecologist will recommend that you have your ovaries removed as a preventive measure, once you have finished having children.

MY TREATMENT OPTIONS

As with most types of cancer, treatment is likely to involve several stages and will depend on how far the tumor has progressed and whether the cancer has spread to other organs. The mainstays of treatment are surgery and chemotherapy. The side effects can be severe, so you should discuss the implications with your doctor. Following treatment, you will be given regular checkups to ensure that the cancer has not recurred.

Surgery The surgical option is a total hysterectomy (see p103) that includes a bilateral salpingo-oophorectomy, an operation in

---

DO I HAVE THE SYMPTOMS?

One of the problems with diagnosing ovarian cancer is that symptoms aren't apparent until the disease is well developed. This makes successful treatment more difficult. You might have:

- Lower abdominal pain
- Swelling in the abdomen
- Frequent need to urinate
- Abnormal vaginal bleeding (this is rare).

You may also have general symptoms such as loss of weight, nausea, and vomiting.
See your doctor if you have any of the symptoms above.

"In women who have been taking oral contraceptives long term, the risk of ovarian cancer is reduced by 50 percent."

> "A number of clinical trials are currently under way to try and improve the success rate of treatment."

which your uterus, ovaries, and fallopian tubes are all removed. (Although this is a major operation, it is relatively common —hysterectomy is performed for various reasons on one in five women, most of whom recover without any complications.) However, as with any surgery, there are slight risks involved with having an anesthetic. In addition, bleeding, postoperative infection, or accidental damage to the bladder or bowel are very rare complications. If you are still menstruating, having your ovaries removed will cause instant menopause, and you could experience severe, menopausal symptoms. If this happens, discuss your treatment options with your doctor.
Chemotherapy You are also likely to be given chemotherapy, either before the operation to reduce the size of the tumor, or afterward to kill off any remaining cancer cells.
Other options Radiation therapy is not often used to treat ovarian cancer but it is an option if the cancer recurs after surgery and chemotherapy, or has spread to other organs in the body, such as the liver or lungs.

Several clinical trials are in progress to try and find different therapies and combinations of chemotherapies to improve the success rate of treatments.

HOW CAN I HELP MYSELF?
Because doctors have very little understanding of what causes ovarian cancer, it is difficult for them to recommend any lifestyle changes that might have a protective effect against the disease. However, it is estimated that in women who have been taking oral contraceptives long term, the risk of ovarian cancer is reduced by 50 percent. You may want to discuss this with your doctor, if you are currently using other contraceptive methods.

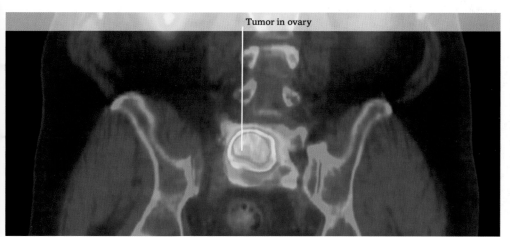
Tumor in ovary

Sites of cancer
This scan combines CT and PET (positron emission tomography) to get an accurate picture of ovarian cancer in this woman. The tumor (green) can be seen clearly on the surface of the ovary (red).

Uterine disorders

Problems with the uterus—which include infections, inflammation, and tumors—are common. Not all of these disorders are serious, but getting prompt treatment is important, particularly if you plan to get pregnant. Anything that affects your uterus may also affect your fertility.

Pelvic inflammatory disease

This is a common cause of pain in the pelvic and abdominal areas. However, pelvic inflammatory disease (PID) can often be present for some time without causing obvious symptoms.

WHAT IS IT?
PID is an inflammation of the uterus, fallopian tubes, and ovaries that is usually caused by a sexually transmitted disease (see pp114–19). If left untreated, PID can cause permanent scarring of the fallopian tubes, leading to infertility.

WHAT NEXT?
Your doctor will examine you and take a vaginal swab to diagnose the infection. A laparoscopy (see below) to examine your pelvic region may also be recommended.

MY TREATMENT OPTIONS
PID is treated with drugs to fight the infection. Your doctor may also suggest that you take painkillers Ask about any possible side effects.
Oral antibiotics You'll probably be prescribed oral drugs, unless your condition is severe.
Intravenous antibiotics If PID is making you seriously ill, perhaps because your immune system is compromised, you'll receive IV medication in the hospital.

HOW CAN I HELP MYSELF?
Practice safer sex and use condoms for protection against STDs. If you use an IUD, consider other contraceptive methods.

AM I AT RISK?
The risk factors include those for contracting STDs (see pp114–19). Other possible risk factors are having recently had an IUD inserted and the termination of a pregnancy.

DO I HAVE THE SYMPTOMS?
Symptoms vary depending on the severity of the infection, but may include:
- Severe pain in the pelvic region
- Pain during intercourse
- Heavy, painful periods
- Bleeding between periods
- Fever and feeling unwell.

See your doctor without delay if the symptoms come on suddenly or you feel very unwell.

LAPAROSCOPY
This procedure, performed under general anesthetic, allows a gynecologist to look at—and sometimes operate on—a woman's reproductive organs. Small cuts are made in the abdomen, through which a viewing instrument (called a laparoscope) and a probe to manipulate the internal organs are inserted.

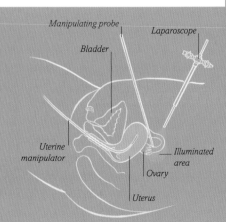

Manipulating probe

Laparoscope

Bladder

Uterine manipulator

Illuminated area

Ovary

Uterus

Fibroids

By the end of your reproductive life, you have a 50 percent chance of noncancerous tumors called fibroids being found in your uterus. These won't give you any problems unless they grow very large or bleed heavily.

WHAT ARE THEY?

Fibroids are abnormal tissue growths that can form on the inner or outer wall of the uterus, or within the muscle layers of the wall. They vary in size from a pea to a grapefruit, and some are attached by stalks. Very large fibroids may distort the uterus.

WHAT NEXT?

If your doctor feels fibroids during a pelvic or abdominal examination and wants confirmation, you may have an ultrasound scan of your abdomen or a transvaginal scan (taken through the vagina). Other examinations could include hysteroscopy (see p100), or a CT or MRI scan.

MY TREATMENT OPTIONS

Unless your fibroids cause problems or you're being investigated for infertility, you probably won't need treatment. Fibroids depend on estrogen for their growth, so after menopause they start to shrink and no further action is necessary.
Gonadotropin-releasing hormone (Gn-RH) agonists
These drugs, such as leuprolide, stimulate the pituitary gland (see pp318, 330) so that your ovaries produce less estrogen and progesterone, and you experience a temporary menopause. This effect disappears once the drugs are discontinued, but your fibroids may return.

Synthetic androgens A male hormone, such as danazol, can help shrink fibroids, but it also reduces the size of your uterus and stops your periods. Such drugs have other unpleasant side effects, such as weight gain, headaches, unwanted hair growth, and a deeper voice. Discuss the implications with your doctor.

Surgery Fibroids can be removed by laparoscopy (see opposite) or via the cervix, but they often grow back. A hysterectomy (removal of the uterus, see p103) may be considered if the fibroids are large and troublesome. In a newer, highly effective procedure called uterine artery embolization, blood-clotting agents are released into a blood vessel in the uterus to starve the fibroids of their blood supply and make them shrink.

HOW CAN I HELP MYSELF?

You can't do anything to prevent fibroids, but you should report any unusual symptoms to your doctor.

DO I HAVE THE SYMPTOMS?

Many fibroids are found incidentally during a routine pelvic examination or prenatal checkup, but they may cause you:

- Pelvic pressure
- Pelvic pain
- Heavy periods
- Frequent urination
- Constipation
- Backache.

See your doctor if your symptoms are worrying you.

TYPES OF FIBROIDS

Fibroids are classified by where they grow in the uterus. They can develop on the inner surface of the uterus (submucosal fibroids), in the middle of the uterine wall (intramural fibroids), on the outer surface (subserous fibroids), or in the neck of the uterus (cervical fibroid). Sometimes fibroids grow on a stalk (pedunculated fibroids).

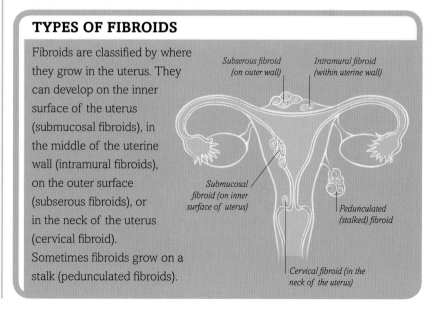

Subserous fibroid (on outer wall)

Intramural fibroid (within uterine wall)

Submucosal fibroid (on inner surface of uterus)

Pedunculated (stalked) fibroid

Cervical fibroid (in the neck of the uterus)

Endometrial polyps

These small growths in the uterus are usually harmless. They do sometimes cause bleeding, though—which needs investigating as it can be a symptom of more serious diseases. You're more likely to have endometrial polyps if you're between 40 and 60 years old.

WHAT IS IT?

An endometrial polyp is a tiny overgrowth of cells that is attached to the lining of the womb (the endometrium). Polyps may be as small as a sesame seed or as large as a golf ball, and you may have one or more. The most common type sits on top of a thin stalk.

WHAT NEXT?

To investigate polyps, your doctor may send you for a transvaginal (through the vagina) scan.

This may be combined with hysterosonography, in which saline is injected into your uterus to expand it for a better view. Another procedure for investigating abnormalities in the uterus is hysteroscopy (see box below).

MY TREATMENT OPTIONS

If your polyps are very small and are not causing symptoms, you may not need treatment. The polyps may even disappear spontaneously. Otherwise, the only way to get rid of polyps is by removing them surgically. (Unfortunately, polyps do sometimes grow back, when they may require further surgery.)

If a polyp is protruding into your cervix, it may be possible for your doctor to pull it off using a long pair of tweezers. If this is not an option, you may need one or both of the following procedures.

Curettage This procedure involves removing the polyps by scraping them off with a long loop-shaped instrument. If a polyp is found during a hysteroscopy investigation (see left) it will probably be removed there and then by curettage.

Hysterectomy Polyps that are removed by curettage are always sent for laboratory analysis. Very occasionally this reveals precancerous cell changes that cause concern. In such cases, and depending on your age, you may need a hysterectomy (see p103).

HOW CAN I HELP MYSELF?

To eliminate other disorders, report unusual bleeding to your doctor.

AM I AT RISK?

Women taking HRT (see p137) or tamoxifen have a higher than normal risk of endometrial polyps. Other factors include high blood pressure, obesity, and a history of cervical polyps.

DO I HAVE THE SYMPTOMS?

It's possible that you have no symptoms, but usually at least one of the following is present:
- Irregular periods
- Bleeding between periods
- Heavy periods
- Infertility
- Bleeding after menopause.

See your doctor if any of these symptoms persist. They can be the symptoms of other problems, too. Bleeding after menopause needs prompt investigation.

HYSTEROSCOPY

Gynecologists use a device known as a hysteroscope, which is inserted through the vagina and cervix, to closely examine the inner lining of the uterus. The cavity of the uterus is filled with a gas or fluid to make viewing easier. During a hysteroscopy, tissue samples can be collected for further tests, and polyps and fibroids (see p99) can be removed.

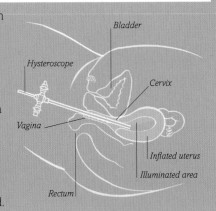

Bladder

Hysteroscope

Cervix

Vagina

Inflated uterus

Illuminated area

Rectum

Endometriosis

Although this condition is common, it is a bit of a mystery, as doctors do not know exactly why it occurs. The symptoms vary widely, which sometimes makes endometriosis difficult to diagnose.

WHAT IS IT?

In endometriosis, tiny fragments of the lining of the uterus (the endometrium) go astray and turn up in other parts of the body. The endometriotic tissue may attach itself to any nearby organs, such as the ovaries, bowel, or bladder. This tissue is affected by the menstrual cycle in the same way as the uterine lining. When a period occurs, the stray tissue bleeds, too—but because it is trapped in the body, it swells up and causes pain.

LOCATION OF ENDOMETRIOSIS

Stray endometriotic tissue most commonly attaches itself to the areas shown below.

Around the ovaries and fallopian tubes

On the outside of the uterus

In the intestines and the bowel

In the bladder

In the vagina

Around the cervix

Eventually, scar tissue may build up. You are more likely to develop endometriosis if you delay pregnancy until you are in your 30s, or if you never become pregnant. The condition usually eases up when you become pregnant and then disappears entirely when you reach menopause.

Endometriosis can often be confused with other conditions that cause pelvic pain, such as pelvic inflammatory disease (PID; see p98), or inflammatory bowel disease (IBD; see pp310–11).

WHAT NEXT?

Your gynecologist will give you a pelvic examination and you may have an ultrasound or MRI scan. Sometimes laparoscopy is also needed (see p98).

MY TREATMENT OPTIONS

Your doctor will consider your age and the severity of your symptoms when deciding on treatment. If you are prescribed medication, ask your doctor about possible side effects.

Oral contraceptives The standard treatment for many years has been birth control pills, which can be quite effective.

Gonadotropin-releasing hormone (Gn-RH) agonists are drugs that act on the hormones in your body, and they are now the main treatment. When injected, they lower estrogen levels, stop menstruation, and shrink the stray tissue. You may need repeat injections if your symptoms return, although this may not be for years.

DO I HAVE THE SYMPTOMS?

Most women have a range of symptoms, with pain being the most common. You may have:

- Painful periods (dysmenorrhea; see p91)
- Pain during intercourse
- Lower abdominal pain during ovulation, bowel movements, or urination
- Irregular periods (oligomenorrhea; see p90) or heavy periods (menorrhagia; see p91)
- Constipation and/or diarrhea
- Infertility.

See your doctor if your symptoms are severely disrupting your life.

Surgery If medication doesn't work, surgery is an option. The stray tissue may be destroyed with a laser during laparoscopy. If you want to become pregnant, your gynecologist will be careful to remove the tissue without damaging your reproductive organs. If you do not desire future pregnancy, a hysterectomy, including removal of your ovaries (see p103), may be best.

HOW CAN I HELP MYSELF?

You can take over-the-counter analgesics for the pain. Taking a warm bath or putting a heating pad or hot-water bottle over your pelvis can help to reduce cramping pain. Some women find joining a support group enormously beneficial.

Adenomyosis

This is a less common version of endometriosis (see p101). Adenomyosis isn't dangerous but it causes a lot of discomfort.

WHAT IS IT?

Adenomyosis occurs when stray pieces of the lining of the uterus (the endometrium) become embedded within the muscle fibers of the uterine wall. This tissue bleeds during menstruation, causing very heavy periods and abdominal pains.

WHAT NEXT?

Your doctor will take your medical history, carry out a pelvic examination, and possibly send you for an MRI or ultrasound scan of your uterus. Adenomyosis is very difficult to diagnose. Some of the symptoms are similar to those of other disorders of the uterus, for example polyps (see p100) or fibroids (see p99). These other conditions may have to be ruled out first. The only certain way of confirming the diagnosis is to examine the tissues of the uterus after hysterectomy (see opposite).

MY TREATMENT OPTIONS

Your treatment will depend on how close you are to menopause, because adenomyosis disappears when you stop having periods. Ask your doctor about any side effects when discussing your options.

Anti-inflammatory drugs, such as ibuprofen, help control the pain and may be the best treatment if you're nearing menopause.

Hormone treatments such as oral contraceptives may ease pain and bleeding. The progesterone-coated Mirena IUD (see pp132, 135) can provide relief by stopping your periods completely.

Surgery If you have very severe pain and are very far from menopause, your gynecologist may recommend surgery to remove your uterus (see hysterectomy, opposite).

HOW CAN I HELP MYSELF?

A hot-water bottle on your pelvis may help to lessen severe pain.

DO I HAVE THE SYMPTOMS?

You may have adenomyosis but no symptoms. However, one or more of the following symptoms is more usual:

- Heavy or prolonged menstrual bleeding, possibly containing blood clots
- Severe, piercing pelvic pain
- Bad cramps during your period
- Pain during intercourse
- Bleeding between periods.

See your doctor if any of these symptoms interfere with your everyday life.

DO I HAVE THE SYMPTOMS?

The main symptoms of both acute and chronic endometritis are:

- Lower abdominal pain
- Vaginal bleeding
- Vaginal discharge
- Fever.

See your doctor if you have any of these symptoms and if you also feel unwell.

Endometritis

This condition (not to be confused with endometriosis, see p101) can affect women of any age, both before and after menopause. Endometritis may develop over time or appear quite suddenly.

WHAT IS IT?

Endometritis is an inflammation of the lining of the uterus (the endometrium), usually following an infection of the genital tract.

Chronic endometritis This form of the infection develops gradually. Chronic endometritis can be a major part of pelvic inflammatory disease (see p98), which is itself usually the result of a sexually transmitted infection (see pp114–19). Sometimes, tuberculosis can also lead to chronic endometritis.

Acute endometritis The type of infections that cause acute endometritis, when symptoms develop very rapidly, are most likely to be a complication of gynecological procedures. These could include the insertion of an IUD (see p132), termination of a pregnancy, and delivery of a baby, especially by cesarean section.

WHAT NEXT?
Your doctor will ask about your symptoms and how long you've had them. It is very important to find out whether you have acute or chronic endometritis, so that the appropriate treatment can be given. Your doctor will also give you a physical examination to establish if there is any abdominal tenderness. He or she and will probably do some blood tests and take a vaginal swab. Laboratory analysis of the swab will reveal which infective organisms are causing the condition.

MY TREATMENT OPTIONS
Endometritis is treated with antibiotics. Your doctor will decide which medications are best for you after taking into consideration whether you've just had a baby and how ill the condition is making you.

Most cases of mild endometritis are successfully treated with a course of oral antibiotics. If you're very ill, you may need to go to the hospital for intravenous antibiotics. These are usually combined with—or followed by—a course of oral antibiotics. Ask your doctor about any likely side effects.

HOW CAN I HELP MYSELF?
To reduce the risk of infections, use condoms if you are sexually active. If you use an IUD, consider other methods of contraception.

Endometrial hyperplasia

This condition is most common in women who have reached menopause. Sometimes, endometrial hyperplasia can lead to cancer of the uterus (see p104).

WHAT IS IT?
Endometrial hyperplasia is an overgrowth of the tissue lining the uterus. This can be due to hormone imbalances at menopause or because of drug treatment.

WHAT NEXT?
Your doctor will examine you and may recommend a transvaginal scan (through your vagina). A tissue sample may be taken to look for precancerous cell changes.

MY TREATMENT OPTIONS
Treatment depends on what the biopsy reveals and may involve drugs or surgery. Ask your doctor about any likely side effects.

Hormonal therapy If there are no signs of cell changes, you'll probably receive hormonal therapy to remove the excess growth.
Hysterectomy If there are abnormal cell changes, or if you've reached menopause, your doctor may recommend a total hysterectomy (see below) to prevent cancer developing in the future.

HOW CAN I HELP MYSELF?
Get symptoms checked at an early stage to reduce the risk of cancer.

DO I HAVE THE SYMPTOMS?

Symptoms can apply to many other disorders of the uterus and may include:
● Bleeding between periods
● Heavy menstrual bleeding.
See your doctor if you have a noticeable change in your periods.

WHAT IS A HYSTERECTOMY?

A hysterectomy is an operation to remove the uterus and cervix. It is used to treat conditions such as cancer and endometriosis. Sometimes the fallopian tubes and ovaries are also removed. Removal of both ovaries causes immediate menopause.

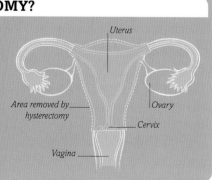

Uterus
Area removed by hysterectomy
Ovary
Cervix
Vagina

Cancer of the uterus

DO I HAVE THE SYMPTOMS?

The symptoms depend on whether or not you've reached menopause:
- Premenopause: increasingly heavy periods, bleeding between periods, or bleeding after sexual intercourse
- Postmenopause: renewed bleeding, which may vary from spotting to heavier bleeding.

See your doctor if you have any abnormal bleeding. Bear in mind that irregular bleeding is a common symptom of many noncancerous conditions.

Uterine cancer is the most common gynecologic cancer in the US. If detected at an early stage, it can often be treated successfully.

WHAT IS IT?

This cancer usually develops as an abnormal growth in the lining of the uterus (the endometrium). Far more rarely, cancer occurs in the muscle wall of the uterus.

WHAT NEXT?

If your doctor suspects cancer, he or she will give you a pelvic examination, and may take a small tissue sample from your uterus for testing. You may need further tests such as a transvaginal scan (through your vagina) to look closely at your uterus, ovaries, and fallopian tubes.

Larger tissue samples may need to be taken by dilation and curettage (D & C) or a hysteroscopy (see p100). If uterine cancer is detected, you will have more tests to determine what stage it has reached (see box right).

MY TREATMENT OPTIONS

Treatment depends on the stage the cancer has reached. Talk to your doctor about the side effects, which may be severe.

Surgery Removal of the uterus (see hysterectomy p103), is the usual treatment. You may also have lymph nodes in your pelvic area removed at the same time.

Radiation therapy You may have radiation therapy after surgery to ensure that any remaining cancerous cells are destroyed.

Chemotherapy Treatment with cancer fighting drugs may be recommended if the cancer has spread to your lymph nodes.

HOW CAN I HELP MYSELF?

Be aware of the danger signs and do not delay in reporting unusual symptoms to your doctor.

THE FOUR STAGES OF UTERINE CANCER

Tests that analyze tissue samples of the uterus and lymph nodes reveal that there are four stages of uterine cancer as it grows and spreads. It is important for doctors to identify which stage the cancer has reached in order to decide the best treatment.

Stage I
The cancer is found only in the wall of the uterus

Stage 2
The cancer has spread to the cervix

Stage 3
The cancer has spread to the pelvic region, perhaps including lymph nodes

Stage 4
The cancer has spread to the bladder or rectum, and possibly also to distant tissues beyond the pelvic region, such as the lungs and liver

AM I AT RISK?

Your risk of developing uterine cancer increases if you have:
- Become overweight
- Reached your late 50s
- Never had children
- High blood pressure
- Taken estrogen-only HRT
- Had breast cancer and have been treated with tamoxifen for more than two years.
- Endometrial hyperplasia (see p103), which can turn cancerous.

Uterine prolapse

Pregnancy and childbirth take their toll on your body. In many women the muscles and ligaments that hold the uterus in place become too stretched to provide support.

WHAT IS IT?

In uterine prolapse the uterus drops down into the vagina. This displacement may be very slight, but in severe prolapse the uterus may appear outside your vulva.

WHAT NEXT?

Your doctor can diagnose a prolapse by physical examination.

DO I HAVE THE SYMPTOMS?

With a mild prolapse you may have no symptoms, but if the condition is more severe, you'll have some or all of the following:

- A feeling of heaviness or pulling in your pelvis
- Urinary incontinence: urge (needing to get to a toilet in a hurry) or stress (leaking when you cough or jump) or both
- Low back pain
- Difficulty with bowel movements
- A sensation of sitting on a small ball
- Pain during intercourse.

See your doctor if you have any of these symptoms, particularly if they are disrupting your life.

AM I AT RISK?

Risk factors for uterine prolapse include one or more vaginal births, being menopausal, doing a lot of heavy lifting, chronic cough (for example, in COPD; see pp240–1), obesity, and constipation.

MY TREATMENT OPTIONS

If the symptoms aren't too annoying, your doctor may suggest self-help measures (see right). You may need treatment if you are in great discomfort.

Vaginal suppository You will be fitted with a ring suppository, which is inserted through your vagina to hold your uterus in the right place. The suppository will need to be replaced at intervals.

Surgery If you have a severe prolapse, you'll probably need surgery. This might include reinforcing weakened supporting tissues with mesh to keep the uterus in place. If you don't intend to have any more children, or you have reached menopause, your doctor may suggest that you have a hysterectomy (see p103), to remove the uterus.

HOW CAN I HELP MYSELF?

The following self-help measures can help you prevent or reverse mild uterine prolapse.

Lose weight if you're overweight.
Give up smoking if you smoke.
Get treatment for any chronic condition that causes coughing.
Avoid lifting heavy objects.
Avoid constipation—eat fiber, fruit, and vegetables, drink water, and get exercise (see also p303).
Strengthen your pelvic floor muscles with a regular daily routine of exercises (see p341).

PROLAPSE OF THE UTERUS

Compare a normal uterus (below left) with a prolapsed uterus (below right). With a prolapse, the uterus drops into the upper half of the vagina. This causes the bladder to bulge into the front vaginal wall and the rectum to bulge into the back vaginal wall.

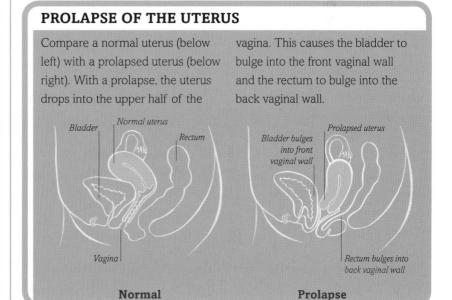

Bladder Normal uterus Rectum Bladder bulges into front vaginal wall Prolapsed uterus

Vagina Rectum bulges into back vaginal wall

Normal   **Prolapse**

Cervical disorders

The cervix is the lower part, or "neck," of the uterus. Muscles in the cervix keep it closed during pregnancy and allow it to expand in childbirth. Sometimes, the surface cells of the cervix show abnormal changes, which may develop into cancer. If detected early, cervical cancer is usually curable.

Cervical dysplasia

This condition is also referred to as cervical intra-epithelial neoplasia (CIN). Although cervical dysplasia can be an early warning of cancer, in most women the condition doesn't go on to become cancerous.

WHAT IS IT?
In cervical dysplasia, the cells of the cervix show abnormal changes. Most cases are caused by the human papilloma virus (HPV, see pp117, 366), which is transmitted by sexual intercourse. In mild dysplasia cells often return to normal. Severe dysplasia may develop into cancer if left untreated.

WHAT NEXT?
The condition is usually only picked up by a Pap smear test. If your smear reveals precancerous changes, your gynecologist will let you know. He or she will examine your cervix through a viewing instrument called a colposcope, and may take a sample of tissue from the most abnormal looking area. The tissue will be sent to a laboratory for testing and assessment.

MY TREATMENT OPTIONS
Treatment depends upon the severity of the condition. You may not need any treatment at all if you have only mild dysplasia—although you'll be monitored every six months to check for further cell changes. In more severe cases, you'll need treatment to remove or destroy all affected cells:
Cryosurgery This rare procedure uses extreme cold to freeze the affected cells, which will slough off. New, healthy cells are regenerated.
Laser therapy The affected cells are destroyed by laser treatment.

DO I HAVE THE SYMPTOMS?
You may have no symptoms (see cervical cancer, opposite). This is why having an annual Pap smear is so important.

Surgery There are two surgical methods for treating cervical dysplasia. In the loop electrical excision procedure (LEEP), a thin wire emitting low-voltage, high-frequency radio waves cuts away the affected area under local anesthetic. In a cone biopsy, a cone-shaped section of cervical tissue is removed, usually under general anesthetic.

HOW CAN I HELP MYSELF?
Always go to your routine Pap smear test appointments.

AM I AT RISK?
The following are possible risk factors:
- Unprotected sex before the age of 18
- Unprotected sex with mutiple partners
- Smoking.

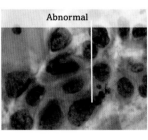

Healthy | Abnormal

Dysplasia
These two Pap test samples, seen under a microscope, show a comparison between normal and abnormal cervical cells.

Cervical cancer

Cancer of the cervix is one of the most common cancers in women worldwide—and one of the most readily prevented. Pap smear screening, introduced nearly 50 years ago, has dramatically reduced the number of cases; the HPV vaccine should reduce them further (see p117).

WHAT IS IT?

In cervical cancer, the cells of the cervix become severely abnormal. The disease is caused by the human papilloma virus (HPV) (see pp117, 366), which is transmitted by sexual intercourse. However, of the many types of HPV, only a few cause cancer. If left untreated, cervical cancer can spread to other organs in the pelvis, such as the bladder.

DO I HAVE THE SYMPTOMS?

There are no symptoms during the early stages of cervical cancer, but once it has started to spread you may experience:

- Unusual vaginal bleeding, such as after intercourse, between periods, or after your menopause.
- A heavy, watery vaginal discharge, which may be blood-stained and foul-smelling.
- Pain during intercourse.

See your doctor immediately if you experience any of the above symptoms.

WHAT NEXT?

Many cases of cervical cancer are detected at a regular Pap smear. If your test reveals abnormal cells, your gynecologist will examine your cervix through a viewing instrument called a colposcope and take a sample of tissue. This may done by a punch biopsy, in which the doctor removes a small, circular section of cervix, or a cone biopsy, in which a cone-shaped area of the cervix is removed. You may have additional tests such as a chest X-ray, a CT, or an MRI scan.

MY TREATMENT OPTIONS

Treatment depends on whether the cancer is confined to the outer layer of the cervix (noninvasive) or has invaded deeper layers (invasive). Your doctor will advise you on the best treatments, taking into account your age, your general health, and your own preferences.
Noninvasive cancer Surgery, ranging from minor to major procedures, is the mainstay of therapy. Your options include cone biopsy; laser surgery; loop electrical excision (LEEP), which uses radio waves; and cryosurgery, which uses extreme cold. Removal of the uterus (hysterectomy, see p103) is sometimes performed).
Invasive cancer Surgery, radiation therapy, and chemotherapy are the options for more advanced cancer.

AM I AT RISK?

One or more of the following will increase your risk of contracting cervical cancer:

- Unprotected sex before the age of 18
- A large number of sexual partners
- Having one or more STDs, such as chlamydia
- A weakened immune system
- Smoking.

Hysterectomy is the standard treatment, provided the cancer hasn't spread to the pelvic walls. Radiation therapy, given through your pelvis or internally via a tamponlike applicator, may be used before or after surgery, or combined with chemotherapy. Chemotherapy may be the only option in advanced cancer. Ask your doctor about the side effects of the treatments.

HOW CAN I HELP MYSELF?

Use safe-sex methods to cut down on the risks of HPV infection.
Pap smears Get your regular Pap smear tests.
Vaccination A vaccination against cervical cancer has been developed, which the manufacturer recommends be offered to females aged between 9 and 26 years.

"It's estimated that over a 10-year period, cervical screening by means of Pap smears has saved thousands of lives in the US."

Vaginal disorders

Your vagina connects the outside of your body to your cervix and uterus. The soft, moist folds of skin that line the vagina's thick, muscular walls produce secretions that help to keep it clean and protected against infection. Problems with the vagina are common but rarely serious.

Vaginitis

This condition, which causes itching and irritation, can affect any woman at any age. Vaginitis can be embarrassing and uncomfortable, but it's harmless and will go away with treatment.

WHAT IS IT?

Vaginitis is the inflammation of the lining of the vagina. It may be due to an infection, allergic reaction, or dryness resulting from low levels of estrogen after menopause (atrophic vaginitis). It often occurs with vulvitis (itching of the vulva).

DO I HAVE THE SYMPTOMS?

You may have all the following symptoms, or just one or two:
- Burning
- Itching
- Soreness
- Vaginal discharge
- Unpleasant vaginal odor, often fishy
- Pain during intercourse.

See your doctor or sexual health clinic if your self-help measures don't bring relief.

Common infections that bring on vaginitis include the yeast *Candida albicans*, which causes yeast (see opposite), and a microorganism called *Trichomonas vaginalis*, which causes trichomoniasis (see p119).

WHAT NEXT?

Your doctor will take a vaginal swab to check for infection. You may also need your urine tested for glucose to exclude diabetes mellitus (see pp320–5), which can sometimes lead to yeast infections of the vagina.

MY TREATMENT OPTIONS

Your doctor will recommend a treatment depending on what is causing your vaginitis. Ask about the side effects of any drugs.
For bacterial infections, you'll be prescribed antibiotics.
For fungal infections, you may be prescribed antifungal drugs to be taken either by mouth or as a vaginal cream or suppository.
To relieve itching, rub a cream onto your vulva. Your pharmacist can advise you on what to buy.
For atrophic vaginitis, you may be prescribed moisturizing cream, or a cream, tablets, or vaginal ring containing estrogen.

AM I AT RISK?

You may be at risk of developing vaginitis if you:
- Use perfumed or scented bath products, sanitary protection, or detergents
- Use intimate deodorants
- Have recently taken a course of antibiotics
- Are diabetic
- Eat a diet that is high in carbohydrates
- Sit around in a wet bathing suit or workout clothes, or wear jeans that are too tight.

HOW CAN I HELP MYSELF?

There are various self-help steps you can take to deal with vaginitis.
Avoid scented products, such as bath products, detergents, scented sanitary protection, and intimate deodorants.
Take care of your genital region by keeping yourself clean, dry, and cool, and wearing cotton underwear and loose clothes.
Eating live yogurt or taking acidophilus or probiotics can also help. Some women swear that inserting a tampon coated with plain, live yogurt really works.

Yeast infections

Many women develop an uncomfortable vaginal itching accompanied by a thick, white discharge, especially during their childbearing years. This is vaginal yeast—a nonserious but sometimes recurrent disorder.

WHAT IS IT?
Yeast infections are caused by a yeast known as *Candida albicans*, which lives naturally in the vagina and is normally kept in check by "good" bacteria. If the bacteria are killed by antibiotics or spermicides, *Candida* can flourish unchecked. The bacteria can also be disrupted when the levels of female sex hormones change—for instance, before a period, during pregnancy, or as a result of taking the contraceptive pill. Intercourse with a partner who is infected with *Candida* can also lead to yeast infections.

WHAT NEXT?
If you're unsure about the discharge and itching, consult your doctor. He or she may give you a pelvic examination and take a swab of the discharge.

MY TREATMENT OPTIONS
Your doctor may suggest antifungal suppositories, creams, or pills. Some of these products are available over the counter. Ask your doctor or pharmacist about any side effects.

DO I HAVE THE SYMPTOMS?
You may have developed vaginal yeast if you have:
- A vaginal discharge that has a "cottage cheese" appearance
- Vaginal and vulval irritation.
See your doctor if you are worried about the symptoms or if self-help measures don't work.

HOW CAN I HELP MYSELF?
Wash your vagina with water only, and avoid spermicides and scented sanitary napkins and tampons. Keep the outer vaginal area clean, and stay cool and dry by wearing cotton underpants and loose clothing.

Dyspareunia (painful intercourse)

Thousands of women suffer from pain when they have sex. It may be embarrassing to ask for help, but treatment can work wonders.

WHAT IS IT?
The causes of dyspareunia can be medical or psychological, such as having had the following:
- Sexual abuse or rape
- Pelvic surgery
- Radiation or chemotherapy
- Reproductive organ infection
- Endometriosis, ovarian cysts, PID, uterine prolapse, fibroids.

WHAT NEXT?
Your doctor will ask about your sex life and medical history, and give you a pelvic examination. You may have an ultrasound test before discussing treatment.

MY TREATMENT OPTIONS
Your doctor may recommend the following. Ask about any possible side effects.
Medications Painkillers may be injected into the site of the pain.
Hormone therapy If you're postmenopausal, you may be prescribed estrogen in a cream, pill, or vaginal ring.
Desensitization Exercises to relax your vagina and pelvic floor may help to reduce the pain.
Counseling Talking to a sex therapist may help.

DO I HAVE THE SYMPTOMS?
Your pain might occur:
- With any type of penetration, including tampons
- Under certain conditions, such as with particular partners
- After pain-free intercourse
- During thrusting movements
- As a burning or aching pain.
See your doctor if you have any of the above symptoms.

HOW CAN I HELP MYSELF?
Avoid scented bath products and douching, since they can cause irritation and deplete your body's natural lubricants.
Try changing sexual positions.

Vaginismus

If your vagina tightens painfully when you have sex or try to insert a tampon, you are suffering from vaginismus, a condition that affects many women. This disorder can cause untold distress, but the good news is that it's treatable.

WHAT IS IT?

Vaginismus occurs when your vaginal muscles contract against your will. This is usually caused by a subconscious fear of penetration, following such events as difficult childbirth or sexual assault.

A woman who is suffering from vaginismus finds sexual intercourse either impossible or very painful. The impact on her emotional health and relationships can be profound. What should be a pleasurable and loving act feels like violation. Feelings of dread, guilt, shame, and failure make the problem worse, especially if she is unable to talk about her problem.

DO I HAVE THE SYMPTOMS?

The involuntary symptoms of vaginismus may include:
- Spasm of the muscles around the vagina
- Fear of pain
- Real pain
- Intense fear of penetration
- Loss of sexual desire.

See your doctor if you have any of these symptoms.

WHAT NEXT?

Despite the embarassment, it's very important to see your doctor and be totally frank about your symptoms. Your sex life will be discussed in complete confidence. Your medical history and a physical examination, which could also be painful, will determine whether you require further tests. Your doctor will check for physical reasons, such as an infection or thinning of the vagina, that cause pain and therefore spasm.

MY TREATMENT OPTIONS

Your doctor will discuss treatment options with you, which may include the following.

Vaginal dilators You can try to retrain the muscles around your vagina gradually with a set of vaginal dilators—four smooth cones of increasing width and length. You can ask your partner to help you with this. Insert the smallest cone when you're relaxed; when you can do this without pain, move up a size. When you're confident with the largest cone, you may find you are ready to try sexual intercourse.

Drug treatment You may need antibiotics to clear up an infection, or hormone drugs for vaginal thinning.

AM I AT RISK?

Several predisposing factors increase your risk of vaginismus:
- A vaginal or pelvic injury
- Dyspareunia (painful sex) (see p109)
- Bad early sexual experiences
- Sexual assault, abuse, or rape
- Aftereffects of childbirth
- Religious or cultural taboos about sex
- Strict upbringing during which sex was never discussed.

Discuss the side effects with your doctor.

Counseling Talking to a sexual health therapist or counselor can often be helpful.

HOW CAN I HELP MYSELF?

You'll need plenty of patience, self-belief, and a supportive partner.

Know your body Have a warm bath and relax on your bed. Touch yourself around your vaginal opening. If you tense up, stop, relax, and slow your breathing. Then try again. After a few days of doing this exercise, try inserting a finger—or ask your partner to insert his or her finger. Next, try a tampon. Finally, attempt intercourse.

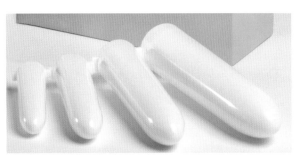

Vaginal dilators
Dilation therapy for vaginismus involves using four penis-shaped dilators of different sizes to retrain the vaginal muscles.

VAIN

Vaginal intra-epithelial neoplasia (VAIN) is a symptomless condition in which there are changes in the lining of the vagina. It is more common in women who are over 50. Rarely, VAIN may lead to vaginal cancer (see below).

WHAT IS IT?
In VAIN, abnormal cells are found in the skin lining the vagina. The condition is not fully understood, but infection with the human papilloma virus (see p117) may be a factor. In a very small number of women, the abnormal cells become cancerous. The severity of VAIN depends on the depth to which the cells are affected.

WHAT NEXT?
If VAIN is suspected, your doctor will use a viewing instrument called a colposcope for a magnified view of your vagina. A tissue sample may be taken at the same time.

MY TREATMENT OPTIONS
Mild cases of VAIN sometimes revert to normal without treatment. For more severe VAIN, you may need one of the following.
Ablation destroys the abnormal vaginal cells, either by laser or by loop electrical excision procedure (LEEP) under a local anesthetic.
Surgery may be used to remove the area of abnormal tissue. Sometimes, in severe cases, a larger area of surrounding vaginal tissue also has to be removed.

DO I HAVE THE SYMPTOMS?

VAIN does not cause symptoms, and is detected by chance during other investigations, such as a Pap smear (see p106-7).

Radiation therapy is reserved for treating recurrences, or if the condition is widespread. It is performed internally, using an applicator similar to a tampon.
Chemotherapy Cancer fighting drugs may be used in the form of a cream to be applied internally.

HOW CAN I HELP MYSELF?
Early detection is important, so keep up your routine Pap smears.

Cancer of the vagina

Vaginal cancer is a rare disease that is most likely to affect women between 50 and 70.

WHAT IS IT?
The cause of this cancer is unclear. In the most common type, called squamous cell cancer (see p359), tumors tend to appear in the upper part of the vagina.

WHAT NEXT?
If cancer is suspected you'll have an internal examination, a Pap smear, and investigations with a viewing instrument called a colposcope. Your doctor will also take a tissue sample for analysis.

MY TREATMENT OPTIONS
Your doctor will discuss the most appropriate treatment depending on your age, tumor size, and whether it has spread.
Radiation therapy This is the usual treatment for most women. It may be applied externally through the pelvis, or internally via a tampon-like applicator inside the vagina.
Surgery removes the tumor and surrounding tissue, keeping as much of the vagina as possible. Occasionally, a larger part or all the vagina is removed and a new vagina made from other tissues.
Chemotherapy Intravenous cancer fighting drugs may be the

DO I HAVE THE SYMPTOMS?

You may have one of these:
- A blood-stained vaginal discharge
- Postcoital bleeding
- Pain
- Problems passing urine
- Rectal pain.
See your doctor at once if you have any of these symptoms.

only option for very advanced, or recurrent, vaginal cancer.

HOW CAN I HELP MYSELF?
Early detection is important, so keep up your routine Pap smears.

Vulvar disorders

A woman's external sex organs, together known as the vulva, aren't susceptible to many disorders, but things do occasionally go wrong. This area is highly sensitive, and problems such as pain and itching can be uncomfortable. Don't ignore any symptoms because you feel embarrassed to see your doctor.

Vulvodynia

At some time in their lives, about one in 10 women may suffer from vulvodynia. The name of this disorder means "pain in the vulva," and the pain can be so severe that having sex or even sitting down causes extreme discomfort.

WHAT IS IT?

Vulvodynia is a raw, burning pain that could be caused by a range of problems. Doctors don't know the cause for certain. Possible sources of the pain may include injury or irritation of nearby nerves, vaginal infection, local allergies, muscle spasm, and reduced estrogen levels if you are postmenopausal.

WHAT NEXT?

This condition is often difficult to diagnose. Your doctor may want to refer you to a gynecologist who will try to rule out any conditions that cause the same symptoms— for example, a sexually transmitted infection (STI) or skin condition.

You may also have a tissue sample taken from the affected area for investigation. This might reveal chronic inflammation.

MY TREATMENT OPTIONS

Even if all treatable medical conditions have been discounted, there are still a number of options. Your doctor will discuss the most appropriate treatment for you. Ask him or her about possible side effects.

Medications You may be prescribed a low dose of an antidepressant such as amitriptyline, or an anticonvulsant drug such as gabapentin, both of which can be helpful in treating pain. You may also be offered a local anesthetic ointment to use before intercourse to relieve any discomfort. Estrogen cream may also help to alleviate the pain.

Biofeedback You will be taught to relax your pelvic muscles, which will help reduce the pain.

Physical therapy A range of different therapies, including massage and transcutaneous

electrical nerve stimulation (TENS), may also be recommended by your doctor.

HOW CAN I HELP MYSELF?

These options may help to reduce the symptoms of vulvodynia.
- Cold compresses on the area
- Avoid tights and nylon pants
- Avoid hot baths
- Avoid washing the vulvar area too enthusiastically
- Take antihistamines
- Get regular exercise
- Use lubricants before intercourse.

> **DO I HAVE THE SYMPTOMS?**
>
> It can be difficult to pinpoint the symptoms of vulvodynia, listed here, and the pain may be constant or intermittent (it can last for months or even years):
> - Burning, soreness, and rawness in the genital area
> - Sitting is uncomfortable
> - Having sex is impossible
> - The pain can't be alleviated
>
> **See your doctor** if the discomfort that you feel fits one or more of these different symptoms.

"Over recent years, a number of specialized clinics have been set up to treat and investigate this particular condition."

Bartholin's gland cyst

At the base of your vagina is a pair of glands, called Bartholin's glands, which secrete a fluid that helps keep your vagina moist and lubricated during sexual intercourse. Occasionally the ducts leading from the glands become blocked, which causes swelling.

WHAT IS IT?

Bartholin's glands are the size of a pea, and normally you cannot see them. If the duct opening out of one or both of the glands is blocked, a fluid-filled swelling called a Bartholin's cyst forms. The cyst can vary in size. It may remain small and painless, but it may swell up to the size of a lime and cause great discomfort if it gets infected. A painful abscess (an area of pus surrounded by inflamed tissue) may form as a result of the infection.

WHAT NEXT?

Your doctor will probably take your medical history and do a pelvic examination.

MY TREATMENT OPTIONS

Most cysts respond to self-help treatment or antibiotics; sometimes no treatment is needed at all.
Drainage of the cyst Your doctor may drain a large cyst under local anesthetic.
Marsupialization In this procedure a permanent drainage hole is made in the cyst to prevent frequent recurrence.
Removal of the gland In very rare cases the gland is removed.

HOW CAN I HELP MYSELF?

Most Bartholin's cysts occur for no apparent reason, and once a cyst develops you can try these options:

DO I HAVE THE SYMPTOMS?

With a small, uninfected cyst, you may be symptom-free. Usually only one gland is affected, so symptoms will be on one side of the vaginal opening:
- Tender or painful lump on one side of your vulva
- Discomfort, especially when you're walking or sitting
- Pain during intercourse
- Fever

See your doctor if you think you have an infected Batholin's gland.

Warm baths Taking a warm bath several times a day can sometimes help the cyst to burst and drain, easing the symptoms.
Analgesics You can buy over-the-counter remedies to relieve pain.

Vulvitis

Most women at some point in their lives are affected by vulvitis. This very common condition causes severe itching and soreness of the vulva. It has many of the same symptoms as vaginitis (see p108).

DO I HAVE THE SYMPTOMS?

If you experience inflammation and itching of the outer genital area, consult your doctor.

WHAT IS IT?

Vulvitis is an inflammation of the vulva that produces itching, rawness, soreness, or a burning sensation. It can have variety of causes, including infections such as thrush (see p109), genital herpes (see p116), warts (see p117), pubic lice, or scabies. Vulvitis may also be an allergic reaction to soaps or detergents.

WHAT NEXT?

Your doctor will probably take your medical history and do a physical examination.

MY TREATMENT OPTIONS

Your doctor will recommend the treatment best suited to you:
Emollients help ease itching.
Drugs applied to the vulva will help treat the specific cause. Ask about any possible side effects.

HOW CAN I HELP MYSELF?

These simple procedures may help prevent vulvitis:
Avoid contact of the vulva with bubble bath, soap, perfumes, personal deodorants, and so on.
Avoid tight garments that may chafe or overheat the area.

Sexually transmitted infections

The infections described here are usually passed from one person to another through sexual contact. Not all of them have obvious symptoms, especially in women. If you suspect that you have been at risk, see your doctor. Early treatment of sexually transmitted infections (STIs) saves later complications.

Gonorrhea

While less common than it used to be, gonorrhea is still a risk for anyone having unprotected sex. Men may have symptoms such as pain on urinating, but many women have no symptoms.

WHAT IS IT?
Gonorrhea is caused by a bacterium that is passed on through sexual contact, whether vaginal, anal, or oral. The infection can spread throughout the pelvic area and may even affect the joints.

DO I HAVE THE SYMPTOMS?
You may feel perfectly well with a gonorrhea infection, but symptoms can appear suddenly. They include:
- A vaginal discharge; burning feeling in the vagina and urethra
- A frequent need to urinate
- Anal irritation or discharge
- Bleeding between periods or heavier periods.

See your doctor if you have any of the above symptoms.

WHAT NEXT?
If you or your partner suspect you have an infection, visit your doctor or sexual health clinic. The doctor or nurse will take a swab sample from the cervix, or any other area likely to have been infected, and send it for tests. Test results are generally ready in a couple of days. If you do have gonorrhea, you may be tested for other STIs.

MY TREATMENT OPTIONS
You should get treatment as soon as possible. Gonorrhea can have serious complications (see right).
Antibiotics The infection is usually cleared up with a single dose of antibiotics. This can be given orally or as an injection.
Surgery If you have a pelvic abscess associated with pelvic inflammatory disease (see right), it may need to be drained.
Your partner Any partner you have had in the last three months should be treated, too.

HOW CAN I HELP MYSELF?
Practice safe sex by using condoms, especially if you have many partners. If you are infected, avoid sex until your doctor gives you the all-clear.

AM I AT RISK?
You are at risk of contracting gonorrhea if you have unprotected sex and genital contact with an infected partner. If gonorrhea is left untreated, complications can arise.
- Gonorrhea can cause pelvic inflammatory disease (PID, see p98); symptoms include pelvic pain, fever, vaginal bleeding, and pelvic abscess
- It can spread to the abdominal cavity and the liver, and cause perihepatitis (inflammation of the tissues surrounding the liver)
- It can spread via the bloodstream and lead to arthritis.

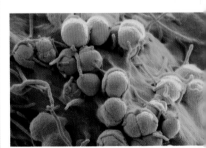

Gonorrhea
This magnified image shows gonorrhea bacteria (colored red) infecting a human cell.

Chlamydia

A woman can have chlamydia without knowing it, since the infection often causes no symptoms.

WHAT IS IT?

This bacterial infection can frequently go undetected for years, unless it leads to complications, such as pelvic inflammatory disease (see p98) and infertility. Once diagnosed, it's easily treated.

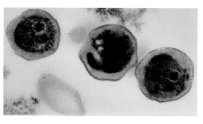

Chlamydia bacterium
Chlamydia trachiomatis (black areas) can cause serious damage if untreated.

WHAT NEXT?

If you suspect you have chlamydia, visit your doctor or sexual health clinic, where they'll take a sample swab from your cervix. The results are usually ready in 24 hours.

DO I HAVE THE SYMPTOMS?

There are often no specific symptoms of chlamydia, but the following can be signs of the infection:

- Discharge from the vagina
- A frequent need to urinate
- A burning pain while urinating
- Lower abdominal pain.

If you experience any of the above symptoms, ask for a chlamydia test from your doctor or sexual health practitioner.

MY TREATMENT OPTIONS

Make sure both you and your partner are treated.

Antibiotics Chlamydia is treated with antibiotics. You will have a follow-up test in three to four months.

HOW CAN I HELP MYSELF?

Practice safe sex by using condoms, especially if you have many partners. You can buy home testing kits to check for chlamydia, if you need reassurance.

AM I AT RISK?

Chlamydia is a risk at any age, but it's most common in young women aged 15–25. You're at risk if you have unprotected sex or genital contact with an infected partner.

Syphilis

If left untreated, syphilis gradually progresses through three distinct phases. After the early stages, an infected person may show no further symptoms for many years.

WHAT IS IT?

Syphilis is a bacterial infection caught through sexual contact. A sore, or chancre, is usually the first symptom. Other symptoms (see right) develop a few weeks later, and then often disappear. Third-stage syphilis, which causes widespread damage, may develop up to 20 years later.

WHAT NEXT?

If your doctor suspects syphilis, he or she will examine you and take a blood sample and a swab of any sore to be sent for testing.

MY TREATMENT OPTIONS

Treatment in the early stages for both you and your partner avoids serious complications later:

Antibiotics Syphilis is treated with antibiotics, given by injection. Ask your doctor about side effects.

HOW CAN I HELP MYSELF?

Practice safe sex by using condoms, especially if you have many partners.

DO I HAVE THE SYMPTOMS?

The initial symptoms include:

- A painless sore on the vulva, anus, tongue, or lips.

Secondary symptoms include:

- Fever and aches and pains
- Rash
- Swollen lymph nodes in the groin
- Hair loss
- Flat warts on the vulva.

Third-stage symptoms include:

- Blindness
- Stroke and heart disease
- Paralysis.

Genital herpes

This disease is caused by the same virus that produces cold sores. Genital herpes, which is one of the most common STIs, tends to recur and needs to be controlled by careful management.

WHAT IS IT?

Herpes is caused by a strain of the herpes simplex virus, which is known as HSV2. A few days after infection, painful blisters may appear on the genitals, together with itching and burning sensations, and a feeling of general ill health (see below). These symptoms usually disappear in two to three weeks, but the virus remains permanently in the body. This means that further episodes of herpes may occur, and that the infected person can pass on the virus to a partner at any time. Some people only have one attack, while others have frequent recurrences. Usually, the symptoms are milder in recurrent attacks and last for a shorter time.

WHAT NEXT?

If you suspect you have herpes, go to see your doctor as soon as possible. He or she will examine your genitals, take a sample of the fluid from the blisters, and send it away for testing. If your symptoms have disappeared, the doctor will take a blood test.

MY TREATMENT OPTIONS

Over-the-counter medication for cold sores won't treat genital herpes, so always go to your doctor. He or she will prescribe the best course of treatment. Make sure your partner is evaluated, too. There are many ways to relieve herpes. Discuss possible side effects with your doctor.

Ointment Anesthetic ointment on blisters helps pain and itching.
Medication Antiviral medication is used during the initial attack. If you are prone to severe recurrent attacks, you can also take antivirals daily as a preventive measure to reduce the number and severity of the attacks.

HOW CAN I HELP MYSELF?

Bathing the area with a salt solution, taking cool showers, and wearing loose clothing can help relieve the pain and discomfort of blisters. If you have an attack of herpes, avoid even protected sex until all the symptoms have gone.

DO I HAVE THE SYMPTOMS?

The following may occur:
- Painful blisters usually on the vulva but can occur anywhere
- Headache
- Fever and feeling unwell
- Aches and pains
- Swollen lymph nodes in your groin
- A burning sensation while urinating.

Talk to your doctor if you have one or more of these symptoms.

AM I AT RISK?

You're at risk if you have oral or genital contact with an infected partner or partners.

DISPELLING THE HERPES MYTHS

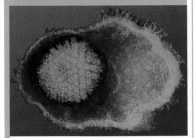

Herpes virus
This common virus infects a cell, then makes a copy of itself so it can go on to infect other cells.

- Myth: herpes is forever. While it is true that the virus remains in your system, it isn't true that outbreaks can't be treated or even prevented entirely. Antiviral drugs can reduce the likelihood of flare-ups.
- Myth: herpes makes you infertile. No, herpes, can't make you infertile. If you're pregnant and have herpes, medication can be prescribed. And if you give birth while having an outbreak, you'll be given a planned cesarean delivery so that your baby won't be infected.
- Myth: herpes gives you cancer. There's no association at all between herpes infections and any type of cancer.

Genital warts

Genital warts are the most common STI in the world. They tend mostly to affect women aged 16 to 25. Treatment for them is simple, but they are stubborn and tend to recur. The infection cannot be cured but it can be controlled.

WHAT ARE THEY?

Genital warts are caused by infection with the human papilloma virus (HPV) (see p366). They grow as soft, painless lumps in and around the entrance to the vagina, anus, and the vulva. You may not realize that you have been infected, since the warts can take up to 18 months to appear. Some people have no symptoms at all. However, even if you have no visible warts, you can still pass on the infection to a sexual partner.

HPV has been linked to cervical cancer (see p107). Leaving genital warts untreated may increase your risk of this cancer, but regular Pap smears to detect precancerous changes can help protect you.

WHAT NEXT?

If you think you may have genital warts, visit your doctor or sexual health clinic for an examination. A diagnosis will be made after a physical examination and you may be tested for other STIs as well.

MY TREATMENT OPTIONS

Don't try to treat genital warts with over-the-counter wart medication, as this will not work. Instead, talk to your doctor about the best treatment option for you with the fewest side effects. You should also make sure your partner is treated. Regardless of the type of treatment you have, genital warts often reappear.

Cream or liquid This kills the skin cells infected with the virus.

Laser treatment If medication does not work, your doctor may suggest that you have the warts removed by laser.

Vaccine The Gardisil vaccine is available to protect young women from becoming infected with four strains of the HPV virus and with the two strains most likely to cause cervical cancer. It is recommended that young women, age 11 to 26, have the series of three injections before they become sexually active. It is estimated that women who have the vaccine reduce their chances of developing cervical cancer by about 70 percent.

HOW CAN I HELP MYSELF?

The main thing you can do to reduce your risk of contracting the HPV virus that causes genital warts, and of preventing the recurrence of warts, is to always practice safe sex with your partner.

DO I HAVE THE SYMPTOMS?

Warts vary in size and shape from tiny lumps to cauliflower-like growths. They usually:

- Occur singly or in groups inside the vagina, on the cervix, and around the area of the anus (in men, they appear on the anus, the foreskin, the penis shaft or head)
- Feel itchy.

See your doctor if you are worried that you or your partner may have genital warts.

Abstain If your partner or potential partner has visible genital warts then you should avoid sexual contact. However, since the virus has a long incubation period, it's possible to become infected by a new partner who does not show any signs of the infection but who is a carrier of the virus.

Use a condom For up to three months after an infection, using a condom every time you have sex can help prevent reinfection, and give you protection against other STIs. However, since a condom may not cover all affected areas, it isn't a guarantee of complete protection against genital warts.

AM I AT RISK?

You're at risk if you have sexual or skin-to-skin contact with an infected partner.

"This highly prevalent STI is best avoided by practicing safe sex with a new partner, even if he shows no obvious symptoms."

Hepatitis B

Hepatitis, or inflammation of the liver, can occur for a number of reasons. The most common causes are viral infections, of which there are several different types. The hepatitis B virus is spread through sexual contact.

WHAT IS IT?

The hepatitis B virus is transmitted to the liver by direct contact with contaminated blood and bodily fluids, such as semen, saliva, and vaginal fluids. In most cases, hepatitis B causes a short-term, or acute, infection that may or may not produce symptoms (see right). Hepatitis often clears up within about three months. However, if the liver inflammation lasts for more than six months it is regarded as a chronic, or long-term, form of the illness, and there may be permanent liver damage.

If you have hepatitis B and are pregnant, you can pass it on to your child while giving birth, so all pregnant mothers are now tested for the infection. Babies are vaccinated immediately after birth against hepatitis B.

WHAT NEXT?

If you think you may be suffering from hepatitis B, visit your doctor who will do a blood test. You may also be given a test to check your liver function.

MY TREATMENT OPTIONS

Talk to your doctor about the best treatment option for you with the fewest side effects.

Lifestyle There's no specific treatment for acute hepatitis, but rest and a healthy diet with no alcohol can help.

Medication For chronic hepatitis, antiviral medication may help to prevent more liver damage.

DO I HAVE THE SYMPTOMS?

There may be no symptoms; if they do develop they can include:
- Mild fever
- Aches and pains
- Fatigue
- Loss of appetite
- Nausea and/or vomiting and diarrhea.

Talk to your doctor if you have symptoms that concern you.

Vaccination If you think you have an increased risk then you should be vaccinated.

HOW CAN I HELP MYSELF?

Practice safe sex methods and avoid anything, such as tattooing, that may involve dirty needles.

AM I AT RISK?

You're at risk of contracting hepatitis B if you have unprotected sex, or share needles with an infected partner, or if you have an open wound and come into contact with infected blood. If you're planning to travel to a country where hepatitis B is common, or to stay in a high-risk area for more than three months, then you may be at an increased risk through contact sports, or having medical or dental treatment where the equipment may not be sterile.

WHAT HAPPENS IN HEPATITIS

Hepatitis caused by a viral infection can be acute or chronic. Acute infection comes on suddenly and causes short-term inflammation of the liver. In chronic hepatitis, the inflammation of the liver lasts for six months or more and may continue for several years. For more information on hepatitis, including those forms that are not spread by sexual contact, see p296.

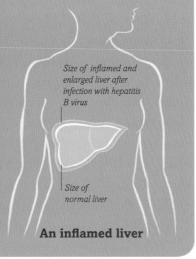

Size of inflamed and enlarged liver after infection with hepatitis B virus

Size of normal liver

An inflamed liver

Trichomoniasis

Trichomoniasis is a relatively common genital tract infection, which is usually, though not always, transmitted sexually. It's not normally serious and can affect both men and women of any age, but it is often easier to diagnose the condition in women.

WHAT IS IT?

Trichomoniasis is caused by a small organism called *Trichomonas vaginalis* and affects your vagina and urethra (the tube that carries urine from the bladder to the outside). Women's symptoms can start either a few days after infection or can take up to a few weeks to develop. The most easily recognized symptom is a frothy, smelly, yellow vaginal discharge. However, about half of women

with the infection don't experience any symptoms at all, so you can be infected and not realize it. The organism may be found when you have your routine Pap smear.

If you're pregnant and are infected, you run a slightly higher risk of having a preterm baby.

WHAT NEXT?

If you suspect that you have trichomoniasis, you should visit your doctor or sexual health clinic, where they will take a swab from your vagina for testing. Tests for other STDs may be carried out at the same time.

MY TREATMENT OPTIONS

Trichomoniasis is usually treated very quickly and easily. You should also make sure that your partner is tested and treated if necessary.
Antibiotics This is the usual form of treatment. Most cases are treated with the antibiotic metronidazole (Flagyl), which is very effective. You will need to take it twice a day for five to seven days, or as a single, concentrated dose. However, it may make you feel nauseous and you may vomit. If you vomit, tell your doctor, since it could be that the treatment is not working properly. If you're on the contraceptive pill or patch and are prescribed metronidazole, check with your doctor to see if your contraception will be affected. If so, you'll need to take extra

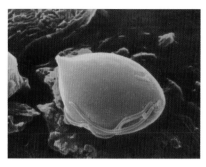

Trichomoniasis
The microorganism that causes trichomoniasis infects cells in the vagina and urethra.

AM I AT RISK?

You are at risk if you have unprotected sex with an infected partner.

precautions. If you are pregnant, you will be unable to take the single concentrated dose of metronidazole.
Follow-up You may need a follow-up test if you still have symptoms after finishing the full course of antibiotics.
Avoid alcohol You must not drink alcohol while you are taking metronidazole or for at least 48 hours after finishing the course. Drinking alcohol while you are taking this medicine can cause severe side effects.

HOW CAN I HELP MYSELF?

Abstain from sex while taking medication, or at the very least use a condom, to avoid reinfection.

DO I HAVE THE SYMPTOMS?

There may be no symptoms, but you could have:

● Inflammation and itching around the vagina
● Profuse, greenish yellow, and smelly vaginal discharge
● A burning sensation when urinating
● Discomfort during intercourse
● Pain in the lower abdomen.

See your doctor or visit your sexual health clinic if you experience any of these symptoms.

"Always practice safe sex and use a condom."

HIV infection and AIDS

Worldwide, human immunodeficiency virus (HIV), which can lead to acquired immunodeficiency syndrome (AIDS), is one of the most feared diseases of modern times. However, early diagnosis and access to the right treatment can greatly improve the outlook of people who are infected with HIV.

DO I HAVE THE SYMPTOMS?

The first symptoms of HIV infection usually appear within six weeks and may include:

- Fever
- Fatigue
- Aches and pains
- Rash across the chest.

The infection goes into a dormant phase and you may feel well. But if left untreated, HIV lowers the immune system and the following may develop:

- Weight loss
- Night sweats
- Persistent diarrhea
- Persistent swollen glands
- Herpes infection, such as cold sores
- Yeast infections of the mouth and vagina.

Once the immune system has been severely damaged, which can take up to 10 years, infections and cancers occur:

- Tuberculosis
- Pneumonia
- Kaposi's sarcoma (a form of skin cancer)
- Lymphoma (cancer of the lymph nodes).

WHAT IS IT?

HIV attacks the immune system, weakening the body's resistance to illnesses such as infections or cancers. HIV infection can be transmitted via blood, semen, vaginal fluids, and, to a certain degree, through breast milk. The virus enters the body more easily by anal sex than by vaginal intercourse. Once the virus is in the bloodstream, it enters special white blood cells called CD4 cells, which are responsible for fighting infections. HIV destroys these cells rapidly. Although the body can replace the CD4 cells, eventually the virus reduces the numbers of cells to such an extent that the immune system eventually fails, which leads to the development of AIDS. Particular illnesses are associated with AIDS, and a person is said to have AIDS if she or he has developed one of these illnesses (see Do I have the symptoms, left.)

WHAT NEXT?

If you think you've been exposed to HIV infection, you should visit your doctor who will do a blood test to check for antibodies against the virus. If the test is negative, you may be advised to take another test three months later, because the antibodies can take a long time to develop. If the test is positive:

- You'll be referred to an HIV clinic, where you'll receive counseling and treatment from health-care professionals
- You must tell your sexual partner, who should also be tested for the virus
- You'll need a Pap smear at least once or twice a year, since HIV positive women are at high risk of developing cervical cancer.

MY TREATMENT OPTIONS

The HIV virus can change its form (mutate) fairly easily. This means that no vaccine to prevent HIV has

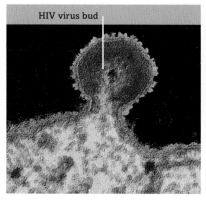

HIV virus bud

HIV virus
This HIV virus particle is "budding" out from the human body cell in which it has developed. Now it will infect other cells.

AM I AT RISK?

Anyone who has unprotected sex, especially with many different partners, may be at risk of contracting HIV. People at particularly high risk are those who have unprotected anal sex, or use intravenous drugs and share or reuse needles. Infection through contaminated blood transfusions is now rare.

been successfully developed, because every time the virus mutates a different drug has to be used against it.

Medication Fortunately, over the last 15 years, antiviral drugs have been developed to keep HIV-infected people from progressing on to AIDS. In many people, these drugs have reduced the virus to almost invisible levels in the body. Some of the drugs do have side effects, such as nausea.

However, antivirals are not a miracle cure for HIV, and can only help keep the disease under control. In many countries, people have no access to such medication.

HOW CAN I HELP MYSELF?

Most importantly, anyone diagnosed with HIV should always use a condom during sex (see also box, right). Eating well, getting plenty of exercise, and stopping smoking, drinking, or taking drugs can help to improve general health.

PREGNANCY AND HIV-INFECTED WOMEN

In a pregnant woman, HIV is readily transmitted through the bloodstream to the unborn child. However, over the years, HIV medications have progressed and are now extremely effective in preventing HIV from reaching the baby. In all parts of the world, it has been suggested that pregnant women should be tested routinely for HIV infection; and in many countries, HIV testing for pregnant women is already compulsory.

AVOIDING HIV INFECTIONS

Prevention is difficult, but blood testing for HIV is reliable and readily available. If you have a new partner, it is usually recommended that you do not have sex until he or she has had a negative HIV test.

- Even if a new partner has a negative HIV test, you should use a condom, because it can take up to three months after infection for a test to reveal a positive result
- Avoid having sex with many different partners
- Never share a needle with anyone to inject drugs
- Avoid practices such as tattooing unless you are sure that only sterile, disposable needles will be used
- If you're a health-care provider and stick yourself with an HIV positive needle, or if you're sexually assaulted by an HIV positive person, you should take HIV medications immediately to reduce your chances of becoming infected.

HIV VIRUS PARTICLE

An HIV particle has an outer membrane with 72 tiny protein spikes and two strands of genetic material—RNA—in the core.

A spike attaches to a body cell and the virus enters the cell. Here the virus reproduces. The new viruses break out to infect other cells.

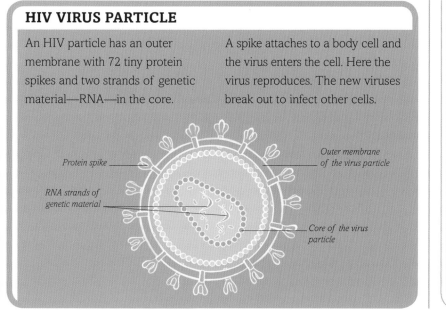

Protein spike

RNA strands of genetic material

Outer membrane of the virus particle

Core of the virus particle

Infertility

Once you've decided the time is right to have a child, it's easy to start worrying if you don't become pregnant right away. But many couples take a few months to conceive, especially if they are over age 30, when fertility declines. If you have problems conceiving, either you or your partner may need help.

DO I HAVE THE SYMPTOMS?

If you have not conceived after trying for a year, see your doctor to discuss possible problems.

WHAT IS IT?

If a couple fails to conceive after a year of well-timed intercourse without using contraception, they may be said to have a problem with fertility. The cause may be found in either the man or the woman—the chances are roughly equal. Some couples have no difficulty conceiving their first child but encounter problems when they try to increase their family. This is known as "secondary infertility."

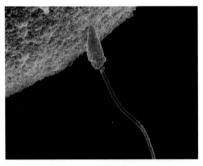

A sperm fertilizing an egg
Out of an ejaculation of semen containing up to 300 million sperm, just one sperm fertilizes a ripe egg in the fallopian tube.

There are many reasons why it may be difficult to conceive. The causes could include the following:

- Failure to ovulate, when no eggs are released by the ovaries
- Tubal infertility, where the fallopian tubes are blocked or damaged and the egg can't travel to meet a sperm
- Cervical mucus that destroys the sperm or is too thick for the sperm to pass through
- Sperm factors, such as too few sperm, abnormally shaped sperm, or sperm that fail to swim well. Blocked sperm ducts are another cause of infertility but this condition is rare.

WHAT NEXT?

It's advisable to see your doctor if you haven't conceived after a year of trying. However, if you are over 35 you should seek advice after six months. This is because the older you get, the less fertile both your and your partner become. You may have the following investigations:

- A blood test to check your levels of the hormone progesterone. If levels are high, you are ovulating normally
- A test on a tissue sample from the lining of your uterus to

REASONS FOR INFERTILITY

Both male and female factors account for fertility problems, with the causes split fairly equally between the sexes.

Other causes
Ovulation problems
Problems with the sperm
Problems with the fallopian tubes
Cervical mucus problems

check for abnormalities that may be stopping a fertilized egg from becoming implanted
- A hysterosalpingogram (HSG) test. This easy test checks that your fallopian tubes aren't blocked. A dye, which absorbs X-rays, is injected into your uterus through your cervix and travels up into the fallopian tubes. The tubes are monitored on a fluoroscope (X-ray) screen to see if the dye has filled them and is passing through into the pelvic area. If it has, it proves

that the tubes are not blocked. This test also shows abnormalities such as fibroids (see p99)

- A laparoscopy (see p98) may be done to examine your fallopian tubes, ovaries, and uterus. This can reveal such problems as endometriosis (see p101), scar tissue, or pelvic inflammatory disease (see p98)
- An analysis of your partner's semen may be done to check the number and appearance of his sperm, and to see how fast they are moving. The test also checks the seminal fluid to see if it's thin enough and has the right acid balance for the sperm.

If the test results are all negative, your fertility problems will be described as "unexplained infertility." The good news is that about half of couples with unexplained infertility will eventually conceive on their own. But if the tests reveal any possible problems, your doctor will refer you to a fertility specialist.

MY TREATMENT OPTIONS

There are a number of treatments possible for fertility. Ask your doctor about the side effects.

Clomiphene These pills can help improve ovulation.

Hormone injections If clomiphene doesn't work, you may be given injections of follicle-stimulating hormone (FSH) and luteinizing hormone (LH) to "kick start" the ovaries.

Surgery If your fallopian tubes are blocked, your doctors may suggest surgery to unblock them.

IN VITRO FERTILIZATION (IVF)

IVF is one of the most widely used fertility treatments. In this procedure, eggs are removed from the woman and mixed with her partner's sperm in a laboratory, so that fertilization takes place outside the body. One or more fertilized eggs are then returned to the uterus.

If all goes well and an egg implants in the lining of the uterus, a normal pregnancy is likely to follow. Success rates with IVF depend on the woman's age. In women under the age of 40, 50 percent have a successful pregnancy following several cycles of IVF.

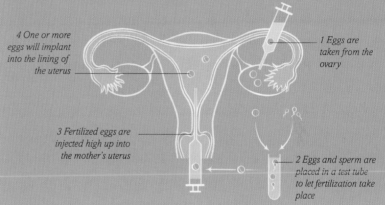

4 One or more eggs will implant into the lining of the uterus

1 Eggs are taken from the ovary

3 Fertilized eggs are injected high up into the mother's uterus

2 Eggs and sperm are placed in a test tube to let fertilization take place

---

In vitro fertilization (IVF) Some doctors recommend this treatment (see box above).

Improving your partner's sperm If your partner's sperm is the problem, he can get treatment to improve its quality.

- Blocked sperm ducts can be treated surgically, or by taking sperm directly from the testes
- If the sperm can't be improved, a sperm may be injected directly into an egg. This is done outside the uterus and the embryo is put back into the woman's body using in vitro fertilization (see box above).

Egg and sperm donation If other options fail, egg and sperm donation might be your next step.

HOW CAN I HELP MYSELF?

You can buy a kit that detects changes in your hormone levels, which indicate if you are ovulating. This information will also tell you the best time to have sex.

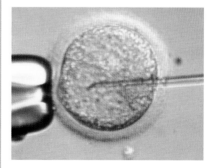

IVF
A human egg being fertilized by IVF. A micro-needle on the right injects the sperm while the egg is being held steady by a pipette on the left.

Complications of pregnancy

During the nine months of pregnancy, every woman worries about the things that could go wrong. However, for the majority of women—and their developing babies, too—all goes according to plan and without problems from conception to birth. But occasionally, complications do arise.

Miscarriage

Miscarriage occurs in about 15 percent of all pregnancies, most commonly during the first 12 weeks. Having a miscarriage doesn't mean that you can't have a successful pregnancy next time.

WHAT IS IT?

A miscarriage is the spontaneous loss of a baby before 24 weeks. There are a number of factors that may cause miscarriage, including genetic abnormalities in the fetus or a disorder of the uterus such as fibroids, but often the reason is unknown. You may be at increased risk if you are:

- Over 35 years old
- A heavy smoker
- Pregnant with twins or more.

If you've had a miscarriage, the emotional impact can be devastating and it is natural to feel grief. You may be advised to see a counselor to help you come to terms with your loss. Although you can start having sex again once symptoms such as bleeding (see right) have cleared up, your doctor will probably advise you to wait for a couple of menstrual cycles before trying to conceive again.

WHAT NEXT?

If you experience bleeding during early pregnancy it may not mean you are having a miscarriage, but you should still see a doctor without delay. He or she can run some tests, including an ultrasound scan, to see whether or not the pregnancy is continuing normally. If everything is well and the pregnancy is quite advanced, a fetal heartbeat will be picked up. This scan can also reveal other causes for the bleeding, such as an ectopic pregnancy (see opposite).

MY TREATMENT OPTIONS

In a complete miscarriage, the fetus is expelled naturally from the uterus. Provided the bleeding has stopped within 7 to 10 days, you'll need no further treatment.

Surgery If you have persistent or heavy bleeding, you'll need a D&C (dilation and curettage) procedure, which is usually performed under a general anesthetic, to clear the uterus of any remaining pregnancy tissue.

Tests If you have three or more miscarriages in a row, your doctor will run some tests to find out if there's a specific cause.

HOW CAN I HELP MYSELF?

Do a lifestyle and diet check. The risk of miscarriage is higher in women who are seriously underweight or overweight.

DO I HAVE THE SYMPTOMS?

The most common symptoms of a miscarriage are:

- Vaginal bleeding
- Cramping pains in the lower abdominal area
- Sudden cessation of pregnancy symptoms such as sore breasts and nausea

Call your doctor immediately if you experience bleeding and/or cramping. If the bleeding is very heavy, you should go to the hospital immediately.

> "As soon as you are ready, both emotionally and physically, you can start to try for another baby—usually after a couple of cycles."

Ectopic pregnancy

About 1 percent of all pregnancies end in the first few weeks because of a complication known as ectopic pregnancy. The condition needs urgent diagnosis and medical attention.

WHAT IS IT?

An ectopic pregnancy occurs when the egg implants outside the uterus, usually in the fallopian tube, but sometimes in the ovary, abdominal space, or cervix. In many cases the pregnancy results in a spontaneous miscarriage. However, if an ectopic pregnancy continues undiagnosed, it can rupture the fallopian tube and lead to a life-threatening situation.

An ectopic pregnancy is quite difficult to detect at first, since the symptoms are usually the same as for a normal early pregnancy, such as nausea and vomiting, tender breasts, frequently going to the bathroom, and missed periods. But if you experience any bleeding and a sharp and stabbing pain in your abdomen, especially on one side, it may suggest an ectopic pregnancy and should see your doctor immediately.

Any woman can be at risk of having an ectopic pregnancy, but you may be at an increased risk if you've had:

- Pelvic inflammatory disease (PID), see p98
- Endometriosis (see p101)
- Chlamydia (see p115)
- Pelvic surgery
- A previous ectopic pregnancy
- IUD usage.

WHAT NEXT?

Your doctor may do a urine test to confirm that you're pregnant. If he or she thinks you may have an ectopic pregnancy, you will have an ultrasound scan to investigate your uterus and fallopian tubes.

DO I HAVE THE SYMPTOMS?

- Lower abdominal pain on one side
- Vaginal bleeding
- Shoulder pain

See your doctor immediately if you suspect an ectopic pregnancy. If it is left untreated it can be life threatening.

MY TREATMENT OPTIONS

As soon as an ectopic pregnancy is diagnosed, action is usually taken. Your doctor will explain what needs to be done and discuss the side effects.

Medication If the ectopic pregnancy is diagnosed before the fallopian tube ruptures, you may be given the drug methotrexate to stop the pregnancy from proceeding. The embryonic tissues will be absorbed by your body.

Surgery If the fallopian tube ruptures, you must have surgery immediately to remove the ectopic pregnancy. If the tube is damaged, it will need to be repaired or, if repair is not possible, completely removed. You'll still have a good chance of having a normal pregnancy with one fallopian tube.

HOW CAN I HELP MYSELF?

Ectopic pregnancies are thought to be more likely in women who use an IUD for contraception (see pp132–3). You may want to discuss this with your doctor and perhaps choose a different method.

ECTOPIC OR "TUBAL" PREGNANCY

Once an egg is fertilized, it usually passes down the fallopian tube into the uterus, where it implants into tissue and begins to develop. In an ectopic pregnancy, however, the fertilized egg implants itself in tissue outside the uterus, most often in the fallopian tube. This may happen because the egg can't reach the uterus, perhaps due to a blockage in the fallopian tube.

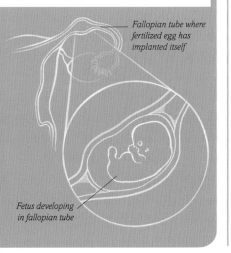

Fallopian tube where fertilized egg has implanted itself

Fetus developing in fallopian tube

Chromosomal abnormalities

In each cell of our body, there are threadlike structures called chromosomes. These are made up of genes that control how cells work. Abnormalities in chromosomes or a faulty gene may result in a disorder in the fetus.

WHAT IS IT?
We each have 23 pairs of chromosomes. Sometimes eggs and sperm carry the incorrect number of chromosomes, or a defective gene, which causes abnormalities in a developing baby. The most common genetic disorder is Down syndrome.

DO I HAVE THE SYMPTOMS?
Only special tests, either on the fetus or on a baby after birth, can reveal chromosomal disorders.

Babies born with chromosomal abnormalities may have only mild problems and many lead normal lives. Others need lifelong care.

WHAT NEXT?
If your doctor thinks that your baby may be at risk of a chromosomal disorder, because of your family history or your age, he or she is likely to offer you the option of special tests, including amniocentesis (see below).

MY TREATMENT OPTIONS
If blood tests or ultrasound scans reveal abnormalities in your baby, you may be offered counseling.

HOW CAN I HELP MYSELF?
Joining a family support group can provide help and advice.

AMNIOCENTESIS TEST
Amniocentesis is a procedure used to obtain a small sample of the amniotic fluid that surrounds the baby in the uterus. This is done around weeks 16 to 18 of your pregnancy. Cells shed from the fetus into this fluid are tested for chromosomal or genetic disorders. The test carries a small risk of miscarriage.

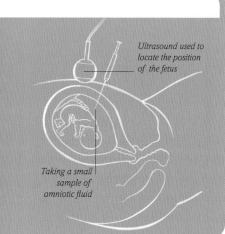

Ultrasound used to locate the position of the fetus

Taking a small sample of amniotic fluid

Incompetent cervix

This complication, which is unlikely to occur before about the 14th week of pregnancy, can be a cause of miscarriage.

WHAT IS IT?
The cervix—the neck of the uterus—normally stays tightly closed during pregnancy to keep the fetus in the uterus, and opens during childbirth. An incompetent cervix is one that starts to open too early. Often there are no warning symptoms, so the fetus can just fall out. You may be at an increased risk of this disorder if you've had:
- Multiple dilations and curettage procedures (D & Cs)
- Cervical or uterine surgery.

WHAT NEXT?
If you do experience such a miscarriage, you'll be monitored closely during your next pregnancy

DO I HAVE THE SYMPTOMS?
Most women don't know that they have an incompetent cervix until after a miscarriage.

with pelvic examinations and ultrasound scans.

MY TREATMENT OPTIONS
If your cervix is seen to be opening, your doctor can place a

stitch like a purse string around it, to sew it shut (a procedure called cerclage). It is done around the fourth month of pregnancy. The stitches are cut out late in pregnancy to allow delivery.

HOW CAN I HELP MYSELF?
If you have a cerclage, you should avoid strenuous activity and rest as much as possible for the remainder of your pregnancy.

INCOMPETENT CERVIX

An incompetent cervix can be successfully held shut with stitches (cerclage) to keep the baby in the uterus. The stitches are left in place until just before the end of pregnancy. They are removed, without the need for an anesthetic, to allow for a normal vaginal birth.

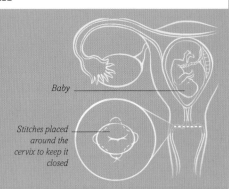

Baby

Stitches placed around the cervix to keep it closed

Gestational diabetes

Diabetes can develop temporarily when you're pregnant. This is called gestational diabetes and usually occurs in late pregnancy. If you are already diabetic (see p320) and are contemplating pregnancy, it's important to ensure that your condition is as well managed as possible beforehand.

WHAT IS IT?

Gestational diabetes occurs when there is too much glucose in your blood and your body cannot produce enough insulin to control it. This can happen in pregnancy because hormones produced by the placenta counteract the effect of insulin. You may be at an increased risk of developing gestational diabetes if you have a family history of diabetes, you are an older mother, or if you are very overweight. Some women who have gestational diabetes later go on to develop permanent diabetes.

WHAT NEXT?

All pregnant women have routine urine tests between 24 and 28 weeks to check their glucose levels. If a urine test suggests that your glucose levels are high, you will be given a blood glucose test. If that shows significantly raised levels of glucose in your blood, it means that you are probably diabetic.

MY TREATMENT OPTIONS

If you have been diagnosed with gestational diabetes, you will probably be asked to reduce the sugar in your diet and eat more fiber and carbohydrates.
Tests Your doctor will regularly test your glucose levels. You may

DO I HAVE THE SYMPTOMS?

Often, there are no specific symptoms but you may notice:
● Constant thirst
● A need to urinate more frequently
● Extreme fatigue
See your doctor as soon as possible to have your glucose levels checked.

also be asked to do frequent blood and urine tests yourself at home.
Insulin injections If your blood glucose levels remain high you may need daily insulin injections. Your doctor or nurse will teach you how to do this correctly.

HOW CAN I HELP MYSELF?

Healthy eating, regular exercise such as swimming and walking, and keeping your weight down will help to stop you from developing permanent diabetes later in life.

"Gestational diabetes usually disappears after childbirth."

Preeclampsia (toxemia)

This potentially serious condition affects 5–8 percent of pregnant women annually in the US. The causes of preeclampsia are not fully understood, but the disorder can affect both the mother and her baby.

WHAT IS IT?

In preeclampsia, a pregnant woman develops high blood pressure, together with fluid retention and sometimes protein in the urine. The condition may be linked to problems with the placenta, but doctors are still uncertain. If preeclampsia is not treated, it may develop into eclampsia, a highly dangerous condition that can cause convulsions and coma, and at worst be a threat to life.

WHAT NEXT?

Preeclampsia is likely to be diagnosed during your routine checkups, when your blood pressure is taken and your urine is tested as a matter of course. If you have severe symptoms (see box, right), you will probably be admitted to the hospital for observation. If your symptoms are mild, your doctor may just recommend that you have more frequent checkups than normal.

MY TREATMENT OPTIONS

If you still have several weeks of pregnancy to go, your doctor may order bed rest, possibly in the hospital. In severe cases, women who are near their birth date will have labor induced. Preeclampsia usually disappears after delivery.

DO I HAVE THE SYMPTOMS?

This condition is usually characterized by:
- High blood pressure
- Protein in your urine
- Edema (swelling of tissues, often in the feet and ankles)
- Disturbed vision and headaches
- Pain in your stomach, sometimes with nausea or vomiting.

See your doctor or midwife immediately if you suddenly develop the last three symptoms.

HOW CAN I HELP MYSELF?

For mild preeclampsia, you can try resting as much as possible, lying on your side. You should also drink lots of fluids.

Abruption

This disorder is a common cause of bleeding in late pregnancy. Abruption can be dangerous to both mother and baby and calls for swift medical treatment.

WHAT IS IT?

Normally, after your baby is born, the placenta, or afterbirth, peels off the wall of the uterus and is delivered through the vagina in the final stage of labor. However, occasionally, the placenta partially separates from the uterus wall before delivery. This causes bleeding, which may be vaginal but can also be concealed inside the uterus. If the bleeding is very heavy, this is an emergency situation that needs immediate attention at the hospital. What causes abruption of the placenta is still unknown, but high blood pressure, smoking, excessive alcohol drinking, and cocaine usage may all increase a woman's risk.

WHAT NEXT?

Diagnosis is usually by physical examination and an ultrasound scan. The heartbeat of the fetus will also be monitored.

DO I HAVE THE SYMPTOMS?

The symptoms may include:
- Dark red vaginal bleeding
- Severe abdominal pain
- Uterine contractions.

See your doctor immediately if you think you have any of these symptoms.

MY TREATMENT OPTIONS

The treatment depends on the amount of bleeding, how many weeks pregnant you are, and whether the fetus is showing signs of distress. If the placenta has separated only a small amount and bleeding is slight, bed rest may stop the bleeding and allow your pregnancy to continue as normal. If the condition is serious, the baby needs to be delivered right away, probably by cesarean section. You may need to have a blood transfusion to replace lost blood.

HOW CAN I HELP MYSELF?
Do a lifestyle check and cut out anything, such as smoking, that could put your pregnancy at risk.

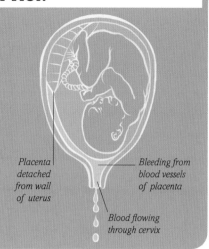
Premature delivery

Babies born before the 37th week of pregnancy are considered to be premature. Provided these early babies are normally developed for their age, they often do very well with special care.

WHAT IS IT?
Sometimes, a woman goes into labor weeks before her baby is due. The cause of premature labor is often unknown, although in some cases there is a link to lifestyle factors such as smoking, drug abuse, and excess alcohol drinking. Occasionally, the membranes surrounding the baby rupture early, which can be caused by an infection in the pelvic area. Women expecting more than one baby also have a high chance of going into premature labor.

WHAT NEXT?
If you start getting contractions or your water breaks, you'll be admitted to the hospital where they will run some tests and monitor you carefully.

MY TREATMENT OPTIONS
If your baby is still so immature that birth would be risky, you may be given intravenous drugs to stop the contractions, and you will have to rest in bed. If the birth is imminent, you'll be given steroid injections, which help to prepare the baby's

immature lungs for the outside world. Often, premature babies are delivered normally through the vagina. However, if the baby appears to be distressed during labor, you will have a cesarean section for fast delivery.

HOW CAN I HELP MYSELF?
You can reduce your risk of premature labor by following a healthy diet, exercising regularly, stopping smoking if you are a smoker, and not taking drugs.

"If you don't have an infection in your uterus and the baby is doing well, you will be given medication to stop the contractions."

Placenta previa

This is an abnormal positioning of the placenta that is potentially dangerous to mother and baby. However, careful monitoring usually keeps the situation under control and the baby is usually born with no ill effects.

WHAT IS IT?
In early pregnancy it is not unusual for the placenta to be placed low in the uterus. As the pregnancy progresses, and the uterus expands, the placenta usually repositions itself near the top of the uterus. It is then delivered after the baby in the final phase of labor. In placenta previa, the placenta remains low in the uterus throughout pregnancy and may cover part or all of the cervix (see box below). This condition can cause a lot of bleeding before or during delivery of the baby.

You may be at an increased risk of developing placenta previa if:
- You've had previous surgery on your uterus, including a cesarean section
- You've had uterine fibroids or surgery to remove fibroids
- You are over age 35
- You have had several previous pregnancies
- You are expecting more than one baby.

WHAT NEXT?
Placenta previa is usually first diagnosed during a routine ultrasound scan. You will then be monitored to see if the placenta migrates upward in your uterus as your pregnancy progresses. If you experience sudden, unexpected bleeding, you may have to go into the hospital immediately for observation or treatment.

MY TREATMENT OPTIONS
Your treatment depends on the severity of the bleeding and how far your pregnancy has progressed.
Bed rest If you have had light bleeding, you'll be advised to rest in bed and to avoid any vigorous activities, including having sex. If

PLACENTA PREVIA

There are three types of placenta previa: where the placenta covers the whole cervix as shown below; where the placenta covers only part of the cervix; and where the placenta is located just near the edge of the cervix.

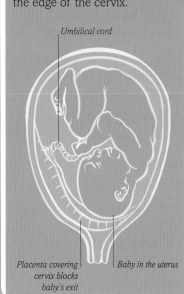

Umbilical cord

Placenta covering cervix blocks baby's exit   *Baby in the uterus*

DO I HAVE THE SYMPTOMS?

The most common symptom is:
- Vaginal bleeding, ranging from spotting to heavy blood loss, with no abdominal pain

See your doctor or midwife immediately if you start to have bleeding at any time during pregnancy. If you have severe bleeding, your baby may need to be delivered immediately.

the bleeding has been heavy then you'll be admitted to the hospital and may be given intravenous drugs to prevent premature labor (see p129).
Cesarean section If the bleeding is very heavy or won't stop, you may need to have your baby delivered immediately. You may also need to have a blood transfusion to replace lost blood.

Cesarean section is usually the only delivery option if you have placenta previa, regardless of the severity of the condition. Even if your pregnancy has been proceeding without any problems, you are likely to be delivered by cesarean at 38 weeks. A vaginal birth, even if the placenta is not completely blocking the cervix, carries a high risk of causing uncontrollable bleeding.

HOW CAN I HELP MYSELF?
You can't do anything to prevent placenta previa. If it is diagnosed, stay alert for any signs of bleeding.

Multiple births

If you are expecting more than one baby, you may be at a slightly higher risk of problems than women expecting a singleton. However, your prenatal care team will make sure that you have any extra attention you need.

WHAT IS IT?

Multiple births can mean twins, triplets, and, rarely, even more. The babies may be either identical (produced from one fertilized egg that splits) or nonidentical (produced when separate eggs are fertilized by different sperm). Some multiple pregnancies happen naturally, and may run in families. However, increasingly, the conception of twins or more is due to the use of treatments for infertility (see pp122–3). These procedures result in more than one egg at a time reaching maturity and being released from the ovary.

WHAT NEXT?

Multiple pregnancies are diagnosed by an ultrasound scan in early pregnancy. Usually the babies can be seen by the end of the second month. The chances are that your pregnancy will go well, but because of its complexity you may be at an increased risk of:

- High blood pressure
- Diabetes (see p127)
- Preeclampsia (see p128)
- Abruption (see p128)
- Premature labor (see p129).

Throughout your pregnancy you'll be monitored very closely and possibly put under the care of a specialist in multiple births. You will have more frequent checkups and scans than usual, especially in the later stages of pregnancy, to make sure that the growth and position of the babies are normal.

DO I HAVE THE SYMPTOMS?

If you are carrying more than one baby you may:
- Get lots of morning sickness
- Look extra large for your dates
- Feel very tired but be unable to sleep properly
- Rapidly gain weight in the first trimester.

See your doctor if your symptoms of early pregnancy are worse than you expected.

MY TREATMENT OPTIONS

Most multiple babies are delivered early, often by cesarean section. The vaginal birth of twins is possible in many cases, depending on their positions (see box below).

HOW CAN I HELP MYSELF?

If you are pregnant with more than one baby, you need to make sure your body can cope with the strain:

Healthy diet Eat more, for your developing babies.

Calcium intake Increase your calcium intake by eating more dairy products

Supplements Take iron supplements to prevent anemia

Physical exercise Avoid strenuous physical activity after 24 weeks. Walking or swimming may be fine, but check with your doctor.

Rest Get as much rest as you can.

DELIVERY OF TWINS

In a twin birth, if the baby closest to the birth canal is lying head downward, you may be able to try for a natural delivery. If the second baby is also head downward, he or she is likely to arrive without complications less than 30 minutes after the first one. However, if the second baby turns out to be in the breech position (bottom first), delivery by cesarean section may be necessary. You may be given an ultrasound scan during labor to check the babies' positions.

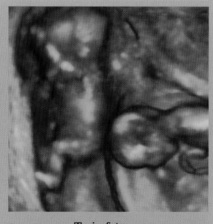

Twin fetuses
This color 3-D ultrasound scan shows nonidentical twin fetuses at 16 weeks. Each baby has its own placenta.

Contraception

Many different contraceptives are now available and some are more reliable than others. Usually, the main responsibility for contraception falls on the woman. When deciding which method to use, you need to take various things into consideration, including your lifestyle, relationships, and any health issues.

NATURAL METHODS

Natural family planning This method is based on your menstrual cycle. It involves being able to identify your body's natural fertility signs, such as changes in your temperature and cervical mucus, on each day of your menstrual cycle, so you avoid sex when you are most fertile. When used correctly it may be effective, but is best used if you are in a long-term relationship and wouldn't mind having an unintended pregnancy.

Advantages
- No hormones or devices involved
- No side effects
- Can be used to plan a pregnancy.

Disadvantages
- No protection against STDs (see pp114–21)
- Requires a regular menstrual cycle
- Must be taught by a professional
- Daily records must be kept
- Not very reliable.

Withdrawal Your partner withdraws his penis before ejaculating. Since sperm can leak out beforehand, this method is not reliable.

BARRIER METHODS

Condoms have been available for many years, and although they are not 100 percent perfect, they are reasonably effective for preventing pregnancy and protecting against STDs. There are now two types of condoms, male and female. The male condom is usually made from latex, a form of rubber, and fits over an erect penis. Its effectiveness rates range from 88–95 percent; of course, this assumes that a couple uses the method correctly.

A male condom must be used early in sexual activity: the first drop of semen that comes from the penis, which can appear during foreplay, contains millions of sperm that can result in a pregnancy.

The female condom, made from polyurethane, is placed in the vagina. If used correctly, it is as effective as a male condom.

Advantages
- Protection against pregnancy
- Protection against STDs
- No side effects
- Easily available and used only when having intercourse.

Disadvantages
- Can split or slip off during intercourse
- Some people are allergic to latex
- Can be used only once.

Intrauterine devices (IUDs) or coils, and Intrauterine system (IUS) IUDs are small T-shaped devices. The old type were made of copper and have been available for many years. Originally called Copper Ts, they are now called Paragards. They prevent sperm from traveling up into the fallopian tubes to reach the egg. Inserted into your uterus by your doctor, an IUD stays in place for several years.

An IUS—commonly called Mirena—is a newer, progesterone-coated plastic device. The progesterone is slowly released and deactivates the sperm as they enter the uterus so they cannot travel up the fallopian tubes. An IUS lasts for five years. Like an IUD, an IUS is inserted into your uterus by your doctor. Your doctor will review your medical history before prescribing any hormonal contraception. An IUS may not be appropriate if you think you are pregnant.

Advantages
- Your periods are lighter, or stop, although Paragards are associated with heavier periods

"Condoms are widely available, and protect against sexually transmitted diseases (STDs)."

- Very effective at preventing pregnancy
- Last for several years.

Disadvantages
- Sometimes difficult to insert
- No protection against STDs
- Side effects may occur.

Diaphragms and cervical caps

The diaphragm is a dome-shaped device made from rubber that covers the cervix to prevent sperm from entering the uterus. It is inserted before having intercourse either immediately, or up to two hours beforehand. After intercourse the diaphragm must be left in place for at least six hours, or overnight. It can then be removed, washed, and used again.

Diaphragms are designed to be used with spermicidal creams or gels (see p134). If you have sex more than once with a diaphragm in place, you should add more spermicidal gel into the vagina. If used correctly, their effectiveness ranges from 85–95 percent.

A cervical cap is somewhat smaller than a diaphragm, and fits right over the cervix. It should be filled with a spermicide prior to use, and may be left in place for several days. Caps are slightly less effective than diaphragms.

Advantages
- Only need to be used while having intercourse
- May help prevent STDs and cervical cancer
- Easy to use
- No health risks.

YOUR CONTRACEPTIVE BARRIER METHODS

Some contraceptives are more effective than others. One of the major factors you have to consider is how reliable your preferred method needs to be. With any barrier contraceptives, always use a spermicide as well. If you use a diaphragm or cap, it will need to be checked regularly by your doctor or a nurse to maintain the correct fit.

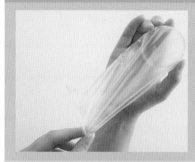

Female condom
Lightly lubricated for easier use, this sheath contains two rings that help to keep it in place inside the walls of the vagina. It must inserted before intercourse, and used only once. Female condoms are thought to be 95% effective if used correctly.

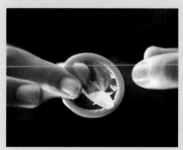

Male condom
This sheath should be unrolled carefully over an erect penis before intercourse (the roll of rubber should be on the outside, not the inside). Any air at the end should be squeezed out. Male condoms can provide reliable contraception if used carefully.

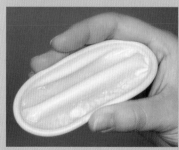

Diaphragm
This dome of thin rubber has a metal spring in the rim. It fits diagonally across the front wall of the vagina so that the cervix is covered during intercourse. The diaphragm is thought to be about 90% effective when used with a spermicide.

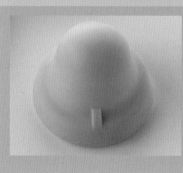

Cervical cap
The cap, smaller and more rigid than a diaphragm, is held in place by suction over the cervix. Caps are usually used by women who can't use diaphragms because of a prolapse or cystitis. Used properly with a spermicide, caps are thought to be 85% effective.

Disadvantages

- May increase risk of cystitis (see pp336–7) and pelvic inflammatory disease (see p98)
- May cause serious inflammation
- May cause an allergic reaction
- Diaphragms and caps are available in different sizes, so you'll need to be fitted for the correct size by your doctor or a nurse.

Spermicides There are several chemicals, known as spermicides, that are known to kill sperm, but are not toxic to vaginal tissue. They are available over the counter in a gel, cream, pessary, and foam form. Used in conjunction with barrier methods, they give added contraceptive protection; some experts believe that if a woman inserts a spermicide and a man uses a condom, they will achieve about 97–98 percent protection from pregnancy. Some experts also believe that spermicides protect against HIV transmission; however, the evidence here is less clear.

Advantages

- Widely available over the counter
- Can increase the effectiveness of diaphragms and caps.

Disadvantages

- Can cause allergic reactions
- No protection against STIs
- Not reliable if used alone in protecting against pregnancy.

HORMONAL CONTRACEPTIVES

Birth control pills first appeared in the early 1960s, and are one of the most popular forms of

> ## "If taken correctly every day, the pill is thought to be 99 percent effective."

contraception. If taken correctly, they are 99 percent effective. There are many types of pill. The combined pills all contain the hormones estrogen and progestogen, which stop the ovaries from producing eggs. They also thicken the mucus in the cervix, so sperm has difficulty in reaching the egg, and they make the lining of the uterus thinner so it doesn't accept a fertilized egg readily. You need to take a pill daily; if you forget to take one, you probably won't have a failure, but if you forget on two days, use a back-up method of contraception for the rest of the month. If the combined pill is not suitable, you may be prescribed the mini pill, which contains just progestogen. It also has fewer side effects than the combined pill.

Advantages

- Protection against pregnancy
- Your periods are usually lighter, shorter, and less painful
- Some pills can help reduce PMS (see pp92–3)
- May help against acne
- May help with perimenopausal symptoms (see p136).

Disadvantages

- No protection against STIs
- You may have minor side effects when starting them
- Sometimes, serious side effects, such as heart attacks, deep vein thrombosis, or strokes, can occur as a result of taking the pill. Heart attacks and strokes mainly

happen to smokers, which is why older smokers should not take the birth control pill.

Injections You may prefer an injection of long-acting progestogen. Depo-Provera is an injection of a synthetic progesterone, which prevents ovulation and is effective for three months. It is 99 percent reliable, and only requires you to have an injection four times a year.

Advantages

- Protection against pregnancy for 12 weeks
- You don't have to remember to take daily pills.

Disadvantages

- Possible breakthrough bleeding
- Weight gain.

Implants If you prefer a very low-maintenance hormonal method, you could try an implant, called Implanon. This is a piece of plastic, about the size of a matchstick, that is coated with progestogen and works in a similar way to the injection. It's inserted beneath the skin of your upper arm under local anesthetic by your doctor or nurse, and provides three years of contraception. Your doctor must take it out either at the end of three years, or if you decide you would like it out sooner.

Advantages

- You don't have to remember to take daily pills.

Disadvantages

- Your periods may be irregular

- You may have mood swings and tender breasts.

Patches Adhesive skin patches have recently become available, and work in much the same way as the combined pill. The patch is attached to a non-hairy part of your skin and lasts for seven days. After three weeks there's a break for a week, and during this time you will have a period.

Advantages
- You only need to remember to replace the patch once a week
- Your periods are usually regular, lighter, and less painful
- Menstrual regulation.

Disadvantages
- Visible on the skin and there may be some skin irritation
- Possible breakthrough bleeding.

PERMANENT METHODS

Sterilization If you don't wany any more children, you can be sterilized. During the procedure, which is carried out under general anesthetic, your fallopian tubes are cut or blocked with rings or clips. There are no changes in your sex hormone levels, or in your femininity afterward.

Advantages
- Very effective.

Disadvantages
- No protection against STIs
- Not usually reversible
- Not as easy an operation to perform as male sterilization.

Male sterilization This procedure, called vasectomy, is as reliable as female sterilization and carries fewer potential health risks than female sterilization.

YOUR OTHER CONTRACEPTIVE METHODS

If contraceptives are to work effectively, they must be used correctly. Birth control pills, condoms, and diaphragms, which rely on being taken daily or used immediately before intercourse, will not work if they stay in a drawer, while an IUD, for example, will be effective all the time for up to five years.

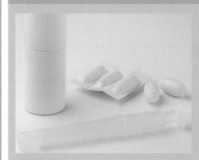

Spermicide
Some spermicides are recommended for use with barrier methods. Others are used alone; they are inserted into the vagina as near to the cervix as possible with an applicator, and are about 70% effective if used correctly.

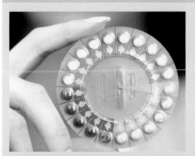

Birth control pills
If taken at approximately the same time every day, the pill will give maximum contraceptive effect— about 99%. The first course of pills is started on the first day of a period, or on the fifth day after bleeding starts.

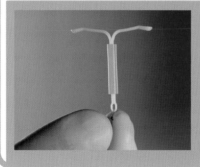

IUS
The progesterone-covered plastic IUS device is inserted into the uterus through the cervix by a doctor or nurse. As long as it is replaced every five years, an IUS is thought to be more than 99% effective (see p132).

FEMALE STERILIZATION

A usually permanent method of contraception, in which the fallopian tubes are sealed with clips, cut, removed, or blocked with plugs. This procedure can be performed laparoscopically (see p98), during another open abdominal procedure, for example, Caesarian section, or hysteroscopically (see p100). This method has a very small failure rate.

Menopause

Menopause is when our fertility comes to an end and menstruation stops. It is a perfectly natural part of getting older. This time of life brings many hormonal, physical, mental, and emotional changes, some of which can be challenging. The good news is that plenty of help is available.

DO I HAVE THE SYMPTOMS?

All women will experience menopause differently. You may have several symptoms, or you may find that you are relatively unaffected by it. Of all the various symptoms that women experience the most common ones include:

- Hot flashes and night sweats
- Irregular periods and/or heavy bleeding
- An inability to sleep at night
- Vaginal dryness and discomfort during intercourse
- A loss of sex drive
- Bladder problems, such as incontinence and urinary tract infections (e.g. cystitis; see pp336–7)
- Mood swings, depression, and anxiety
- Poor concentration
- Short-term memory problems
- Feeling tired and lethargic
- Dry and itchy skin
- Thinning hair
- Weight gain
- Headaches
- Palpitations.

See your doctor if your symptoms are causing problems.

WHAT IS IT?

Menopause is the stage in your life when your ovaries stop working. Having released an egg each month since you reached puberty, they now cease to do so. At the same time, they also stop producing both estrogen and progesterone. It is the drop in the level of these hormones in your bloodstream that gives rise to the symptoms of menopause. As a result of these changes, you stop having periods and can no longer conceive.

Menopause usually happens gradually. A few years before, perhaps as early as your 40s, you may notice that your periods become irregular and bleeding is heavier. This stage is called perimenopause and usually lasts about four years.

Some women can go through menopause without experiencing any problems at all, while others suffer from one or more symptoms, such as hot flashes, night sweats, and insomnia (see box, left). Hot flashes are often worse during the perimenopausal stage, but then, within two years of their last menstrual period, many women notice a significant improvement and experience fewer hot flashes.

About 20 percent of women never experience hot flashes, but if you have had a sudden menopause—for instance, after having your ovaries removed—your symptoms may be more severe. Few women get every menopausal symptom, but certain risk factors, such as smoking and being overweight, can make your symptoms worse.

Once you have gone for a full year without having a period, you are said to be "menopausal," or "postmenopausal." Until this time you should continue to use your chosen method of contraception. If you have gone for a year without a period, but then start bleeding again, you should see your doctor. It's important to make sure there is nothing abnormal happening in your uterus that is causing you to bleed.

Although some women have menopausal symptoms much

"Women experience menopause differently and you may not suffer from any symptoms at all."

"POSTMENOPAUSAL ZEST"

The anthropologist Margaret Mead described this syndrome, whereby women feel much better once they have passed through menopause. Particularly in societies that revere older women as wiser and more experienced, menopausal symptoms seem much less bothersome.

Many of the medical disorders and conditions in this book are likely to get better after you have passed through menopause. These include fibroids (see p99), endometriosis (see p101), and heavy bleeding (see p91). If you have always been worried about getting pregnant, you can now stop worrying and enjoy a hassle-free sex life, which is good news since you can hopefully expect to live 30 or more years beyond menopause!

earlier than others, the average age of menopause is about 51. Most women have reached menopause by the age of 59. There are some exceptions:

- If your ovaries are removed surgically, you will have an instantaneous menopause
- If you have chemotherapy or radiation therapy treatment, your periods usually stop, but they normally start again after finishing treatment
- If you smoke you are more likely to go through menopause about one to two years earlier than nonsmokers
- About 1 percent of women will go through menopause before the age of 40. If you think that you may be experiencing an early menopause you should visit your doctor for advice.

After menopause, lower levels of estrogen and progesterone in your body may increase the likelihood of some long-term health problems. These include:

- Osteoporosis, or bone thinning (see pp260–2)
- Heart disease (see pp162–74)
- Stroke (see p196).

If you are suffering from any unexplained symptoms or feel concerned about these health problems, then talk to your doctor.

WHAT NEXT?

If you are having uncomfortable menopausal symptoms, or want to know if you are still fertile, talk to your doctor. He or she may be able diagnose menopause by your symptoms, age, and patterns of your period. Sometimes doctors use hormone tests, but none of these is definitive. They include a follicle-stimulating hormone (FSH) test to measure the level of FSH—the hormone that stimulates ovulation—in your blood.

MY TREATMENT OPTIONS

There are many ways to deal with menopausal symptoms, from lifestyle changes to hormone replacement therapy (HRT) and complementary therapies (see pp139, 140). Your doctor can advise you on the best course of treatment. You may find one particular treatment that suits you, although many women get good results by using a combination of therapies together with self help (see pp139–40).

Hormone replacement therapy (HRT) This is the most effective way to treat the symptoms of menopause, including hot flashes, night sweats, vaginal dryness, and infections of the urinary tract.

The therapy works by replacing some of the hormones that your body stops producing during and after menopause. It usually means you take a combination of estrogen and progestogen (synthetic progesterone).

IS HRT RIGHT FOR ME?

HRT may be ideal for your particular symptoms and your doctor may suggest that you follow this treatment. However, there are circumstances when HRT isn't appropriate, including if:

- You've had breast cancer or cancer of the uterus
- You've had a heart attack or angina
- You've had deep vein thrombosis (DVT)
- You have liver disease
- You have abnormal vaginal bleeding.

If you've had your uterus removed in a hysterectomy (see p103) you can take estrogen-only HRT so long as you don't have any contraindications. This therapy was commonly offered to any woman thought suitable for HRT until the 1970s; at that point, researchers found that women with a uterus were more likely to develop uterine cancer if they only took estrogen. To make HRT more closely resemble the the natural menstrual process, during which the ovaries make both estrogen and progesterone, progestogen was added to the hormone medication. The increased risk of uterine cancer disappeared.

HRT was extremely popular in the 1980s and 1990s, and was used not only for the treatment of symptoms of menopause, but also to reduce the risks of heart disease and osteoporosis. However, some studies done in the UK and the US, and released in 2002 and 2003, showed that women who take HRT with the combination of estrogen and progesterone for more than five years have a slightly increased risk of breast cancer, heart disease, and stroke. Many experts feel that the increased breast cancer risk is greatest after taking HRT for more than five years, and that in otherwise healthy women with moderate to severe menopausal symptoms, the benefits may exceed the risks. Women considering HRT should

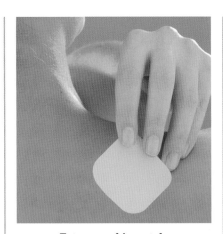

Estrogen skin patch
The skin patch slowly releases estrogen into the bloodstream, which helps relieve menopausal symptoms.

discuss their risks and benefits carefully with their doctors.

Combined HRT comes in many forms. You can choose from pills that are taken orally, adhesive skin patches that are placed on your stomach, chest (not breasts), back, upper arm or buttocks, implants, and skin gels. Vaginal creams, suppositories, and vaginal rings, which are applied or inserted into your vagina, are particularly effective if you are suffering from problems such as vaginal dryness. All these different forms are also available in many different combinations of estrogen and progesterone and in different strengths. So if one type of HRT doesn't seem to agree with you, you can try another. There is truly no "one size fits all" for this type of therapy.

There are many benefits, but also some side effects when taking HRT, so you should discuss these with your doctor before you start the therapy. The benefits include the following:
- Relief from hot flashes and night sweats
- Relief from vaginal dryness
- Improved quality of sleep
- Potential delay in the onset of Alzheimer's disease (see pp184–5)
- Reduced risk of osteoporosis (see pp260–2)
- Reduced risk of colon cancer.

You may also suffer from some of the side effects when taking HRT and these include:
- Tender breasts
- Heavier periods
- Water retention
- Weight gain
- Depression
- Irritability.

Taking HRT long term is also associated with certain medical conditions, which include:
- Breast cancer
- Cancer of the lining of the uterus and ovaries
- Deep vein thrombosis
- Heart disease
- Gallstones
- Stroke.

If you do decide to take HRT then you will need to see your doctor for regular checkups to make sure there are no problems and side effects.

Vaginal therapy If you only have problems with vaginal dryness, topical lubricants and moisturizers are readily available over the

"Hormone therapy is one of the most effective ways to treat menopausal symptoms."

> **"Herbal remedies may offer an alternative treatment for relieving the symptoms of menopause."**

counter. However, for many women these really aren't sufficient to relieve dryness and pain with intercourse, so vaginal estrogen creams, suppositories, and rings are available by prescription. The amount of estrogen absorbed from vaginal tablets and rings is minuscule; most oncologists will allow their breast cancer patients to use vaginal estrogens for moisture. If you use HRT patches or oral tablets, you may need to supplement them with vaginal therapy.

Antidepressants These may be prescribed for women who prefer not to take hormonal therapy, but for whom natural self-help remedies don't work.

Commonly used antidepressants include drugs known as selective serotonin reuptake inhibitors (SSRIs) and serotonergic noradrenergic reuptake inhibitors, both of which can be helpful in relieving menopausal symptoms. Women who have had breast cancer, and for whom treatment with estrogen is not appropriate, may find significant relief with these medications. However, the exact role of these drugs on menopause has yet to be clarified and they are not FDA-approved for this indication.

Natural therapy Herbal remedies may offer an alternative to conventional treatments for menopausal symptoms, and can sometimes be used in addition to mainstream medicine.

There is some data that shows that preparations of black cohosh, which is a member of the buttercup family, may be helpful in alleviating mild hot flashes. Two other commonly suggested herbal remedies are *Vitex agnus castis* and sage. However, you should be cautious about self-dosing with any herbal remedy. Very few such remedies have been subjected to rigorous clinical trials; some trials have found these products to be equally effective as placebo. If you are on other medication, always check with your doctor before taking any additional remedy. He or she will work with you to find the best treatment for your particular needs, taking into account your individual symptoms and the possible side effects of each treatment.

HOW CAN I HELP MYSELF?
If you're reluctant to use either hormonal or herbal therapies to relieve menopausal symptoms, there are plenty of nonmedical options you may be more comfortable with.

Lifestyle habits Often, simple lifestyle habits are helpful. For example, to help relieve hot flashes and night sweats:

- Wear light clothing made of natural fibers, such as cotton
- Dress in layers that are easy to remove if a flash comes on
- Get regular exercise
- Reduce stress with relaxation techniques
- Eat a balanced diet

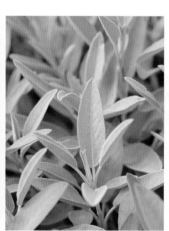
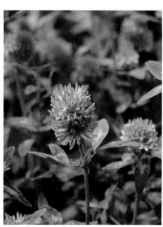
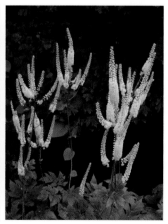

Herbs for hot flashes
Three herbs that may help reduce hot flashes are sage (far left), red clover (center), and black cohosh (left). Herbal remedies aren't regulated the same way as drugs, so make sure you buy them from a reputable supplier and always follow the manufacturer's advice on dosage.

- If you are suffering from night sweats, do all you can to keep your bedroom cool
- Avoid nightclothes and bed linen made from nylon or polyester
- Avoid known triggers, such as red wine and spicy foods.

Soy-based foods If none of these lifestyle habits help, try adding soy-based foods to your diet (see Food therapy, opposite). However, some specialists do not regard soy as particularly helpful if you are already taking estrogen replacement therapy.

Other lifestyle measures The following medication-free, self-help measures may relieve symptoms such as irritability, anxiety, depression, and mood swings:

- A diet high in vitamin B, zinc, and magnesium (see pp52–5)
- 30 minutes of strenuous exercise to release endorphins (the body's natural stress-relieving chemicals)
- Relaxation techniques, such as yoga (see below) or meditation.

"Regular weight-bearing exercise, such as walking and dancing, is great for reducing your risk of osteoporosis."

To improve your quality of sleep:
- Go to bed at a regular time every night
- Avoid exercising at night
- Have a warm milky drink before you go to sleep.

To help relieve skin dryness:
- Avoid using soap, which dries out your skin
- Avoid direct sunlight
- Wear sunscreen
- Make sure your diet includes vitamins A, B, C, and E as well as potassium, zinc, magnesium, iron, calcium, and essential fatty acids (see pp52–5).

HOW TO PREVENT OSTEOPOROSIS

Osteoporosis is a greater risk in menopausal women. To reduce your risk of fracture:
- Stop smoking

- Keep your alcohol consumption within reasonable limits
- Do regular weight-bearing exercise, such as walking, running, and dancing
- Eat a well-balanced diet
- Eat foods that are rich in calcium and vitamin D (see p262)
- Ask your doctor about taking supplements of calcium and vitamin D. It is recommended that menopausal women have 1200 mg of calcium daily and 800-1000 IU of vitamin D.

HOW TO PREVENT HEART DISEASE

Another health risk that increases after menopause is heart disease (see pp160–74). To reduce this risk:
- Maintain a healthy body weight
- Eat a healthy diet that is low in saturated fats and rich in fruits and vegetables
- Get regular aerobic exercise, ideally every day, but at least three to four days a week for 30–40 minutes minimum
- Stop smoking
- Have the level of cholesterol in your blood checked. If your cholesterol level is very high, then you may need to take medication to lower it
- Get your blood pressure checked regularly. You may need medication to lower it (see pp161, 170).

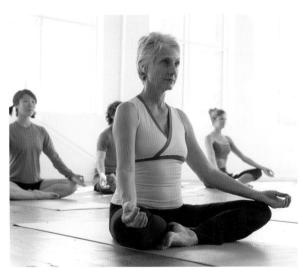

Relaxation techniques
Holistic practices such as yoga are ideal for helping to deal with the range of issues that menopause can bring, from emotional to physical and mental. Yoga aims to harmonize mind and body to help you achieve an equilibrium.

Phytoestrogens and menopause

A number of foods contain chemical compounds that act like estrogen. Called phytoestrogens, these compounds may help reduce menopausal symptoms, although the medical evidence to support this is inconclusive, and Phytoestrogenss have not been proven to reduce the risk of diseases such as osteoporosis and heart disease. Two of the main groups of phytoestrogens are isoflavones and lingnans. These should be eaten as part of a healthy, well-balanced diet (see pp52–5).

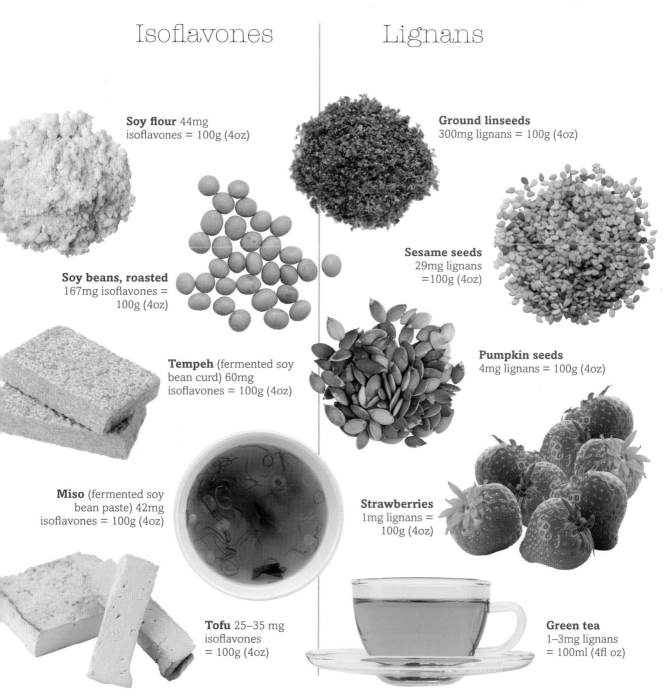

Isoflavones

Soy flour 44mg isoflavones = 100g (4oz)

Soy beans, roasted 167mg isoflavones = 100g (4oz)

Tempeh (fermented soy bean curd) 60mg isoflavones = 100g (4oz)

Miso (fermented soy bean paste) 42mg isoflavones = 100g (4oz)

Tofu 25–35 mg isoflavones = 100g (4oz)

Lignans

Ground linseeds 300mg lignans = 100g (4oz)

Sesame seeds 29mg lignans = 100g (4oz)

Pumpkin seeds 4mg lignans = 100g (4oz)

Strawberries 1mg lignans = 100g (4oz)

Green tea 1–3mg lignans = 100ml (4fl oz)

Breast health

Beth Baughman DuPree MD FACS

Breast health

Our breasts are a vital feature of our body and are an important part of our life as a sexual being. Although the appearance of our breasts helps to distinguish us from men, their main purpose is to feed a baby from the time it is born until it is around a year old. If you are able to breast-feed and choose to do so, breast-feeding can bring you great satisfaction and will benefit your baby. However, especially as we age, our breasts can be a source of tremendous anxiety, both in terms of how we look and our health.

CROSS SECTION OF THE BREAST

The breast is supported by the pectoralis major and minor muscles and its shape is determined by the internal suspensory ligaments.

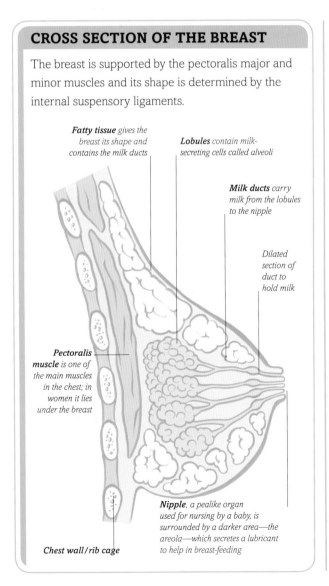

Fatty tissue *gives the breast its shape and contains the milk ducts*

Lobules *contain milk-secreting cells called alveoli*

Milk ducts *carry milk from the lobules to the nipple*

Dilated section of duct to hold milk

Pectoralis muscle *is one of the main muscles in the chest; in women it lies under the breast*

Chest wall/rib cage

Nipple, *a pealike organ used for nursing by a baby, is surrounded by a darker area—the areola—which secretes a lubricant to help in breast-feeding*

THE ANATOMY OF A BREAST

Each breast is made up of four main parts. There are lobules that produce milk, ducts that carry the milk to the nipple, connective tissue that is both fibrous and supportive, and fat. The amounts of fat and fibrous tissue vary, which accounts for differences in breast composition. If you are premenopausal, your breast tissue contains a greater proportion of dense, fibrous connective tissue and less fatty tissue.

HOW YOUR BREASTS CHANGE DURING YOUR LIFETIME

Breasts begin to develop during puberty (when girls are between the ages of 9 and 14) and breast buds develop before the menarche (a girl's first period). The breasts continue to develop and should be fully developed by the time a girl is 17 or 18.

Breasts change in shape and size, depending on the levels of female sex hormones in the body. They usually get larger during puberty, just before the onset of monthly periods, and during pregnancy and breast-feeding. You may become aware of breast pain and general lumpiness at these times.

At various times in your life, you may experience general concern, even anxiety, about the size and shape of your breasts. This in turn affects the way in which you think about your body and yourself, and if you are unhappy with your breast shape and size, this may lead you eventually to contemplate breast surgery (see pp150–1).

> "Our breasts bring us satisfaction when we are nurturing our children and are an important part of our sexual lives."

From a girl's late teens until she has a baby—if this happens—her breasts remain firm and the amount of dense fibrous tissue stays very much the same, unless dramatic weight loss or gain occurs. If this occurs, fatty tissue can increase, causing her breasts to start to sag. As the aging process kicks in, the dense youthful tissue is ultimately replaced by fatty tissue. This is why mammography works so well for the over-50 age group: the fat appears black on a mammogram, which makes it easier for your doctor to spot abnormalities, while dense fibrous tissue appears white, which can hide abnormalities. Your number of pregnancies and length of time you have breast-fed will also influence the final composition of your breast tissue.

THE INFLUENCE OF HORMONES

Your breasts, particularly the ducts and lobules, are constantly being affected by your body's hormonal changes. Every month, estrogen and progesterone prepare your breasts for the possibility of pregnancy and milk production. If you don't get pregnant, the breast tissue returns to its normal state. These hormonal fluctuations can make your breasts feel swollen and tender at certain times of the month. Estrogen can sometimes stimulate other changes in your breasts. For example, it can cause the production of noncancerous, fluid-filled sacs, which are known as cysts. In addition, if you already have precancerous cells in a breast, the estrogen may make them start to divide more rapidly and induce cancer growth.

Your ovaries are the main source of estrogen before menopause, yet your breasts continue to change even after menopause. This is because excess body fat can be converted to estrogen compounds in the adrenal glands as well as in the adipose (fat) tissue itself. In fact, breast changes are very closely related to your body fat content.

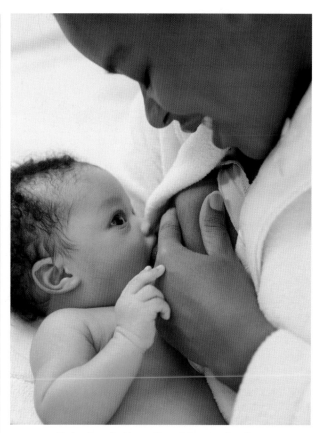

Enjoying the benefits of breast-feeding
If you can and want to breast-feed, do so in the knowledge that breast-feeding is what our breasts were designed for. It can bring you deep satisfaction and offers many benefits to your baby.

THE IMPORTANCE OF BREAST-FEEDING

Our breasts are the most visible sign of our femaleness, but we shouldn't forget that they are also what historically sustained our species. Fear of breast cancer and society's view of breasts as sexual objects often overshadow our appreciation of their amazing life-sustaining function.

Breast-feeding has benefits for both babies and mothers. The benefits for babies include: protection from gastrointestinal trouble, respiratory problems, ear infections, and allergies; improved sleep patterns; and a lowered risk of SIDS (sudden infant death syndrome).

Benefits for the mother include: helping to lose pregnancy weight and reducing postpartum bleeding; helping to bond with the baby; and possibly helping to reduce the risk of breast and ovarian cancer..

Breast pain

Many of us feel the occasional twinge of breast pain from time to time, but it usually subsides quickly and we forget about it until the next time we feel it. For some women, though, breast pain causes considerable discomfort and has an impact on their daily lives. Breast pain can have a number of causes.

Breast pain is very common and is usually linked to the menstrual cycle. The good news is that breast pain on its own is rarely a sign of a more serious condition, such as breast cancer, but if you are worried about it, consult your doctor. Often lifestyle changes (see pp148–9) are enough to help you manage the pain.

WHAT IS IT?

If your breast pain is linked to your menstrual cycle, it's a response to changing levels of estrogen in your body (see p89) and is known as "cyclic" breast pain. If you suffer from this type of pain, you may be more aware of it in the days before to your period. Another sign of cyclic breast pain is that it tends to be generalized, affecting both your breasts, and sometimes radiating out to your arms.

In nearly one-third of women with breast pain, the pain is unrelated to the hormonal changes of their menstrual cycle. This is referred to as "noncyclic" breast pain and is more likely to occur in just one area of your breast, and may be constant or may occur at random intervals. Noncyclic breast pain can have a variety of causes, either related to your breast or to another part of your body. One possible cause is muscle strain, which can mean you feel pain between your breasts and toward your arms.

Other causes of noncyclic breast pain include:
- Being overweight
- Having an overproduction of estrogen
- Having had breast surgery
- Having an inflamed vein in the breast
- Having a breast duct that is abnormally wide
- Infection

Noncyclic breast pain has also been linked to some types of medication, including drugs used in fertility treatments, the oral contraceptive pill, and hormone replacement therapy (HRT) drugs.

If you are a breast-feeding mother, an inflammation of the breast tissue, known as mastitis,

> "Breast pain is rarely the sign of a more serious condition, such as breast cancer."

DO I HAVE THE SYMPTOMS?

The pain you feel in your breast depends on whether it is cyclic or noncyclic:
- If your pain is cyclic, you may feel a pain that affects both breasts, and radiates out toward your armpits. This type of pain becomes more intense before your period
- Cyclic breast pain may be accompanied by swelling and lumpiness
- If your pain is noncyclic, it usually occurs in one breast only and is often localized. The area may feel sore or achy.
- Noncyclic pain can be constant or intermittent.

See your doctor if your pain continues for some time, or if you also notice other changes in your breast.

is a common cause of noncyclic breast pain (see box, p148). Rarely, an acute change in the breast can be mistaken for an infection when it is actually a form of breast cancer known as "inflammatory" breast cancer. This

> ## "Most breast pain is connected with the menstrual cycle and is not a cause for concern."

can develop quickly and without warning (see p153). Although infections in the breast are far more common than cancers, this form of cancer needs to be ruled out quickly since it requires urgent medical treatment.

Occasionally, noncyclic breast pain may be caused by some underlying condition that isn't related to your breast. It is possible that the pain is associated with coronary heart disease (see pp162–73), gastroesophageal reflux (see pp290–1), or gallbladder disease.

Noncyclic breast pain may also be the result of an injury or inflammation in your chest wall or rib joints. More rarely, it may be linked to a cyst or breast cancer (see pp152–7). And occasionally there are times when a doctor cannot find a cause for noncyclic breast pain.

WHAT NEXT?
The first thing you need to do if you have breast pain is to make an appointment to see your doctor.

AM I AT RISK?
You are more likely to experience breast pain if:
- You are premenopausal; most breast pain is associated with the menstrual cycle
- You are over 40 (if the cause is noncyclic).

If you can manage to do so before your appointment, try to keep a diary of the times and occasions when you experience the pain. Once there, your will take your full medical history and will ask you about your experience of the pain. Try to describe the pain as accurately as you possibly can. Your doctor will want to know when and how your symptoms started, how the pain feels, and when and how often you feel it.

Your doctor will also examine your breasts and armpits and may also check your chest wall and listen to your heart and lungs with a stethoscope to determine whether you are suffering from a non-breast-related condition. If your doctor discovers that you are, you will be given the treatment that is appropriate for that condition.

However, if it appears that the pain is definitely coming from your breast, your doctor will try to determine the pattern of the pain, and decide whether it is either cyclic or noncyclic.

If it turns out that you have noncyclic breast pain, your doctor must rule out the possibility of breast cancer. Your doctor will check for any lump or change in your breast tissue. If you are over 35 or have a family history of breast cancer (either parent's side), you will be referred for a mammogram and an ultrasound (see p155).

DECIDING THE CAUSE OF BREAST PAIN

True breast pain comes from the tissue of either breast. If the pain is around an armpit or from your breastbone it is probably musculoskeletal in origin—a muscle strain or an injury or inflammation in the wall of your chest.

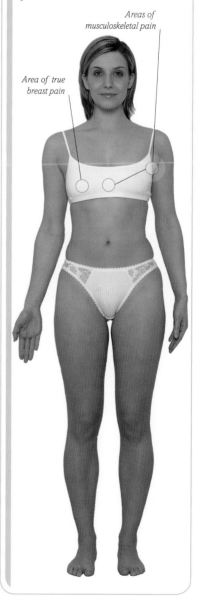

Areas of musculoskeletal pain

Area of true breast pain

MY TREATMENT OPTIONS

Usually, no specific treatment is recommended for breast pain, but if you do need treatment, your doctor will find the best option for you—the one with the greatest benefits and the fewest side effects.

Reassurance If investigations have ruled out the possibility of breast cancer (see pp152–7), reassurance from your doctor is often enough to help you manage the pain and relieve the symptoms.

Medications If your breast pain is particularly severe, your doctor can prescribe one of several different medications. These include danazol (Danocrine), tamoxifen (Nolvadex), bromocriptine (Parlodel), and cabergoline (Dostinex). However, these drugs have significant side effects, so this form of treatment should be overseen by a breast surgeon or a gynecologist who is familiar with the risks as well as the benefits of each medication.

HOW CAN I HELP MYSELF?

For severe noncyclic breast pain, there are several lifestyle changes, together with supplements you can take, that can help you to alleviate your symptoms.

Decrease dietary fat Excess fat in the diet is thought to increase the amount of estrogen that circulates in the body. Estrogen can stimulate the breast tissue and cause pain. Reducing your fat intake—for example, by switching to low-fat or nonfat foods—may significantly reduce the severity of your breast pain.

Take a supplement Evening primrose oil (which contains gamma linoleic acid) may help balance fatty acids in the breast tissue and decrease the sensitivity of the breast ducts to hormones such as estrogen. It is thought that taking the recommended dose of 1.5 grams twice a day for up to three months at a time can alleviate discomfort. Some women swear by taking vitamins E, B_1, and B_6, but placebo trials have indicated that these do not effectively reduce breast pain.

Reduce your caffeine intake Although not proven, it has been suggested that restricting your caffeine intake or not having any caffeine-containing drinks may help reduce breast pain.

Stop smoking If you do smoke, this is yet another reason to stop (see also p64). Ask your doctor to tell you about local support groups that can help you stop smoking.

Support your breasts You may be able to ease the breast pain considerably by wearing a bra that supports your breasts properly. Getting your breasts measured professionally and wearing a well-fitted, firm-support bra can help reduce pain and discomfort. If your breasts are particularly heavy, and your pain is severe, then you may find that wearing a bra at night makes a difference.

Lose weight If you are overweight

MASTITIS

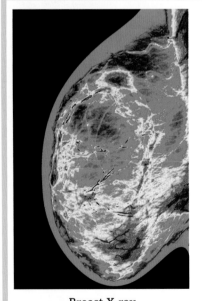

Breast X-ray
This specially colored breast X-ray shows inflamed breast tissue caused by mastitis

Mastitis is a painful inflammation in one or both breasts and affects one in 10 breast-feeding mothers, often during the first six weeks. Redness spreads from the nipple and is accompanied by swelling, tenderness, and possibly fever and fatigue. Mastitis is caused by an infection in a blocked milk duct. It is usually managed with antibiotics, warm compresses, and standing under a hot shower, Mothers with mastitis shouldn't stop breast-feeding or expressing milk, or the breast will become painfully engorged, encouraging an abscess to develop. Rarely, the abscess needs to be surgically drained.

Eating for breast health

A diet for healthy breasts means eating plenty of vegetables and fiber-rich foods, and choosing cold-water fish for the good fats they contain. Adding flaxseed husks to your diet can help, too. You should also reduce the amount of saturated fats and trans fatty acids you eat (see p172).

Vegetables

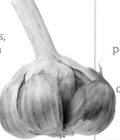

Allium vegetables such as onions, leeks, and particularly garlic, contain sulfur compounds, which may support healthy blood vessels.

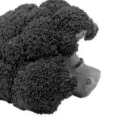

Cruciferous vegetables include cauliflower and broccoli, which are packed with nutrients, including vitamin C.

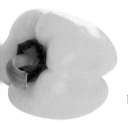

Leafy green vegetables such as spinach and bok choy also contain many essential minerals and vitamins.

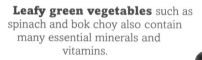

Yellow-orange vegetables such as peppers and carrots are rich in carotenoids that may keep the body's cells healthy.

Beverages

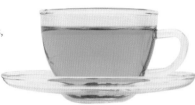

Green tea contains polyphenols and flavonoids, powerful antioxidants that may neutralize damaging compounds in the body.

Fruit

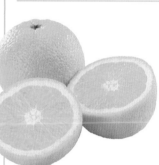

Citrus fruits such as oranges and grapefruit contain carotenoids and flavonoids, which may be immune boosters.

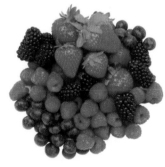

Berries such as raspberries, strawberries, and blueberries are rich in antioxidants.

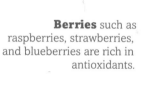

(see pp58–9), you will find that losing weight—using a combination of diet control and increased exercise (see pp56–7)—will help reduce the size of your breasts. When you start to lose weight, the weight loss often occurs first in the breasts.

Direct therapies Alternating hot and cold compresses on your breasts is thought to reduce the discomfort. Another highly effective treatment is to stand under a hot shower. Try to direct the shower head at full strength on to your breast for as long as you can stand it. You may need to do this several times before you feel better and the pain eases.

Reduce stress It is thought that stress and anxiety can contribute to breast pain, so trying relaxation techniques may bring you some relief (see also pp62–3). There is a wide range of relaxation therapies available—for example, yoga and meditation—and you may need to explore several therapies to find one that works for you. Other excellent therapies include acupressure, massage, reflexology, reiki, and Pilates. If there is any part of your life that you experience as stressful, think about reducing it or, better still, eliminating it entirely.

Breast reduction and augmentation

The pressure to look good means that many of us worry about the size of our breasts. Some women think that their breasts are too small and others worry that they are too big. Surgery can make you happier with your body and more content generally, but there may also be serious health reasons for surgery.

Breast reduction

Pain in the shoulder, neck, or back, as well as breasts that are too large, are the main reasons why women choose to have their breasts made smaller. This is one surgical procedure that has the highest patient satisfaction.

Macromastia is the term given for breasts that are too big. If you suffer from this problem, you might well be feeling pain caused by the weight of your breasts pulling on the muscles of your neck, back, and shoulders. You might also have some soreness caused by the skin rubbing under your breasts.

If you decide that surgery is what is needed to make you feel better, you should be aware that, unless your life is seriously affected by the size of your breasts, it is best to wait until you've had children. Although breast-feeding is possible after breast reduction, surgery can block the milk ducts. It is also recommended that women wait until after their breasts are fully developed (age 18 minimum).

The surgery takes between two and four hours (see box, left). As far as possible, the surgeon will try to ensure that you still have sensation in your nipples after the operation. The incisions look like an inverted "T." It's difficult to predict how you are going to scar, but scarring can range from barely perceptible to more defined.

A number of complications might occur, including:

- Fat necrosis—fat cells die and clump together. This may appear as a lump that is found during a breast exam, or a calcium deposit (microcalcifications) on a mammogram
- Microcalcifications on a mammogram that may require biopsy
- Loss of nipple sensation.

SURGERY FOR BREAST REDUCTION

During this procedure, which takes place under general anesthesia, the surgeon makes an incision around the aureola and a keyhole incision. After removing excess tissue, the surgeon transplants the nipple and moves it upward.

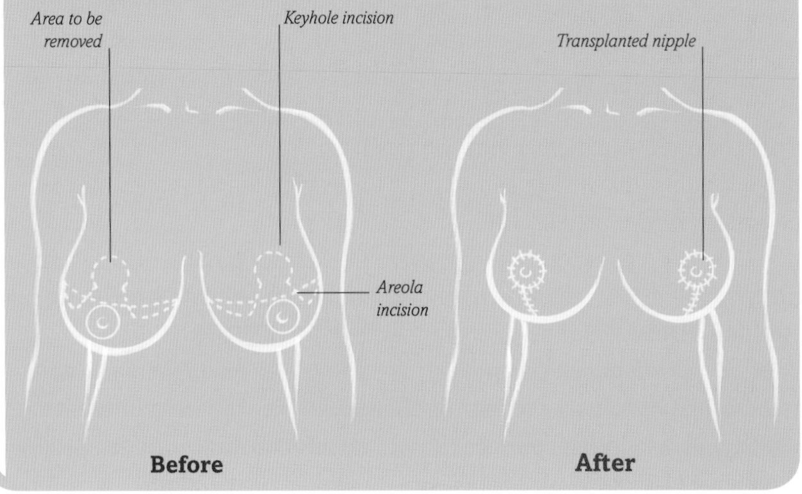

Area to be removed

Keyhole incision

Transplanted nipple

Areola incision

Before

After

Breast augmentation

If you are self-conscious that your breasts are too small or sagging, or if you have lost the volume and size of your breasts after breast-feeding, you may decide that breast augmentation (enlargement) is for you.

The most common reason for breast augmentation is for cosmetic purposes. Medically, the main candidates for breast augmentation are women with genetically underdeveloped breasts (micromastia) and women who have no breast tissue because they have a congenital condition called Poland's Syndrome.

There are other medical reasons for breast augmentation. One is making a woman's breasts symmetrical after she has had a breast removed in a mastectomy. Another is breast reconstruction (see p157).

During surgery (see box, below) the breast is enlarged by adding an implant filled with saline (salt water), silicone gel, or silicone composite gel. Breast augmentation or breast lift (mastopexy) is generally performed as outpatient surgery; an overnight stay is rarely necessary.

A number of complications might occur, including:

- Deflation and/or rupture of the breast implant
- Pain and/or infection
- Changes in sensation in the nipple and breast
- Wrinkling of the implant after a period of time
- Blood or fluid collecting in your breasts
- A feeling of dissatisfaction with the way your breasts look continues after the surgery.
- Calcium deposits in the tissue surrounding the implant
- Delayed wound healing
- Extrusion of the implant, in which the implant emerges through your skin
- Further surgery, which you may need in the event of complication.

ARE BREAST IMPLANTS SAFE?

Breast augmentation has come under tremendous scrutiny, and controversy over the safety of silicone implants has created a stir in both medical and legal communities. The implants were used for breast reconstruction and enhancement between 1962 and 1992, but fear of leakage, formation of calcium deposits, and systemic autoimmune diseases (see pp266-71) resulted in their removal from the market between 1992 and 2006.

Now, however, silicone implants can be used in reconstruction after breast cancer and for enlargement or augmentation in a healthy breast. There are no studies linking breast implants with an increased risk of breast cancer or other breast diseases. The National Cancer Institute has published data to show that there is a lower risk of breast cancer among patients with breast augmentation.

SURGERY FOR BREAST AUGMENTATION

Breast implants may be positioned in front of (below left) or behind (below right) the pectoral muscle. The best place is behind the muscle; this ensures that a woman can feel if she has a breast lump, and that when mammography is done, the breast tissue is not hidden from view.

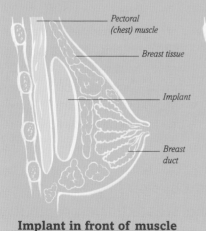

Pectoral (chest) muscle

Breast tissue

Implant

Breast duct

Implant in front of muscle

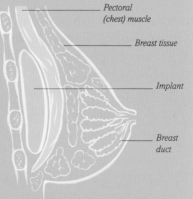

Pectoral (chest) muscle

Breast tissue

Implant

Breast duct

Implant behind muscle

Breast cancer

A diagnosis of breast cancer can paralyze you with fear. Regardless of the outcome, it is a life-changing experience. Knowledge of what can be done to treat this disease is the first step in overcoming the fear. Early detection and treatment can make this disease very treatable and very often curable.

DO I HAVE THE SYMPTOMS?

There are several symptoms of breast cancer (these usually only affect one breast):

- A small painless lump, which may be situated just below the skin or deeper within your breast
- A thickening, ridge, or "gravel-like" area in one breast
- An awareness that your breast feels "heavy"
- A change in the texture of your breast's skin, such as dimpling in the area around the lump, or an "orange-peel" effect (see opposite), which is the result of the skin becoming swollen with fluid
- A change in the way your nipple looks
- A spontaneous, bloody, or clear discharge from one nipple
- A red, oozing, or crusty rash on the nipple itself

See your doctor immediately if you notice any of these symptoms.

Breast cancer is one of the most anxiety-producing conditions that women have to contend with, and many of us have friends who have had the condition. Your likelihood of getting breast cancer increases with age, but there are also other risk factors at play.

There are various ways of assessing your risk, but the one most often used is the GAIL risk assessment model. It can be accessed online. It asks you a series of questions concerning, for example, your age, race, and the age you were when you had your first child. This provides you with useful personal pointers.

The most important thing of all in the treatment of breast cancer is early detection. Women (and far fewer men) die of the disease only when it has spread beyond the breast area, settled in distant organs, and failed to respond to chemotherapy or radiation. If your breast cancer is diagnosed before it has spread, treatment is far more likely to be successful and the cancer is less likely to return later on in your life. The main tool for early detection of breast cancer is mammography, which uses low-dose X-rays to produce two-dimensional images of your breast tissue. When you have a mammogram, each breast is compressed from top to bottom between two plates, and a brief pulse of X-ray produces the image. This is repeated on the area of tissue from your breastbone to your armpit.

Mammograms can often detect lesions years earlier than clinical examination, so although having them regularly won't stop you from getting breast cancer, it may prevent you from dying from it. Studies show that mammograms decrease the chance of dying from breast cancer by 40 percent (see graph opposite).

However, there are differences from country to country as to the age at which you will be offered your first screening mammogram. There are also differences between countries as to how long the intervals between your screening

> "Around 1 in 8 women develop breast cancer; if it is detected early and treated, the possibility of a complete recovery is much higher."

HOW HAVING A MAMMOGRAM COULD SAVE YOUR LIFE

Screening saves lives. A 40 percent decrease in death from breast cancer was found in women who were diagnosed with breast cancer and who participated in mammographic screening in Sweden between 1979 and 1999 (B). The death rate remained the same for women who did not have screening mammograms (A).

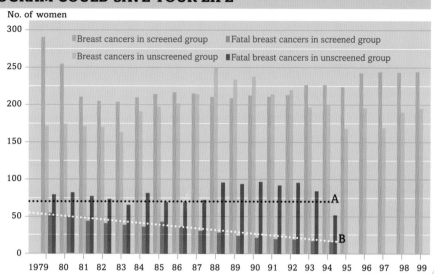

No. of women

Legend:
- Breast cancers in screened group
- Fatal breast cancers in screened group
- Breast cancers in unscreened group
- Fatal breast cancers in unscreened group

mammograms will be. Although screening mammography is key, 20 percent of all breast cancers cannot be picked up by it, so it is vital to get to know your breasts and to check yourself at regular intervals (see p154). The more aware you are of how your breasts normally look and feel, the more easily you can pick up changes early. An annual breast exam by a physician should be another key component of your breast health.

If you discover a lump, whether when you do your own breast exam or via any other method, a surgeon will need to do a breast biopsy (see p155) to decide if your lump is benign, malignant, or needs further investigation.

INFLAMMATORY BREAST CANCER

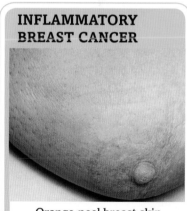

Orange-peel breast skin
The skin becomes swollen with fluid, producing an "orange-peel" effect.

Inflammatory breast cancer (IBC) is a rare cancer that can develop suddenly. Symptoms include: breast turning red, purple, pink, or bruised; orange-peel skin (see above); a thickness in the breast; swelling; warmth; pain, tenderness, or itching; swelling in the armpit; inverted nipple.

AM I AT RISK?

Only 25 percent of all breast cancers occur in women who have one or more family members with breast cancer. Of these women, only six percent are carriers of a specific genetic mutation. Therefore, 75 percent of all breast cancers occur in women who have no family history of it at all. For this reason it is extremely important for you to understand what the risk factors are in your own particular case.

Your chances of developing breast cancer are increased if:
- You are African-American
- You are over 50
- Relatives have had breast cancer
- You had an early menarche or a late menopause
- You had your first child late in life
- You don't have children
- You have had biopsies already
- Atypical cells have been found on a biopsy.

HOW TO BE BREAST AWARE

Examine your breasts yourself every month and maintain this as a practice for life. Breast self-exam is best done in the first week after your period, or in the first week of the month if you're postmenopausal.

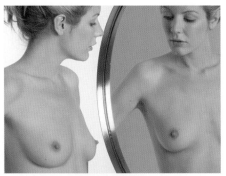

1 Look in the mirror Stand with your arms on your hips, then over your head. Each time look to see if your breasts are the usual shape and size, then check the skin of your breasts for any changes, such as dimpling, pulling in, puckering, or bulging. Is there any redness, soreness, thickening, or swelling? Is the nipple inverted rather than protruding? Has the nipple changed position?

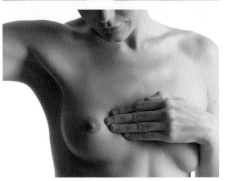

2 Feel your breasts for any changes Use body oil or gel on your hands. Begin with one arm over your head and use firm but gentle pressure with the other hand, gliding the pads of your fingers over your breast. Move your fingers from the top of the breast to the fold below it, moving from the breastbone toward the armpit. Use your right hand to examine your left breast and vice versa. Pay particular attention to the nipple region, feeling for any peculiar changes, such as a pealike or marblelike lump, a thickening or a ridge, or "gravel" in the breast.

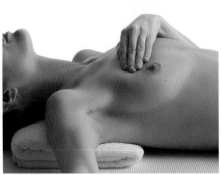

3 Repeat the hand examination lying on your back Place a folded towel beneath your shoulder blade. Check each breast from the armpit to the breastbone and from the collarbone to your abdomen. Squeeze your nipple gently to see if there's any discharge. Green discharge from both breasts when you squeeze the nipple is normal. You only need to worry if: just one breast produces a discharge; the discharge is bloody or a clear fluid; a breast produces a spontaneous discharge (without squeezing); there is a discharge associated with nipple retraction.

IMPROVING YOUR RISK FACTORS

Many risk factors for breast cancer cannot be changed (see p153), but be aware of those that can. The following are some suggestions.
Breast-feed if you have a baby of the appropriate age. It is believed that breast-feeding clears the ductal cells.
Control your weight (see pp58–9), since fat is converted to estrogen compounds in the adrenal glands.
Get exercise (see pp56–7) If you do some cardiovascular exercise for at least three hours each week your risk of developing breast cancer decreases by 20 percent.
Control your alcohol intake (see p65) Your risk increases with the volume you consume.

WHAT IS IT?

Invasive breast cancer is the disorderly or chaotic growth of cells in the ducts or lobules of the breast. These cells have lost their ability to be regulated by the body and so divide uncontrollably. In the process they form tumors, which are also called carcinomas. A carcinoma can destroy the cells in an increasing proportion of normal breast tissue over time. If left untreated it can spread outside the breast to other organs.

Breast cancer does not come about overnight. There are gradual changes in the breast ducts, which can continue to become invasive ductal carcinoma—the most common kind of breast cancer.

WHAT NEXT?

If you have found a lump in your breast, go to see your doctor. He or she will determine which kind of test you need.

A mammogram is the preferred tool for detecting breast cancers early. The smaller and earlier stage the tumor is at diagnosis, the better the chance of curing the cancer. If your mammogram shows an abnormality, you may be given additional diagnostic mammography, breast ultrasound, and, occasionally, breast MRI.

Ultrasound is a noninvasive tool that evaluates the density of your breast tissue and of any masses (lumps) in it. While you are lying on your back with your arm over your head, warm gel is placed on your breast and a "transducer" is gently moved over your breast. Short pulses of electrical energy are transmitted through the transducer that return a signal, which creates an image.

Magnetic Resonance Imaging (MRI) uses the energy of very strong magnets, combined with a contrast medium, to create an image that helps determine the nature of a breast lesion. After the contrast medium has been injected into your blood, you are placed inside the MRI cylinder where the scan is taken. The scan should be performed between days 7 and 14 of your menstrual cycle to eliminate any changes in your breasts that are due to hormonal variations.

A breast biopsy may be needed when a mammogram, ultrasound, or MRI reveals an abnormality, or if a lump is found. It involves removing a small amount of tissue for analysis.

There are four main types of biopsy: fine needle aspiration (FNA), core, vacuum assisted, and open surgical. In FNA a thin needle is inserted and cells are withdrawn. In a core biopsy, a needle is inserted several times to obtain tissue. In a vacuum-assisted biopsy, the device is inserted once and several samples are removed. An open-surgical biopsy requires an operation for either an incisional biopsy (a piece of breast tissue is removed) or an excisional biopsy (the entire lesion is removed).

A biopsy might reveal one of the following results:

● A benign lesion that does not need to be surgically removed and does not increase your risk of developing breast cancer

● A lesion that is not cancer but requires surgical removal since it is considered precancerous

● Lobular neoplasia or lobular carcinoma in situ (LCIS). This is not actually cancer, but it increases the risk of you developing it later

● Ductal carcinoma in situ (DCIS). This is the very earliest stage of breast cancer, where the cancer cells are confined to the ducts.

● Invasive mammary carcinoma. This is breast cancer that has invaded the surrounding tissue of the breast.

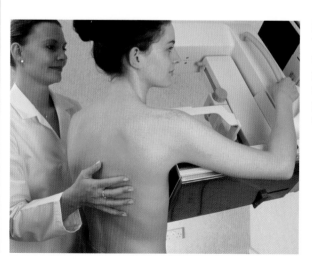

Mammography
The breast is compressed between a plastic cover and the X-ray plate so that X-rays pass through the breast and onto the plate.

MY TREATMENT OPTIONS

First your tumor will be "staged" to see what stage of development it is at. There are several staging tests that may be performed: bone scan, liver function tests, chest X-ray, and possibly a PET (positron emission tomography). Your doctor will then develop your treatment plan based upon the stage and the grade (what your tumor looks like and how quickly it divides) of the tumor. He or she will tell you about which different treatment options are open to you and together you will be able to decide what is the best course of action for your particular case.

Lumpectomy (see right) may be the appropriate treatment for you. During this procedure the breast is conserved and the surgeon removes only the tumor (lump) plus some surrounding normal tissue.

Your doctor also has to check if the tumor has spread outside of the breast. The standard procedure for doing this is by removing and examining (evaluating) the "sentinel" lymph nodes in your armpit. This can be done at the same time as you have the lumpectomy. The sentinel nodes are the first in line to be attacked by any cancer cells that have spread from the tumor. If the sentinel nodes reveal that the cancer has spread, then the surgeon will remove additional lymph nodes as well. Removal of the lymph nodes can cause lymphedema, or swelling of your arm, which can occur months or years after treatment.

After a lumpectomy you will have about six weeks of radiation therapy and then your doctor may prescribe oral medication to help prevent the cancer from returning. If you have large breasts, you may not notice a difference in the shape of your breast after a lumpectomy, whereas if you have small- or medium-sized breasts, the procedure may change their shape.

Chemotherapy is generally given after surgery. However, in some cases, such as inflammatory breast cancer, the first course of treatment is chemotherapy, as well as for

LUMPECTOMY

In a lumpectomy, the surgeon makes an incision in the breast and removes the tumor and some surrounding tissue. Some of the lymph nodes from the armpit are also removed through a separate incision.

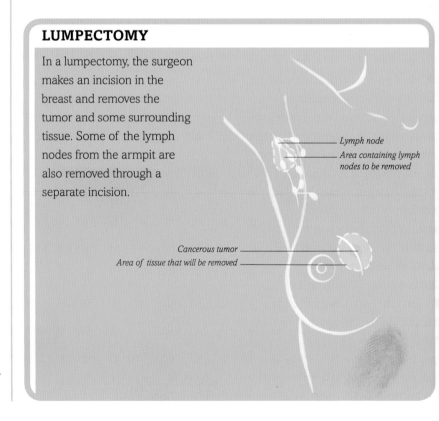

Lymph node

Area containing lymph nodes to be removed

Cancerous tumor

Area of tissue that will be removed

advanced tumors that are too large to be removed. This is done in order to shrink them. During chemotherapy, special drugs are given intravenously in the hospital, or by mouth. There are many different chemotherapy drugs and combinations of drugs, and they all have different side effects. You usually have a rest period of a few weeks between treatments to recover from the side effects. Chemotherapy lasts from four to six months and you may need surgery and radiation therapy afterward.

Mastectomy is surgery to remove the breast tissue, including the "tail" of breast tissue that extends into your armpit (the axillary tail). This allows the breast skin to remain, so that it can be used to reconstruct your breast. During or before a mastectomy you will need lymph node evaluation.

During a mastectomy, the surgeon makes an incision around the nipple and the breast is dissected away from the skin, up to the collarbone, to the breast bone and below to the inframammary fold. The lymph nodes that have the highest risk of cancer in them (sentinel lymph nodes) are removed and evaluated. If the cancer has spread to them, additional lymph nodes are removed.

Breast reconstruction This often begins during the mastectomy surgery. The least invasive method

MASTECTOMY

In a mastectomy, the surgeon makes one incision and removes the tumor and the breast tissue. The lymph nodes in the armpit will also be removed if necessary. The mastectomy leaves a diagonal scar in the chest wall if no reconstruction is performed.

Lymph node in armpit

Cancerous tumor

Area of tissue that will be removed

uses breast implants to reconstruct the mound of your breast. If there's enough skin left after mastectomy, your surgeon can insert these implants immediately. If radiation therapy is anticipated, breast reconstruction may be delayed.

HOW CAN I HELP MYSELF?

Although surgery and medication are the keys to the treatment of breast cancer, there are measures you can take yourself. For instance, being well informed about your particular breast cancer can help allay any fears you may have and help make you feel more positive.

Complementary therapies These therapies complement but do not replace Western medicine. They can help to enhance healing and many cancer patients find them helpful. For example, Reiki, massage, acupuncture, reflexology, yoga, meditation, and other holistic therapies can help you to release fears you might be holding on to when you are first diagnosed. They can help speed recovery and be supportive once treatment is over

Alternative therapies When you have had a breast cancer diagnosis, you are very vulnerable and may be tempted by "treatments" offered as alternatives to Western practice. But there are no effective "alternatives" to surgery, chemotherapy, and radiation therapy.

"Knowing as much as you can about your breast cancer will help you feel more positive."

Heart and circulation

Professor Elsa-Grace V. Giardina MD
Director, Center for Women's Health
Columbia University Medical Center, New York, NY

Your heart

Although your heart is a small portion of your body weight, it is one of your most vital organs. This important pump—the size of a fist—beats continuously, on average, 60–100 times a minute, around 100,000 times per day. Each minute it pumps all of your blood—about 10 pints (5 liters)—around the body via a system of arteries, veins, and capillaries (see p246). This system, together with your lungs, serves to oxygenate your blood, and ensure that every cell in your body receives the oxygen it needs to function.

HOW YOUR HEART WORKS

Your heart weighs approximately 9–12 oz (250–340 g). It is divided into four sections, or chambers, with two chambers on either side. The top two chambers are the right and left atria, and the bottom two are the right and left ventricles.

For your heart to beat normally, electrical impulses make the atria contract. This electrical activity travels to the ventricles, which then contract.

The right side of the heart receives deoxygenated (without oxygen) blood that has traveled, via the veins, from the rest of your body. With every heartbeat, the heart pumps this blood to the lungs, where carbon dioxide is removed and the blood is reoxygenated (see pp230–1). The oxygenated blood then travels from the lungs through your blood vessels to the left side of your heart. From here it travels to the rest of the body through the aorta (the main artery) and other arteries. Blood then returns to the heart via the veins, continuing the cycle.

Valves in the heart—the tricuspid and pulmonary valves on the right and the mitral and aortic valves on the left—control the flow of blood (see opposite). The blood vessels also have valves to ensure that blood flows in the right direction through them.

HOW WOMEN ARE DIFFERENT

When it comes to heart disease, women differ in their risk factors (see p163), their diagnoses (see pp168–9), and their treatments (see pp170–1).

INSIDE YOUR HEART

The heart has four chambers within a muscular structure, the myocardium. The flow of blood is controlled by valves (see opposite).

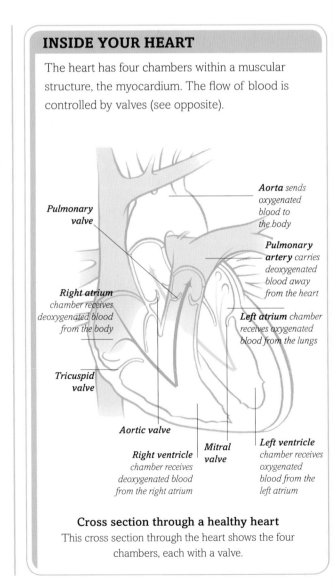

Aorta sends oxygenated blood to the body

Pulmonary valve

Pulmonary artery carries deoxygenated blood away from the heart

Right atrium chamber receives deoxygenated blood from the body

Left atrium chamber receives oxygenated blood from the lungs

Tricuspid valve

Aortic valve

Right ventricle chamber receives deoxygenated blood from the right atrium

Mitral valve

Left ventricle chamber receives oxygenated blood from the left atrium

Cross section through a healthy heart
This cross section through the heart shows the four chambers, each with a valve.

Valves in the heart keep the blood flowing in the correct direction. Atrioventricular valves (mitral and tricuspid) lie between the atria and ventricles; semilunar valves are at the openings of the pulmonary artery and aorta. The valves have cusps or leaflets that open under pressure as the heart contracts to force the blood through. Then the cusps or leaflets shut, closing the valves and stopping the blood from flowing backward.

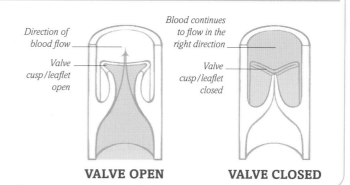

Direction of blood flow

Valve cusp / leaflet open

Blood continues to flow in the right direction

Valve cusp / leaflet closed

VALVE OPEN   **VALVE CLOSED**

BLOOD PRESSURE

Every time your heart beats, it pumps blood into your blood vessels. Blood pressure is the pressure of the blood as it flows through the blood vessels. Your blood pressure is at its highest—known as the systolic pressure—when the heart contracts and pumps blood to the rest of the body. When the heart is at rest, between beats, your blood pressure falls. This is the diastolic pressure.

Your blood pressure should not be higher than 120/80 mmHg (120 is the systolic pressure and 80 is the diastolic pressure). Abnormally elevated blood pressure is defined as 140/90, but in certain conditions, such as diabetes, you doctor may recommend treatment before it gets to that level.

Both your systolic and diastolic pressures are important, and if either one is raised this is known as high blood pressure, or hypertension. Low blood pressure is known as hypotension. There are several ways to measure blood pressure.

Sphygmomanometer The doctor or nurse will wrap a cuff around your upper arm and will inflate the cuff. He or she then listens to your pulse with a stethoscope. When the pulse is first heard, the systolic pressure is measured. The pressure in the cuff is then gradually released and the sound of the pulse becomes faint until it disappears, at which point the diastolic pressure is measured.

Electronic blood pressure machines These devices measure blood pressure electronically. They are often used by patients to monitor their blood pressure at home.

24-hour ambulatory blood pressure monitoring This involves wearing a blood pressure cuff for 24 hours. It measures blood pressure periodically day and night and calculates the average blood pressure for certain periods. This method is useful if your blood pressure is borderline, or to monitor the effect of a medication. It's sometimes used if your blood pressure is thought to be high because you get anxious when a doctor or a nurse measures it. This is known as "white coat hypertension".

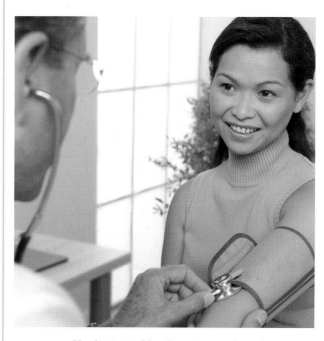

Having your blood pressure taken
This method of checking blood pressure involves using a sphygmomanometer, or cuff that is inflated.

What is coronary heart disease?

Although in the US coronary heart disease (CHD) leads to more deaths in women than in men, there's still a common misconception that it's a disease of men. Women may fear breast cancer more than CHD, yet CHD kills almost ten times more women than breast cancer does.

WHAT IS IT?

Coronary heart disease, or CHD, is a disease of the coronary arteries caused by a buildup of fatty material that can lead to narrowing and blockages in the coronary vessels. The process is called atherosclerosis, and the fatty deposits are known as atheroma.

Once the coronary arteries are narrowed by atheroma, the blood flow to the heart muscle is obstructed, which can cause angina (see p164). A sudden blockage of a coronary artery can lead to a heart attack, or myocardial infarction (see p166).

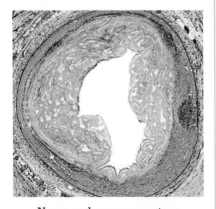

Narrowed coronary artery
Atheroma plaque (yellow area) has almost completely blocked this coronary artery, so blood flow will be obstructed.

DIFFERENCES IN WOMEN

Many women lack the basic awareness that heart disease is their biggest killer and that it can affect them as well as men. In addition, women's symptoms may be different from men's (see p164), so women do not always recognize that they may be having symptoms that could be related to heart disease. Women, therefore, tend to seek medical help later than men.

In addition, because basic cardiac investigations, such as electrocardiograms and exercise tests, tend to be less sensitive and less specific in women compared to men (see pp168–9), making a diagnosis in a woman is more challenging than it is in a man.

Also, since women tend to be protected by their hormones, especially by estrogen, until menopause, CHD is a disease of the older woman. So by the time a woman goes to the doctor or hospital with anginal symptoms, not only is she older, but she is also likely to have more risk factors for CHD, such as diabetes, high cholesterol (hypercholesterolemia; see opposite), and high blood pressure (hypertension).

Women also tend to have smaller coronary arteries than men, so when it comes to treating women with either coronary angioplasty or coronary artery bypass surgery (see pp170–1) the treatment can be more challenging.

DENTAL TREATMENT AND HEART CONDITIONS

The American Heart Association's Endocarditis Committee no longer recommends giving antibiotics prior to a dental procedure except for patients with the highest risk of adverse outcomes. Antibiotics are reasonable for patients with cardiac conditions, including: prosthetic cardiac valve or prosthetic material used in valve repair, previous endocarditis, congenital heart disease, or cardiac transplantation recipients with cardiac valvular disease.

AM I AT RISK?

There are a number of risk factors that increase your likelihood of developing coronary heart disease. These include:

Smoking This significantly increases your risk of coronary heart disease. Smoking reduces the amount of oxygen carried in the blood. It also increases the tendency of the blood to clot by raising the levels of fibrinogen and platelets, both of which are involved in the clotting process of the blood.

High cholesterol (hypercholesterolemia) and high triglycerides Cholesterol and triglycerides are fatty materials made in the liver, mainly from the foods we eat. Present in the membranes of cells, they are essential for healthy functioning. However, there are good (HDL) and bad (LDL) types of cholesterol. Having high levels of LDL, low levels of HDL, and/or high levels of triglycerides all increase your risk of developing cardiovascular disease.

High blood pressure (hypertension) Having high blood pressure increases your risk of CHD as well as your risk of having a stroke (see p196).

Diabetes increases your risk of getting CHD. If you have diabetes it is important that you monitor and keep your blood sugar levels under control.

Being overweight Being overweight can lead to high blood pressure, raised cholesterol, and diabetes, all of which increase your risk of CHD. In particular, it's thought that weight accumulated around your waist increases your risk (see pp58–9).

Lack of exercise Inactivity increases your risk of CHD as well as myriad other conditions (see pp56–7). Regular exercise reduces your risk.

Stress Studies suggest that chronic stress can increase your risk of CHD. In particular, stress can result in high blood pressure, which is a risk factor for CHD.

Being postmenopausal Following menopause (see opposite), women's risk for CHD increases, and by the time of menopause, they may have also developed other risk factors for CHD.

A family history of cardiovascular disease Having a family history of heart disease in first-degree relatives can increase your risk of CHD, especially if you also have other risk factors. It's therefore important to try to modify all your other risk factors to reduce your risk of CHD.

Modify your risk factors

It is imperative that women start modifying their risk factors when they are younger in order to reduce the risk of developing heart disease once they are older. Better awareness and education, more aggressive control of risk factors, as well as early diagnosis and treatment are all desperately needed.

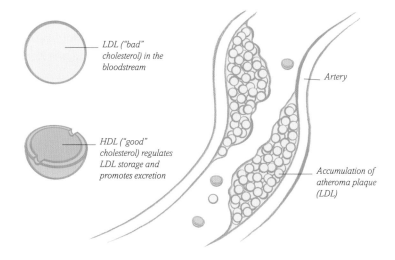

LDL ("bad" cholesterol) in the bloodstream

HDL ("good" cholesterol) regulates LDL storage and promotes excretion

Artery

Accumulation of atheroma plaque (LDL)

HDL ("good") and LDL ("bad") cholesterol

CHD: Do I have the symptoms?

Chest pain is a common symptom in people with CHD. Women, however, may experience other, atypical, symptoms that they may not associate with CHD. That is why it is important for women to be aware of the whole range of possible symptoms so they can seek help at the earliest opportunity.

There is no doubt that CHD is the biggest killer in women: it kills more women in the US than all cancers combined. Women need to be aware of the risk of this potentially fatal disease and realize that it is not just a men's disease. They can help protect themselves by modifying any risk factors they may have, and by learning to recognize the symptoms and seek medical help early. This is the key to successful treatment (see p170).

The main symptom of CHD is chest pain. This is usually described as a heavy, crushing, or squeezing discomfort in the center of the chest. At times, pain or discomfort can also be felt in the arms, neck, or jaw. Chest pain can occur on exertion (angina) or at rest. The chest pain of a heart attack (myocardial infarction) is usually intense and prolonged, and can be associated with sweating, nausea, and vomiting.

Women with heart disease can have various symptoms that are not always typical and can differ from those of men—there are many other symptoms apart from chest pain (see box, opposite).

Angina

It's easy to dismiss chest pain and other less typical symptoms. However, if you have any symptoms that you think may be related to heart disease and you have risk factors, it's best to consult your doctor who can help determine whether the pain is a cause for concern.

WHAT IS IT?

When the heart's blood flow is obstructed due to fatty deposits in coronary arteries, the heart muscle receives insufficient oxygen, which can lead to chest pain, known as angina. When you rest, the heart may be able to manage with a reduced oxygen supply. Angina arises once you increase the heart's oxygen demands, for example, after physical exertion or emotional stress.

WHAT NEXT?

Your doctor will take a medical history to assess your symptoms and any risk factors that you may have. After performing a medical examination, he or she will suggest tests, such as an electrocardiogram (ECG) or a stress test (see p168), to confirm a diagnosis of angina. If your exercise test is positive, your doctor will advise that you have a coronary angiogram to assess whether you have any narrowings or blockages in your coronary arteries.

DO I HAVE THE SYMPTOMS?

The pain is often described as a dull, heavy feeling in the center of the chest that can also extend to the throat, jaw, neck, back, or arms. It usually occurs on exertion—when you walk or exercise, for example—although it can also occur at rest. The pain usually improves when you rest or take medication such as a nitrate spray or a nitrate tablet under the tongue (see p170). If the pain persists, you need to seek medical help.

See your doctor if you have these symptoms.

MY TREATMENT OPTIONS

The treatment your doctor recommends will depend on the extent and severity of your CHD.

Medication Angina can be treated with medications such as nitrates.

Other treatments In some cases, coronary angioplasty and stenting or bypass surgery may be recommended (see pp170–1).

"A heart attack is a medical emergency—if you think you may be having a heart attack, don't delay, seek help immediately."

HOW CAN I HELP MYSELF?

It is important that you start modifying your risk factors from a young age to reduce the risk of developing heart disease when you are older. Modifiable risk factors include stopping smoking, eating healthily, exercising regularly, and having your cholesterol, blood sugar, and blood pressure checked.

ANGINA AND HEART ATTACK SYMPTOMS

Note these symptoms for angina and heart attack (see p166) and if you have risk factors for CHD, do not delay—you must get medical treatment fast.

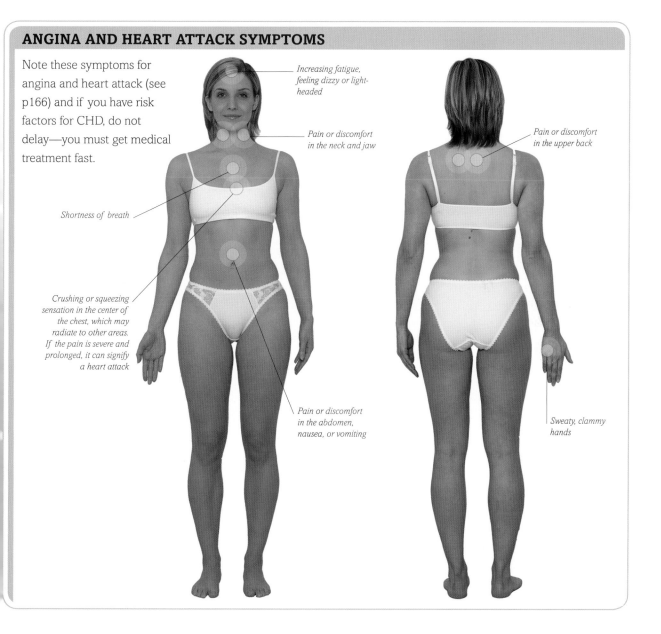

Increasing fatigue, feeling dizzy or light-headed

Pain or discomfort in the neck and jaw

Pain or discomfort in the upper back

Shortness of breath

Crushing or squeezing sensation in the center of the chest, which may radiate to other areas. If the pain is severe and prolonged, it can signify a heart attack

Pain or discomfort in the abdomen, nausea, or vomiting

Sweaty, clammy hands

Heart attack

A heart attack occurs when there is a sudden blockage in an already narrowed coronary artery. Although heart attacks can be fatal, treatments have improved and the degree of damage caused by a heart attack often depends on how quickly a person receives the necessary treatment.

WHAT IS IT?

Narrowing of the arteries occurs over a period of years as fatty deposits gradually accumulate on the arterial walls. A heart attack occurs when a blood clot suddenly forms on the fatty deposits in a coronary artery, blocking the blood supply to the heart.

WHAT NEXT?

A heart attack is an emergency that requires urgent medical attention, so seek help immediately.

MY TREATMENT OPTIONS

Medications for a heart attack mainly include aspirin and clot-busting drugs. Some hospitals offer a primary coronary angioplasty service, in which the person having a heart attack is taken without delay to the cardiac catheterization lab where a coronary angioplasty is performed to unblock the artery responsible for the heart attack (see p170).

HOW CAN I HELP MYSELF?

If you think you are having a heart attack, you should call an ambulance immediately.

DO I HAVE THE SYMPTOMS?

Chest pain that is prolonged often indicates a heart attack. The pain is described as a heavy or squeezing sensation and can spread to the arms, jaw, neck, back, or stomach. It can also be associated with sweating and a feeling of nausea. In women, however, the symptoms may be different (see p165). Women may therefore be unaware that they might be having a heart attack, take longer to seek help, and may be more ill by the time they do. **Get medical help immediately** if you think you are having a heart attack.

Heart failure

Heart failure can be the result of coronary artery disease, valvular heart disease (see p174), high blood pressure (see p161), or cardiomyopathy (disease of the heart muscle). It can also be caused by alcohol excess, certain drugs or toxins, and some infections.

DO I HAVE THE SYMPTOMS?

Common symptoms and signs of heart failure include:
- Breathlessness
- Fluid retention, including swollen legs
- General fatigue.

See your doctor if you have any of these symptoms.

WHAT IS IT?

Heart failure occurs when the heart weakens and its pumping action becomes less efficient. It may be acute, when symptoms come on suddenly, or chronic, when symptoms are milder and build up over time.

WHAT NEXT?

Your doctor, after taking your medical history and examining you, is then likely to arrange certain tests, such as an EKG (see p168), an echocardiogram (ultrasound of the heart, see p169), and a chest X-ray, to help make a diagnosis of heart failure.

MY TREATMENT OPTIONS

There are different treatment options available to treat heart failure. Talk to your doctor about which is the most appropriate for you.

Medication Patients with heart failure will require a combination of oral medications to help the heart pump more efficiently and to reduce fluid overload, which leads to leg swelling and breathlessness. You are likely to need diuretics (water tablets), which will help reduce fluid retention.

Other treatments Depending on the underlying cause of your heart

"There are different treatment options available to treat heart failure, so talk to your doctor about which option is most appropriate for you."

failure, you may be offered other treatments. For example, you may have a pacemaker inserted (see below) to improve the pumping action of your heart. People with pacemakers require regular follow-up to ensure that the pacemaker is functioning correctly. If you are a younger person with severe heart failure, a heart transplantation or a heart mechanical assist device may be an option.

HOW CAN I HELP MYSELF?

Always take the medication that has been prescribed by your doctor. Make an appointment to see your doctor if you feel that your weight is increasing, you are retaining fluid (when the lower legs or ankles swell), or you notice that you are becoming more breathless when you perform your normal everyday tasks.

Palpitations

A racing, or thumping, heart can cause the sensation known as palpitations. Although, often, these aren't a cause for concern and don't require treatment, they can be a sign of a problem with the heart or its blood vessels—known as arrhythmias—and should therefore be investigated.

WHAT IS IT?

Arrhythmias of the heart-occur if the electrical impulses in the heart that coordinate the pumping action don't function correctly so the heart beats too fast, too slow, or irregularly.

DO I HAVE THE SYMPTOMS?

You are experiencing symptoms of palpitations if you feel that your heart is beating too fast, too slowly, or irregularly. **See your doctor** if you have any of these symptoms.

WHAT NEXT?

If you have palpitations that your doctor thinks may be due to an arrhythmia, your doctor may recommend an electrocardiogram (EKG) and a 24-hour monitor (see p168). You will be asked to keep a journal of the times when you experience palpitations. When your doctor analyzes the recording, he or she will check if there was an abnormal heart rhythm at the time you felt the palpitations. Palpitations may also result from anxiety, certain medications, caffeine, or thyroid disorders.

MY TREATMENT OPTIONS

Palpitations may not always require treatment. Your doctor will advise on the most appropriate treatment:
Medication Some people's symptoms subside by taking pills that suppress the arrhythmia.
Pacemakers These are generally used to correct a slow heartbeat. There are a number of different types of pacemakers that can be used

depending on the rhythm abnormality. Pacemaker implantation is normally done under local anesthetic and requires electrical leads to be passed through a vein in the chest to the heart. The electrical leads are then attached to a small pacemaker box, which sits underneath the skin.
Electrophysiological studies and ablation therapy People with troublesome palpitations may be offered an electrophysiological study and ablation therapy. Electrophysiological study involves passing tubes known as electrode catheters into the heart via a vein or artery in the groin. The electrode catheters are positioned in different areas of the heart to try to detect the abnormal heart rhythm. Once detected, ablation therapy can be used to destroy, or ablate, the affected area that is producing the arrhythmia.

HOW CAN I HELP MYSELF?

If you are experiencing symptoms of palpitations (see box, left), it is important that you see your doctor.

CHD: How is it diagnosed?

A diagnosis of CHD will require a number of tests. In women, the diagnosis can be more challenging because women can have more unusual symptoms than men (see pp164–5) and because certain tests can be less sensitive and less specific in women compared to men.

HOW HEART DISEASE IS DIAGNOSED

Simpler tests, such as blood tests, can be done at your doctor's office or a lab. The more complex tests are usually done by a cardiac physiologist in the cardiology department of a hospital, while scans of the heart (CT, MRI, and myocardial perfusion scans) are performed in a hospital or outpatient radiology facility. The tests are then reviewed by a cardiologist. Scans of the heart are usually reviewed by a radiologist specializing in cardiac imaging. The cardiologist will discuss the results with you.

Blood tests These are done to measure your blood sugar, cholesterol, and triglyceride levels. If the results are high, you are at increased risk of heart disease. If you have had a suspected heart attack (see p166), a blood sample will be taken to look for the presence of and to measure specific enzymes, such as Troponin T and Troponin I, that are released into the bloodstream at the time of a heart attack.

Electrocardiogram (EKG) This test is used to record the electrical activity of your heart, including the heart rate and rhythm. During the procedure, sticky pads known as electrodes are placed on your chest, wrists, and ankles. These are connected to a machine that records the readings. The test takes less than 10 minutes, but although the result is available immediately, a cardiologist will need to report on the test. If you have had palpitations, you may need a 24-hour recording to look for evidence of an abnormal heart rhythm, or arrhythmia (see p167).

Exercise test This test combines exercise with an EKG to see how your heart responds to exercise and exertion. During the test an EKG reading is taken while you exercise on a treadmill. Any symptoms of chest pain or undue breathlessness are noted, together with any changes in the EKG reading. Your blood pressure is also recorded. The length of the test depends on how long you are able to exercise for.

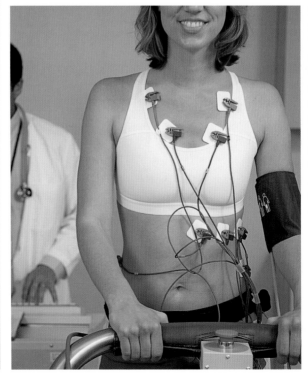

Exercise treadmill test
This woman is exercising on a treadmill with electrodes attached to her chest. The electrodes record the electrical activity in her heart and can detect any changes that occur with exercise. These can indicate that there may be disease of the coronary arteries.

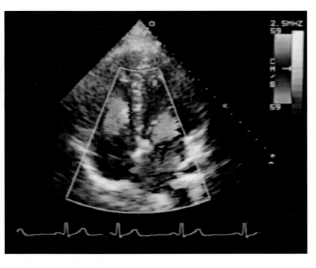

Echocardiogram with Doppler ultrasound
The echocardiogram gives an image of the heart, while the Doppler ultrasound (the colored area within the triangle) shows the blood flow through the valves.

Echocardiogram This is an ultrasound of the heart used to assess the size of the heart, and how well its four chambers and its valves are working. The test takes around 30 minutes.

Stress echocardiogram This is similar to an echocardiogram (see above), but your heart is made to beat faster and stronger using medication injected into your arm. This test assesses how the muscle of the heart responds to stress and exercise.

A stress echocardiogram helps to identify certain areas of the heart that may not be receiving a good blood supply from the coronary arteries. It indicates, therefore, whether there may be narrowings or blockages in the coronary arteries.

Myocardial perfusion scan This two-phase test is used to investigate the function of your heart muscle, both when it is at rest and during exercise. A small amount of radioactive substance (radioisotope) is injected into the bloodstream then, during the first phase of the test, images of the heart at rest are taken using an ultrasound scanner.

During the second phase of the test, you are given a further injection of radioisotope and the function of your heart is reassessed, either after you have exercised on a treadmill (see opposite) or after you have been given an injection of a medication that increases your heart rate (as in a stress echocardiogram; see above). A second set of images is taken, and a direct comparison of the heart muscle at rest and after exercise can be made to help in the diagnosis.

CT (computerized tomography) scans (which include a coronary calcium scoring test and CT coronary angiogram; see p171). These tests involve taking images of the heart and coronary arteries using a CT scanner. The amount of calcium deposits (atheroma) in the coronary arteries can then be measured.

Cardiac MRI (magnetic resonance imaging) scan This test involves taking images of the heart to give a detailed picture of its structure, including its chambers, valves, the muscle of the heart, and the coronary arteries as well as the great blood vessels.

Coronary angiogram This more invasive test is performed by a cardiologist in the cardiac catheterization lab. It is normally performed under local anesthetic and takes approximately 30 minutes but can take longer.

It is used to image the coronary arteries to assess any narrowings or blockages within the coronary vessels. During the procedure, a needle is inserted in one of your blood vessels, either in the groin or in the arm, then hollow plastic tubes, or catheters, are passed along the blood vessel and into your heart. A dye is then injected into the coronary vessels and a series of X-ray images are taken. If you do have narrowings or blockages in the coronary arteries, these are seen as soon as the dye is injected. The cardiologist performing the procedure can discuss the results with you.

"All tests are reviewed by a cardiologist who will discuss the results with you."

CHD: My treatment options

There are various treatments available for CHD. Your treatment will be decided by your cardiologist and will depend on the extent and severity of the narrowings and blockage in your coronary arteries. You may need coronary angioplasty or coronary artery bypass surgery.

Once you have been diagnosed and have had a coronary angiogram, your cardiologist will discuss the best treatment for you. It is likely that you will need a combination of medications or, if there are significant narrowings in your coronary arteries, you may be treated with angioplasty or bypass surgery.

MEDICATIONS

There are a number of medications that may be prescribed by your doctor or by your consultant cardiologist. These medications are divided into different groups, according to what they do. Some drugs relieve the symptoms of angina, others thin the blood, some reduce the level of cholesterol in your blood, and others lower blood pressure. You are likely to need a combination of medications depending on your specific heart condition. When discussing your treatment options, ask your doctor about any possible side effects of the medications.

Medication for angina Nitrate pills or sprays are often prescribed for angina. They dilate the coronary arteries to increase the blood flow in the vessels.

Blood-thinning medications Aspirin thins the blood and reduces the risk of clotting in coronary arteries. Aspirin will also be prescribed after a heart attack.

Lipid-lowering medications If being careful about what you eat (see pp172–3) fails to lower your cholesterol levels enough, you may be prescribed cholesterol-reducing medications, known as statins. If your triglycerides are also elevated, this may influence what type of lipid-lowering medications your doctor recommends. Cholesterol-lowering pills are also prescribed routinely for people with coronary artery disease. There has been some debate about whether statins are as beneficial for women as they are for men, but currently women should be receiving the same treatment as men. Several statins are available, including simvastatin, atorvastatin, rosuvastatin, pravastatin, and fluvastatin. Other cholesterol-lowering drugs include ezetimibe, fibrates, and nicotinic acid drugs. Your doctor will decide which of these is the most appropriate option for you.

Blood pressure medications There are a wide range of medications for lowering blood pressure, including angiotensin-converting enzyme (ACE) inhibitors, angiotensin II receptor antagonists, calcium channel blockers, diuretics, beta blockers, and alpha blockers. Often your doctor will prescribe a combination of medication.

CORONARY ANGIOPLASTY AND BYPASS SURGERY

These are standard treatments for patients with CHD. After a coronary angiogram (see p169), your cardiologist will discuss with you the best treatment.

Coronary angioplasty When blockages have been located on a coronary angiogram, they can sometimes be treated with coronary angioplasty, which is done by a cardiologist in a cardiac catheterization laboratory. During the angioplasty, you have a local anesthetic and a catheter is inserted

"When it comes to treatment of coronary heart disease, often a combination of medications is recommended."

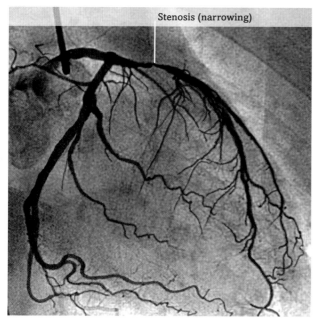

Stenosis (narrowing)

Coronary angiogram
This angiogram of the left coronary system shows a severe stenosis (narrowing) of the left anterior descending artery. This can be treated with coronary angioplasty.

into the heart via an artery in the groin or arm. A very thin wire is passed along the catheter into the coronary artery, and an uninflated balloon is mounted onto the wire. Once the balloon is in place across the narrowed section of artery, it is inflated so that it flattens the fatty material that has caused the narrowing against the wall of the artery. In most cases it is also necessary to use a "stent" (a metal tube) to ensure the artery stays open. The stent is mounted on an uninflated balloon that is passed into the coronary artery, as before. Once in the correct position, the balloon is inflated and the stent expands against the artery wall. The balloon is then deflated and removed, leaving the stent in place.

After coronary angioplasty, you may be able to return home the same day, or you may need to stay in the hospital overnight for observation. You should be able to go back to work about a week later. After the procedure, in addition to continuing to take aspirin, you will also be prescribed clopidogrel, another type of blood-thinning medication. The combination of the two blood-thinning medications helps reduce the risk of clotting in the stent.

Coronary artery bypass surgery
If you have multiple narrowings in your coronary arteries or if the cardiologist decides the narrowings are not appropriate to be treated with coronary angioplasty, you will be referred to a cardiothoracic surgeon for coronary artery bypass surgery. This is done under general anesthetic in the operating room; the operation can take three hours or more.

The surgeon either makes a cut down your breastbone, or may make a smaller incision. Grafts of arteries or veins are taken from the chest, arms, or legs and are sutured (stitched) between the aorta (the main artery in the body) and the coronary arteries, so that the narrowed or blocked areas of the arteries are "bypassed." The number of grafts needed depends upon the number of narrowed or blocked arteries.

After the procedure, you will need to stay in the hospital for seven to ten days. It may take up to three months before you have recovered fully from the surgery and can return to work. After the surgery it is common to feel pain in your chest as well as swelling, discomfort, and pins and needles where the grafts were taken. It is not unusual to feel depressed and emotional in the early weeks after the operation; you may also experience some impairment of your memory. These problems usually improve over the following few months, but you should see your doctor if these symptoms are bothering you.

After both coronary angioplasty and coronary artery bypass surgery, you will need to continue on medication and you will also need to have regular follow-up with your cardiologist. You must also make sure that all your risk factors (see p163) are kept under control to reduce the chance of developing further coronary artery disease. If your anginal symptoms recur, you must seek medical help.

CHD: How can I help myself?

Anyone at risk of CHD (see p163) should take preventive steps to avoid developing it. For women, who typically get CHD later in life when they may have other risk factors, early prevention is key. Fortunately, up to 80 percent of cardiac risk can be reduced with diet and lifestyle changes.

Preventive measures are geared toward preventing the buildup of fatty deposits in your arteries.

WATCH YOUR LIFESTYLE

Follow these simple lifestyle rules for a healthy heart:

Stop smoking Smoking significantly increases your risk of developing CHD (see p163), so stopping is a major step to improving your heart health.

Eat healthily You should make sure you eat a healthy, low-fat diet (see opposite).

Reduce your salt intake Salt raises your blood pressure. You should not eat more than 6 g a day (see p54).

Moderate your alcohol intake A small amount of alcohol is unlikely to cause harm, although you should keep within the recommended weekly allowance. Excessive drinking may increase your risk of CHD (see p163).

Keep fit Keeping active is important in preventing the development of heart disease. This is because exercise helps control your blood pressure and cholesterol and triglyceride levels, helps you maintain a healthy body weight, and reduces stress. If you have diabetes (see pp320–5), a healthy weight helps toward managing your blood sugar levels.

Reduce your stress Learning relaxation techniques can help you to cope with and reduce the harmful effects of long-term stress.

GET CHECKED OUT

In addition to taking steps to improve your lifestyle, it's also important to have your blood pressure and cholesterol and triglyceride levels checked regularly. You can often have high levels of cholesterol and high blood pressure—two major risk factors for developing CHD—yet be symptom-free. Asking your doctor for regular checks can highlight a problem, which can then be treated early.

Lipids Your cholesterol and triglyceride levels can be checked with a simple blood test. If your triglycerides or "bad" cholesterol, or LDL, level (see p163) are high, your doctor will recommend lifestyle changes to lower it (see opposite), and in some cases may suggest medications (see p170).

Blood pressure It's sensible to have your blood pressure checked regularly, at least every year (see pp28–47), and more frequently if you suffer from a condition such as diabetes, have other risk factors for CHD (see p163), or already have heart disease.

Diabetes If you have diabetes (see pp320–5), you are already at an increased risk of developing CHD, so it's even more important to make sure that your diabetes is kept under control and that you take preventive lifestyle measures.

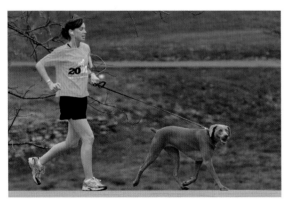

Keeping fit
Being active and building exercise into your weekly routine helps keep your heart healthy. Try to do a 30-minute exercise program at least three times a week.

Foods to eat for a healthy heart

Eating a healthy, low-fat diet, with a minimum of saturated fats (see pp52–5) can help to prevent the buildup of plaque deposits in your coronary arteries. Eating healthily also helps you maintain a healthy weight, which in turn lowers your risk of heart disease as well as of other dangerous conditions such as diabetes.

Soluble fiber

Increases the feeling of fullness, which can help with weight control. RDA of dietary fiber = 30 g

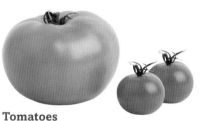

Oats 11 g dietary fiber = 4 oz (100 g)

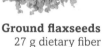

Ground flaxseeds 27 g dietary fiber = 4 oz (100 g)

Oily fish

Provides the heart-healthy omega-3 fatty acids, which may help reduce LDL cholesterol and triglycerides. RDA of essential fatty acids = currently, no amount set

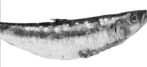

Sardines (canned in oil) 1480 mg (total omega-3 fatty acids) = 4 oz (100 g)

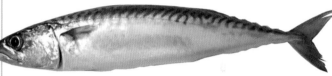

Mackerel (cooked) 1,422 mg (total omega-3 fatty acids) = 4 oz (100 g)

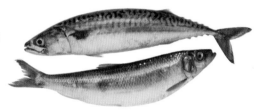

Herring (cooked) 1,729 mg (total omega-3 fatty acids) = 4 oz (100 g)

Antioxidants

Antioxidants (beta-carotene, vitamin C, and vitamin E) may help protect the cardiovascular system from damage. RDA of beta-carotene = none set, vitamin C = 60 mg, vitamin E = 10 mg

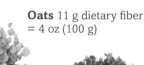

Tomatoes beta-carotene 0.5 mg, Vit C 17 mg, Vit E 1.2 mg = 4 oz (100 g)

Carrots beta-carotene 9 mg, Vit C 5.9 mg, Vit E 1.6 mg = 4 oz (100 g)

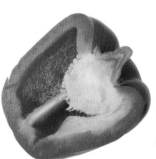

Red peppers beta-carotene 1-2 mg, Vit C 140 mg, Vit E 0.8 mg = 4 oz (100 g)

Magnesium

Important for the function of nerves and muscles. RDA of magnesium = 300mg

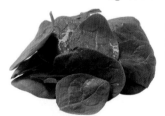

Green vegetables such as spinach (cooked) 34 mg magnesium = 4 oz (100 g)

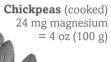

Chickpeas (cooked) 24 mg magnesium = 4 oz (100 g)

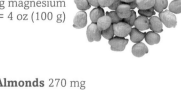

Almonds 270 mg magnesium = 4 oz (100 g)

Valvular heart disease

Your heart valves help control the flow of blood between the four chambers of the heart as well as the blood entering and leaving the heart (see p160). Sometimes a valve can be narrowed or doesn't close fully. Your doctor will be able to hear a heart murmur and you will need to undergo tests.

WHAT IS IT?

Valvular heart disease occurs when there is an abnormality or dysfunction of one or more of the four heart valves. If a valve is narrowed, blood flow will be obstructed. This is known as valve stenosis. If a valve does not close fully, there will be leakage of blood, known as valve regurgitation.

Either problem can be caused by an anatomical abnormality of the valve from birth, as a result of having had rheumatic fever, or simply as part of the aging process.

Valve stenosis or regurgitation can affect the pumping action of the heart. This means that the heart will work less efficiently or may become enlarged, which can result in heart failure.

Endocarditis is a condition that results from infection of heart valves. If the valve is abnormal the risk of endocarditis is greater than in a normal valve.

WHAT NEXT?

It your doctor suspects valvular heart disease, he or she will examine you to check for a heart murmur. You will also need other tests, including an EKG, (see p168), an echocardiogram (see p169), and a chest X-ray.

MY TREATMENT OPTIONS

Patients with mild forms of valvular heart disease may not require any treatment but will need regular follow-up. Some patients require treatment only with

medication, for example diuretics and ACE inhibitors.

Surgery Patients with severe disease and who have symptoms are likely to require surgery, which involves repairing or replacing the existing heart valve using either a metal or a tissue valve. Your cardiologist and surgeon will advise on which is the most appropriate for you. Transcatheter valve procedures are new techniques that are used for treating some valves without the need for open heart surgery. However, they are only available in certain hospitals.

HOW CAN I HELP MYSELF?

If you think you may have the symptoms of valvular heart disease, you should make sure you seek medical help.

VALVULAR HEART DISEASE AND PREGNANCY

Valvular heart disease can get worse during pregnancy, so if you have been diagnosed with this conditon you should consult your doctor if you are planning a pregnancy.

DO I HAVE THE SYMPTOMS?

Symptoms may be minimal, but can include the following:
- Breathlessness
- Chest pain
- Dizzy spells
- Swollen ankles.

See your doctor if you have any of these symptoms.

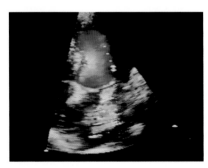

Valve regurgitation
This echocardiogram with Doppler ultrasound (colored area within the triangle) shows a leaking valve (valve regurgitation).

Vascular disease

Varicose veins rarely cause serious complications, but they're at best unsightly, and at worst, uncomfortable. They don't significantly increase your risk of deep vein thrombosis (see pp252–3), but they can cause aching and swollen ankles and can make you more prone to eczema and possible leg ulcers.

Varicose veins

Achy legs are common after you have been standing for a long time, but varicose veins may be to blame.

WHAT ARE THEY?
Varicose veins are enlarged, twisted veins, usually in the leg. Blood runs through superficial veins, then through one-way valves into deeper veins. As the valves become less efficient, blood may flow backward, then pool, enlarging and making the superficial veins visible.

WHAT NEXT?
Your doctor will examine the veins while you are standing. He or she

---

DO I HAVE THE SYMPTOMS?

Visible bulging veins are a clear indication of varicose veins. Other symptoms include:
- Aching or painful legs that continue to ache during rest
- In severe cases, itchy skin and ulceration.

See your doctor if you have symptoms that are painful or concern you.

ANEURYSMS

Aneurysms are rare, occurring where there is a weak area in a blood vessel that balloons out. Most aneurysms are small and symptomless, often going undetected, but the danger is that a larger one may burst, causing a life-threatening hemorrhage. Aneurysms can occur throughout the body but are most common in the aorta, known as an aortic aneurysm. If an aortic aneurysm is found, it will be monitored and surgery may be planned. A burst aortic aneurysm is an emergency; its symptoms include pain or tenderness in the abdomen or chest, a pulselike sensation in the abdomen, and backache.

---

may arrange for a scan to assess the blood flow in the vessels to confirm the diagnosis.

MY TREATMENT OPTIONS
If self-help measures (see below) fail to bring relief, talk to your doctor about the best treatment for you. However, you should be aware that varicose veins can recur after any of the treatments below.
Injections (sclerotherapy) Small veins may be treated with an injection of a chemical, which sticks the vein walls together to stop blood from entering.
Surgery This may be considered for larger varicose veins. Either the vein is tied and cut, or a long vein may be removed, a procedure known as "stripping."

Laser surgery This may be used to treat superficial "thread" veins, but works less well for varicose veins.

HOW CAN I HELP MYSELF?
Several self-help measures may relieve the symptoms.
Compression stockings These help the blood to flow through the veins more efficiently.
Regular exercise This improves your circulation so that blood flows more effectively.
Keeping your weight down This takes pressure off your veins.
Avoiding standing for long periods This can help swelling and aching, as can resting with your legs raised.
Red vine leaf extract This can relieve achy, swollen legs.

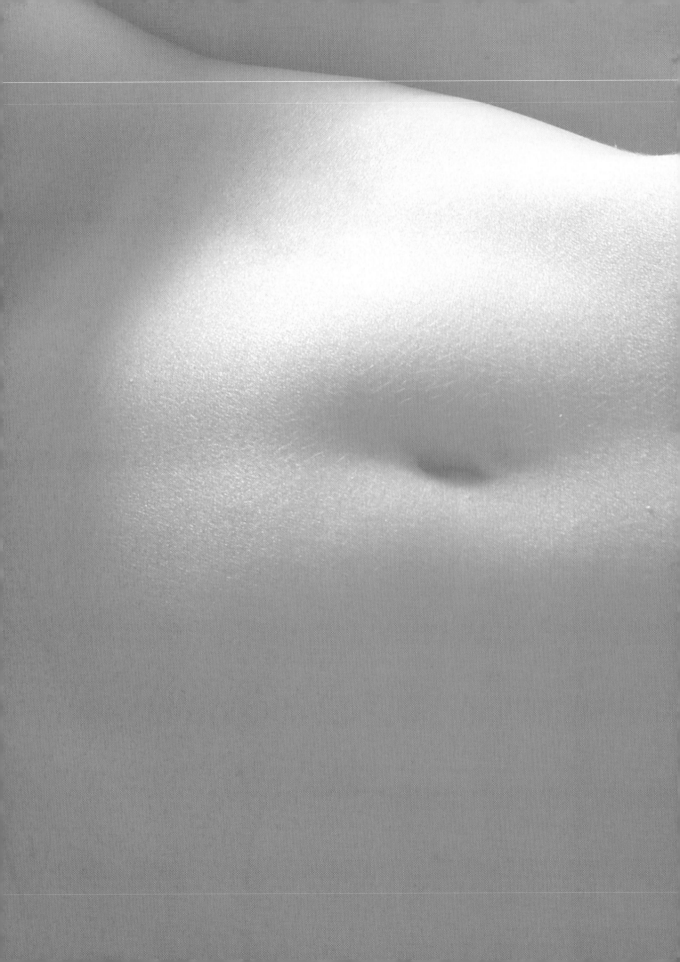

Brain and nerves

Susanna E. Horvath MD FAHA
Division Chief of Neurology, Allen Pavilion
Assistant Clinical Professor of Neurology
Columbia University Medical Center

Your brain and nerves

Your nervous system consists of the central nervous system containing the brain and spinal cord, and the peripheral nervous system—the nerves that link your brain and spinal cord to tissues and organs throughout your body. The complicated network controls everything you do in your daily life. Not only does it keep you functioning and alive, but it also enables you to engage in the complex abstract activities that combine to make you human, such as thought, learning, self-awareness, emotion, and creativity.

THE BRAIN

The adult human brain weighs just over 2¼ lb (1 kg) and is made up of billions of nerve cells called neurons, as well as supporting cells. The largest part of the brain is the cerebrum, which contains gray matter for generating and processing nerve impulses and white matter that transmits nerve impulses. The brain is richly supplied with blood vessels and contains spaces that are filled with cerebrospinal fluid (CSF). This fluid cushions the delicate brain and spinal cord, which are covered by three membranes called meninges.

The areas of the brain perform different functions (see pp18–19). For example, an area called the motor cortex in each cerebral hemisphere controls movement in your

THE STRUCTURE OF THE BRAIN

The side view of the brain shows the cerebral cortex, which is convoluted, the cerebellum, and the brain stem.

A cross section reveals more specialized tissues buried between the two hemispheres (see also pp18–19).

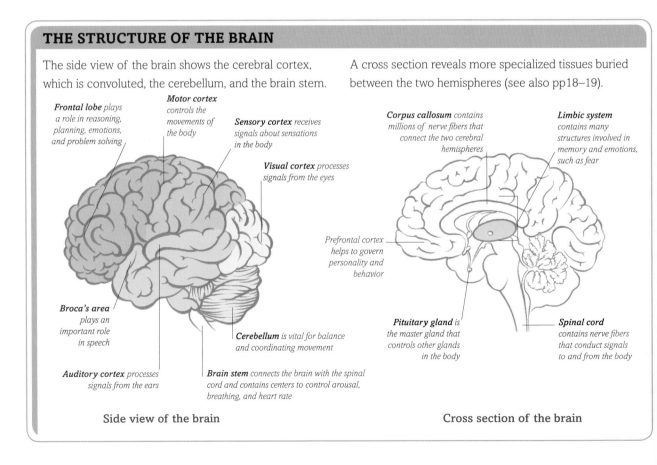

Frontal lobe *plays a role in reasoning, planning, emotions, and problem solving*

Motor cortex *controls the movements of the body*

Sensory cortex *receives signals about sensations in the body*

Visual cortex *processes signals from the eyes*

Broca's area *plays an important role in speech*

Auditory cortex *processes signals from the ears*

Cerebellum *is vital for balance and coordinating movement*

Brain stem *connects the brain with the spinal cord and contains centers to control arousal, breathing, and heart rate*

Corpus callosum *contains millions of nerve fibers that connect the two cerebral hemispheres*

Limbic system *contains many structures involved in memory and emotions, such as fear*

Prefrontal cortex *helps to govern personality and behavior*

Pituitary gland *is the master gland that controls other glands in the body*

Spinal cord *contains nerve fibers that conduct signals to and from the body*

Side view of the brain

Cross section of the brain

> "The brain stem contains nerves important for regulating many basic body functions such as breathing, heart rate, and arousal."

body. The visual cortex at the back of your head processes nervous impulses from your eyes to enable you to see. The location of some other functions—for example, speech—depends on whether you are right- or left-handed.

Scientists have long thought that the brains of men and women were the same. However, it now seems that there are some crucial differences, not only in their structure but also in the way they work (see pp18–19).

NERVE CELLS

Nerve cells are specialized cells that transmit coded electrical signals throughout the brain and the body. They come in all shapes and sizes, but essentially they share similar components (see right). One of the remarkable features of nerve cells is that they can communicate with each other and with other tissues, such as muscles, when their electrical impulses trigger the production of chemicals called neurotransmitters. These chemicals cross tiny gaps called synapses and stimulate impulses in nearby nerve cells. There are a number of different neurotransmitters in the brain and body's nervous systems—for example, serotonin, epinephrine, acetylcholine, and dopamine. Chemical and electrical conduction is fundamental to brain and body function, and many drugs used to treat neurological disorders act by altering these signals.

DISORDERS OF THE NERVOUS SYSTEM

Various symptoms arising from disorders of the brain and nervous systems are very common. They are the cause of between a third and a half of all consultations with family doctors. Common symptoms include:
- Headaches
- Numbness or tingling
- Weakness
- Problems with vision and dizziness.

THE STRUCTURE OF A NERVE CELL

A nerve cell, or neuron, has specialized projections known as nerve fibers, or axons, that carry nerve signals great distances across the body.

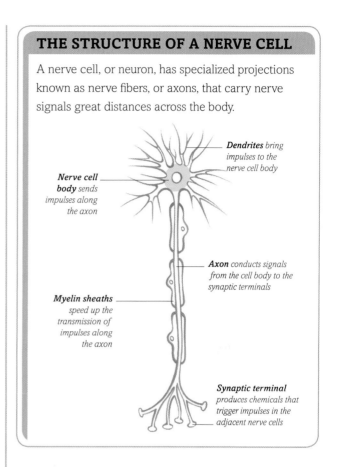

Dendrites bring impulses to the nerve cell body

Nerve cell body sends impulses along the axon

Axon conducts signals from the cell body to the synaptic terminals

Myelin sheaths speed up the transmission of impulses along the axon

Synaptic terminal produces chemicals that trigger impulses in the adjacent nerve cells

Often the symptoms, although distressing, are not due to any serious underlying brain disease.

Careful clinical examination of the head, torso, and limbs can give a great deal of information about the causes of neurological symptoms. Doctors often use computerized tomography (CT) scanning—an X-ray technique that gives cross-sectional images of the brain. Spiral CT scans can yield very detailed images. Magnetic resonance imaging (MRI), a technique that relies on magnetism and radio waves, is particularly useful for looking at the brain and spinal cord. Electrical activity can be measured across the scalp by the technique of electroencephalography (EEG).

Sometimes, a lumbar puncture is needed to take a sample of the cerebrospinal fluid because examination of this fluid is important in the diagnosis of serious disorders, such as meningitis (see p181). Only rarely do doctors take a biopsy from the brain because brain tissue doesn't regenerate.

Headaches

For some women, a headache is one of life's occasional annoyances that may be caused by modern living. For others, though, headaches are regular, unpredictable, and debilitating and interfere with everyday life. Lifestyle changes can often help, and various medications can relieve pain.

Tension-type headaches

About 75 percent of all headaches are tension-type headaches, which last no more than a few hours and which have no serious underlying cause. Nevertheless, if they occur frequently, such headaches can have a detrimental impact on the quality of your daily life.

WHAT IS IT?

No one knows the cause of tension-type headaches. Muscular pain at the back of the neck—for example from poor posture—has been blamed, but there's no evidence to support this. Tension-type headaches may recur, especially if you are depressed or anxious. Women over the age of 20 are most commonly affected.

WHAT NEXT?

See your doctor if the headaches are disrupting your life. You are unlikely to need specific tests.

MY TREATMENT OPTIONS

Your doctor will discuss the best course of action for you.

Analgesics and rest Take simple analgesics, such as acetaminophen or ibuprofen, and lie in a quiet, dark, cool room. Take the recommended dosage but not for more than a few weeks to avoid a medication-induced headache.

Antidepressants Your doctor may prescribe low doses of amitriptyline if the simple analgesics don't work. This antidepressant in low doses

DO I HAVE THE SYMPTOMS?

Tension-type headaches will typically cause:

- A pressing or tightening sensation, usually felt all over the head, that tends to get worse as the day progresses
- Mild or moderately severe pain, but that doesn't force you to stop everyday activities.

See your doctor if you have a severe headache that doesn't respond to self-help measures, or if it is accompanied by other symptoms such as nausea, fever, disturbed vision, or aversion to bright light.

has the alternative and very useful property of preventing chronic pain. Ask about the side effects.

HOW CAN I HELP MYSELF?

It's a good idea to try to identify and deal with any causes of stress. **Get a good night's sleep** to help you cope with stress (see pp60–1). **Try to live your life** on an even keel (see pp50–69). **Relax regularly** (see pp62–3). You may find aromatherapy and acupuncture helpful.

ARE MY HEADACHES SERIOUS?

Not knowing what's causing your headache can be very worrying. The resulting anxiety can, in turn, exacerbate the pain and/or frequency of the headache, which pushes you into a vicious circle. If you're worried about recurrent or severe headaches, make an appointment with your doctor.

A thorough neurological checkup, along with reassurance that nothing is wrong, may be all you need to allay your fears. You might find the headaches start to subside after your visit. In very rare cases, if the examination is inconclusive, your doctor may arrange for further tests, such as a CT or MRI scan.

Meningitis

Rarely, a severe headache may be a symptom of a serious underlying problem. If it's accompanied by fever and a stiff neck, the possibility of meningitis must be considered.

WHAT IS IT?

Meningitis is inflammation of the meninges (the coverings of the brain and spinal cord). It is usually caused by bacteria or viruses.

Bacterial meningitis is a life-threatening disease, but it can be treated successfully if caught early. One type—meningococcal meningitis—may cause a characteristic rash due to bleeding under the skin, which often doesn't appear until the infection has taken hold.

Viral meningitis has milder symptoms, and can sometimes be treated with antiviral agents.

WHAT NEXT?

It's vital that you seek immediate medical help if you suspect you have meningitis because this condition is potentially life threatening if treatment is delayed. In young children, the symptoms may not be as clear-cut as in an adult.

MY TREATMENT OPTIONS

If your doctor suspects bacterial meningitis, you should immediately be given intravenous antibiotics. The infection is confirmed by a lumbar puncture and examination of the cerebrospinal fluid that's taken from the spine. You may be given a different antibiotic drug that fights the particular organism revealed. Ask your doctor about any side effects.

Vaccinations are usually available and these can provide you with lifelong protection against some forms of the disease.

DO I HAVE THE SYMPTOMS?

Meningitis is characterized by a severe headache, along with one or more of the following:
- Photophobia (intolerance of bright light)
- Neck stiffness (inability to bend your head down so your chin touches your chest)
- Fever
- Nausea and vomiting.

See your doctor if your headache is accompanied by any of these symptoms, particularly if they come on suddenly.

HOW CAN I HELP MYSELF?

Recovery from meningitis can take a while, so get plenty of rest, don't rush back to work, and make sure you have lots of support.

Brain tumor

Uncommonly, a headache is a result of a brain tumor. Symptoms vary according to the area of the brain affected, the type of tumor, and its speed of growth.

WHAT IS IT?

Benign (noninvasive) tumors usually grow slowly and can cause problems when their increasing size begins to press on healthy brain tissue. Most malignant (invasive) tumors are secondary—they've spread from a primary cancer elsewhere in the body, often from the lungs, breast, or bowel.

WHAT NEXT?

A CT or MRI scan, as well as various neurological tests, will usually confirm a diagnosis.

MY TREATMENT OPTIONS

Benign tumors can often be removed by surgery, but malignant tumors may require chemotherapy or radiation therapy, depending on the size and stage of the tumor. Ask your doctor about the side effects.

HOW CAN I HELP MYSELF?

After treatment, make sure you have regular checkups and follow-up scans.

DO I HAVE THE SYMPTOMS?

Many of the following symptoms are the result of raised pressure within the skull caused by the brain tumor.
- A headache that tends to be worse when you wake up
- Nausea and vomiting
- Impaired vision or hearing
- Numbness and weakness
- Problems with balance
- Seizures.

See your doctor if you have any of the above symptoms.

Migraines

Migraines are more severe than tension-type headaches (see p180) and can be horribly debilitating. As many as one in five women suffer from them and they are most common between the ages of 25 and 55. But the good news is that migraines become less troublesome after menopause.

WHAT IS IT?

A migraine is an unusually severe headache that is often accompanied by extra symptoms, such as nausea or visual disturbances (see below). No one knows the exact cause of migraines, although some people can identify trigger factors that provoke them (see opposite).

Two main theories describe what happens in the brain as a migraine develops. In the neural theory, a wave of electrical activity starts deep in the brain and spreads over its outer layer.

In the vascular theory, chemicals from the brain stem trigger spasms in the brain's blood vessels, giving rise to an aura (see box, below). Pain comes when the walls of the blood vessels relax. Elements of both theories are probably involved.

WHAT NEXT?

Your doctor will normally diagnose a migraine from your description of the symptoms and may prescribe medicines to prevent and treat your migraines. Ask your doctor about any possible side effects when discussing your treatment options.

MY TREATMENT OPTIONS

Medications are divided into those for prevention and those that treat a migraine once it has started.

Prevention If you can't avoid identified triggers, and if you're experiencing more than a few migraines per month, you may be prescribed medicine to take daily to reduce the frequency of episodes.

- Preventive drugs include beta-blockers, antiepileptics (such as topiramate or sodium valproate), and low doses of amitriptyline. You may have to try several drugs to find the one that's right for you.
- Most women with migraines have them more often during the few days before, or during, their period. This is known as a menstrual migraine. Fewer than 10 percent have migraines solely related to periods. Medication taken during the premenstrual period can help relieve menstrual migraines if your periods are regular. Effective drugs are naproxen, estrogen supplements (some women experience rebound headaches a few days after stopping these), and some of the new triptan drugs, taken for up to five days.

Treatment Various medicines can help treat migraines. You can buy some over the counter, but for others you'll need a prescription.

- Over-the-counter analgesics, such as aspirin or ibuprofen, need to be taken as soon as aura (see box, left) develops
- Nausea medication, such as metoclopramide, combats the nausea. (Some over-the-counter drugs combine analgesics and nausea agents in one pill.)
- Migraine medications, such as the triptan group, are available by prescription as tablets, nasal inhalers, or injections. There are strict limits on how many you can take within a few days since

---

DO I HAVE THE SYMPTOMS?

You may not have all of these symptoms since they vary widely between people.

- A severe, throbbing pain almost always on one side of the head, often behind the eye
- Nausea or vomiting
- Very sensitive to light and noise
- Less commonly, you may have slurred speech, difficulty in finding words, or limb weakness
- 60 percent of people who have migraines experience an

"aura"—from a few minutes to half an hour—before the onset of pain. This may include visual disturbances such as seeing flashing or zigzagging lights, or loss of some of your field of vision. Less commonly, aura involves tingling or numbness, often in one of your hands or around the mouth. A migraine episode may last from a few hours to as long as a few days.

See your doctor if the pain persists and causes you distress.

---

they can have serious side effects, particularly on the heart

- Low-dose oral contraceptives are reported to lessen symptoms in 50 percent of women with menstrual migraines
- Strong opiates may be prescribed if the pain is severe enough to warrant hospital admission.

HOW CAN I HELP MYSELF?
Keep a diary, and you may find out what triggers your migraines. The following advice may help you steer clear of the common triggers.

Avoid excessive stress, such as emotional or work-related stress.

Choose oral contraception carefully. If you have migraines with an aura, avoid the combined oral contraceptive pill, since it has an increased risk of strokes. If you have migraines after starting the combined pill, use a progesterone-only pill or a different method.

Be healthy in your habits. Eat and sleep regularly. Fatigue, lack of sleep, excess exercise, alcohol, and smoke are all known triggers (see Chapter 3, pp50–69.)

Avoid bright or glaring lights, and flashing lights such as strobes. Be aware that even sunlight flickering through trees as you drive by can trigger a migraine (see common types of triggers below).

Foods that may trigger migraines

If you suspect a food is triggering migraine, keep a diary of what you eat and drink. Try to figure out what your particular migraine triggers are and avoid them. Some of the most common foods associated with migraines are shown below. Remember, too, that poor dietary habits, such as skipping meals or dehydration, may also trigger or exacerbate migraines.

Alcoholic drinks

Common triggers include red wine, beer, whisky, champagne

Aged cheese

Common triggers include stilton, camembert, emmental, gruyère, roquefort, gorgonzola, aged cheddar

Chocolate

Common triggers include plain and milk chocolate

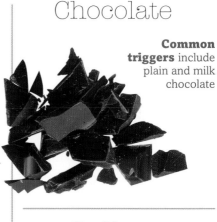

Cured meats

Common triggers include salami, pepperoni, bacon, ham

Fruits: over ripe and dried

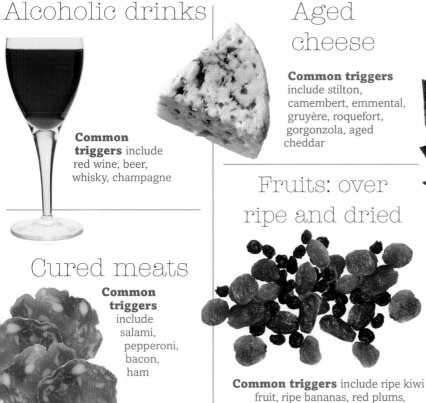

Common triggers include ripe kiwi fruit, ripe bananas, red plums, sultanas, dried apricots

Caffeine

Common triggers include coffee, tea, cola

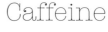
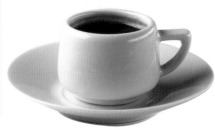

Alzheimer's disease

This degenerative brain disease is not an inevitable consequence of aging. Although the risk of developing the condition—characterized by increasing dementia, including impaired memory and personality changes—increases with age, 9 out of 10 of those over 80 have no symptoms of the disease.

WHAT IS IT?

Alzheimer's disease is a chronic, degenerative condition of the brain cells. It's now the third most common cause of death in the developed world, with more women than men affected.

The first symptom is often an impaired memory for recent events, which can be difficult to distinguish from the normal age-related decline in memory. Often people will tell old stories repeatedly, recalling the story, but not that they have told it already. There may be subtle changes in personality. Someone who was formerly careful with money may spend extravagantly. Previously outgoing people may become quiet and withdrawn.

As the disease progresses, forgetfulness may affect routine activities such as cooking and household chores. Those affected may be aware of their memory difficulties and try to deal with the problem—for example, by writing notes, or by letting someone else manage decisions for them. Sometimes anxiety and frustration over their failing memory results in aggression. Self-neglect is common; sufferers may become uncharacteristically unkempt.

In the late stages of the disease, the changes in memory and behavior are marked. People affected cannot compensate for their memory lapses and become confused. They may not recognize family and friends. They may repeat meaningless words or phrases and perform repetitive behaviors. Paranoid behavior (such as jealousy or accusations of theft) is common. Sufferers may develop false beliefs and visual hallucinations.

In the final stages of the disease, people with this condition cease to recognize even their close family. They commonly lose all speech, although they retain the ability to shout or groan. People in the advanced stages of Alzheimer's disease may refuse to eat, develop unsteadiness, and increasingly lose weight. They eventually become bed-bound. Death often occurs from complications of immobility such as pneumonia and bedsores..

Age is the main risk factor, but it is important to remember that many very elderly people have no hint of Alzheimer's disease. The condition can run in families, which suggests that genetic factors are involved. Sometimes the disease has an early onset (before the age of 65). Early-onset Alzheimer's disease principally

DO I HAVE THE SYMPTOMS?

Many people suffer from increasing absentmindedness as they get older, but this isn't necessarily an early sign of Alzheimer's disease.

See your doctor if your forgetfulness is becoming severe enough to interfere with your ability to live a normal life, or if people who know you well have noticed personality changes or unusual behaviors.

AM I AT RISK?

There are risk factors, some of which can be avoided, but others, such as sex, age, and family factors, are inevitable:

- Being female—the disease is more common in women
- Increasing age—more common over the age of 65
- Genetic factors—the disease sometimes runs in families
- Having diabetes
- Having high blood pressure
- Smoking or drinking alcohol.

> ## "Many people reach a great age without developing Alzheimer's disease."

occurs in families in which the condition is unusually common. Defects in specific genes have been found on genetic testing in some of these families.

There is another, more common genetic influence; recent research has identified the ApoE gene on chromosome 19. Having a particular variant of this gene is a risk factor, but doesn't mean that you'll definitely develop the disease. Only one-quarter of Alzheimer's sufferers have a family history of the disease.

WHAT NEXT?

If you have memory problems, your doctor will start by looking for a treatable cause. These include:

- Vitamin B$_{12}$ deficiency
- Anemia
- Depression
- Sleep disorders
- Medicinal side effects
- Seizures
- Underactive thyroid gland
- Some types of raised pressure in the brain (raised intracranial pressure)—for example, the condition known as normal pressure hydrocephalus
- Certain types of brain hemorrhage. One example is an extradural haemorrhage in which there is bleeding between the membranes covering the brain and the skull. This can occur in elderly people following fairly minor head injuries—for example, after a fall.

Your doctor will examine your physical condition and check your neurological responses. He or she will also test your memory and cognition—for example, by asking you to recall certain names, dates, and number sequences. These tests may not pick up early-stage disease, but the scores are always abnormal in the later stages. You may have a brain scan to see if there's any atrophy (shrinking) of your brain tissue.

MY TREATMENT OPTIONS

As yet there's no effective treatment for slowing, let alone halting, the progression of Alzheimer's disease. Some evidence suggests that people with Alzheimer's have a reduced level of the acetylcholine in their brain. Drugs such as donepezil and rivastigmine may be prescribed to inhibit the chemical's breakdown and so raise its level. Some medications have an effect even in moderate to severe cases. Ask about the side effects if your doctor prescribes them for you.

HOW CAN I HELP MYSELF?

The following measures combined with regular sleep and exercise may help you to maintain good brain health and prevent or delay the onset of Alzheimer's disease:

Stay active The disease is less common in those who are mentally and physically active—doing a crossword or Sudoku each day may help reduce the risk. Socially active people also appear to have a reduced risk.

Maintain a healthy lifestyle Stay fit, don't smoke, and eat a balanced diet. Keep your blood pressure under control and blood levels of sugar and lipids low.

Consider hormone replacement therapy (HRT) Trials suggest that HRT may lower the risk of Alzheimer's, but because it raises the risk of certain cancers it isn't generally prescribed.

EFFECTS ON THE BRAIN TISSUE

The normal brain is scattered with areas of high activity (red and yellow). The Alzheimer's brain shows dark areas of no activity with reduced fully active areas.

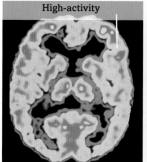

High-activity

Normal brain

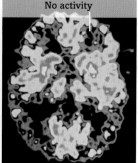

No activity

Alzheimer's brain

Ear disorders

Your ears are responsible for the two senses of hearing and balance. They detect sounds so you can hear what's happening around you, and they help you keep your balance so you can move and stand still without falling over. Ear disorders affect hearing and balance, and can be very disorientating.

Otitis externa

Otitis externa is a common ear condition that can affect anyone. Women are marginally more prone to it than men.

WHAT IS IT?

Otitis externa is an inflammation of the canal that links the external ear (pinna) with the eardrum. It is usually the result of a bacterial, viral, or fungal infection.

The inflammation commonly develops after swimming, which is why the condition is sometimes known as "swimmer's ear." In fact, whenever an ear canal remains wet—for instance, in a hot and humid climate—the moisture increases the likelihood of infection. People who wear a hearing aid or earplugs are also more likely to develop otitis externa. Sometimes, the condition develops after you use eardrops or as a reaction to a chemical in hair dyes.

DO I HAVE THE SYMPTOMS?

You may have otitis externa if one or both your ears are:
● Itchy or even painful
● Producing pus.
See your doctor if you have these symptoms.

WHAT NEXT?

If the condition causes a discharge of pus that blocks an ear canal, don't try to remove it—see your doctor, who will examine your ears with a magnifying instrument called an otoscope. A sample of pus may be taken to find out what kind of organism is causing the infection.

MY TREATMENT OPTIONS

If bacteria are causing the infection, your doctor will probably prescribe antibiotic eardrops. If the infection is severe, you may need an oral antibiotic. Fungal infections are treated with antifungal eardrops, while viral infections are only treated with analgesics.

HOW CAN I HELP MYSELF?

If the ear is inflamed but without pus, you may only need analgesics to ease the pain. Scratching the ear canal can also lead to otitis externa, so be careful when you clean your ears with a cotton swab or put a fingernail inside your ear.

CROSS SECTION OF THE EAR

Most of the functional parts of both ears are hidden within the skull. These delicate and sensitive structures are well protected here, leaving the outer ear to funnel the sound waves to the eardrum.

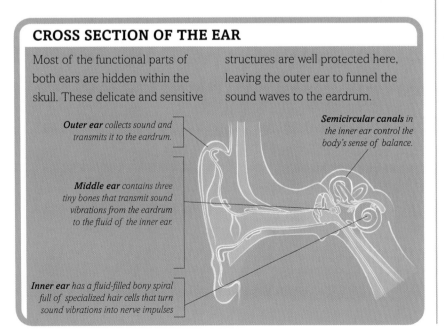

Outer ear collects sound and transmits it to the eardrum.

Semicircular canals in the inner ear control the body's sense of balance.

Middle ear contains three tiny bones that transmit sound vibrations from the eardrum to the fluid of the inner ear.

Inner ear has a fluid-filled bony spiral full of specialized hair cells that turn sound vibrations into nerve impulses

Otitis media

Otitis media affects the air-filled space of the middle part of the ear where the body's three smallest bones—the malleus, incus, and stapes—conduct sounds from the eardrum to the inner ear. The condition is more common among children because their eustachian tubes are narrower, but adults can also develop it.

WHAT IS IT?

Otitis media is an inflammation of the tissues lining the middle ear. It is caused by a viral infection, such as influenza or more particularly the common cold (see p232). It may also be due to a bacterial infection that spreads up the eustachian tube from the throat (see p236).

The condition can bring on a sudden, severe earache that may be accompanied by a fever. As pus and fluid collect around the bones of the middle ear, you may feel a "fullness" in that ear. This may make hearing difficult and can even lead to you experiencing tinnitus (see p188).

Sometimes, the infection causes the eardrum to burst, and a little blood may appear as a discharge. This sounds alarming, but in fact the pain will gradually disappear and the eardrum will heal.

WHAT NEXT?

If your earache is severe, see your doctor immediately. He or she will examine both your ears with a special magnifying instrument called an otoscope. This will help

> ### DO I HAVE THE SYMPTOMS?
>
> You may have otitis media if one or both your ears:
> - Suddenly starts to ache. You may develop a fever
> - Feels "full" and makes hearing difficult.
> **See your doctor** if you have these symptoms.

determine if your eardrum is inflamed or if any pus is leaking from the middle ear into the ear canal.

MY TREATMENT OPTIONS

Your doctor will probably prescribe analgesics to relieve the discomfort. If the infection is caused by a bacterium, you may need to take an oral antibiotic, too. The pain should go away in a matter of days but your hearing may remain affected for a couple of weeks.

HOW CAN I HELP MYSELF?

You can get some relief from the earache by holding something warm, such as a hot-water bottle wrapped in a towel, against the affected ear. Acetaminophen or ibuprofen may help, too.

"Glue ear"

When otitis media (see left) persists or keeps returning, the condition is said to become chronic. "Glue ear" is a form of chronic otitis media. It is common in children under eight but may persist into adulthood.

WHAT IS IT?

In "glue ear" the space inside the middle ear fills with fluid that is thick and sticky, with a gluelike consistency. Inevitably, it causes loss of hearing because the bones of the middle ear can no longer conduct sound from the eardrum to the inner ear.

WHAT NEXT?

You may find that the condition gets better on its own. However, if it doesn't, consult your doctor who will make a diagnosis.

MY TREATMENT OPTIONS

If you need treatment, your doctor may prescribe decongestants to clear your nasal passages, steroids, or antihistamines. If the fluid in your middle ear becomes infected with bacteria, your doctor may prescribe antibiotics.

HOW CAN I HELP MYSELF?

Make sure you take the medications that your doctor prescribes for you. If you need to take antibiotics, make sure you finish the course. Stop smoking if you are a smoker.

> ### DO I HAVE THE SYMPTOMS?
>
> You may have "glue ear" if:
> - You have persistent problems with hearing, especially after colds or ear infections
> - You are a smoker.
> **See your doctor** if you have these symptoms.

Hearing loss

This common symptom may be temporary or permanent. It is likely that your partner or children will notice it before you do yourself.

WHAT IS IT?

Hearing loss may have a number of different causes. These include viral infections (such as mumps or measles), inflammation, excessive prolonged noise (such as rock concerts), a head injury, damage to the blood supply of the inner ear, and certain medication side effects. It may also run in your family.

There are two general types of hearing loss:

Conductive hearing loss is usually temporary and is often caused by otitis media (see p187), a wax blockage of the ear canal, or a ruptured eardrum.

Sensorineural hearing loss is often permanent, resulting from age, noise-related damage to the sensitive hair cells of the inner ear, or brain diseases that affect the auditory nerve pathways.

WHAT NEXT?

If you suddenly lose your hearing, you should seek medical attention immediately because it may be an emergency. Consult your doctor if your hearing loss affects one ear only and is progressive because, although it is rare, it may indicate a brain tumor (see p181).

MY TREATMENT OPTIONS

Hearing loss will probably subside once the underlying cause is treated. However, reduced hearing is very common as we age. If it is caused by old age or family history, your doctor will send you to a specialist to advise you on hearing aids or therapy.

HOW CAN I HELP MYSELF?

Avoid loud noises and use earplugs if needed at work. Many people benefit from a hearing aid (see box).

AM I AT RISK?

You may be at risk of losing your hearing permanently if you are:
- Over 70 years of age
- Often exposed to loud noises
- Suffering from Ménière's disease (see p192) or a neurological disorder such as a brain tumor.

HEARING AIDS

If you have problems hearing, ask your doctor for a hearing test. The results may mean that you need a hearing aid. There are many high-quality, digital, cosmetically acceptable hearing aids to choose from, so it is important to find one that suits you, is easy to use, and improves your hearing. If you have tinnitus you could try a masker, a small electronic device that fits in the ear and produces "white noise" that masks the continuous whistling and ringing sounds of tinnitus.

Tinnitus

An incessant ringing or pulsing noise in the ears can disturb sleep patterns and become a problem. This is tinnitus, a common disorder that affects one in three people.

WHAT IS IT?

Tinnitus is caused by damage to the hair cells in the inner ear. It may be a side effect of anemia (see pp248–9) or of certain drugs, including aspirin.

WHAT NEXT?

See your doctor if you hear noises in your ears that are causing you trouble and distress.

MY TREATMENT OPTIONS

Your doctor may prescribe sedatives or anticonvulsant drugs, such as carbamazepine.

HOW CAN I HELP MYSELF?

Try a tinnitus masker (see box, below). If your tinnitus doesn't respond to drugs, a psychological technique called tinnitus-retraining therapy can alter your response to the increased sensitivity of your hearing (auditory) pathways.

DO I HAVE THE SYMPTOMS?

You may have tinnitus if you experience the following:
- Ringing, whistling, roaring, or buzzing noises in your ears.

See your doctor if you have these symptoms.

Eye conditions

The eye is one of the most highly specialized organs of the body. Its delicate structures are vulnerable to injury, infection, and allergies. Don't delay getting medical help if you have eye symptoms, and seek immediate medical advice if you suddenly experience impaired vision in one or both eyes.

THE STRUCTURE OF THE EYE

The retina layer on the inside of the eyeball contains specialized cells (rods and cones) that convert light signals into electrical impulses.

These electrical signals travel via the optic nerves to the occipital cortex at the back of the brain where they are interpreted.

Vitreous gel, a jellylike substance that fills the main part of the eyeball

Fovea forms the most sensitive part of the retina

Optic nerve transmits signals from the retina to the brain

Choroid layer brings nutrients to the eye

Iris

Cornea helps to focus light rays

Pupil lets light into the eye

Iris controls the diameter of the pupil

Lens focuses light rays on the retina

Macula provides detailed vision

Retina consists of a layer of light-sensitive cells

CROSS SECTION OF EYE

DO I HAVE THE SYMPTOMS?

You probably have a vision disorder if you are having:
- Difficulty distinguishing objects that are either near or far.

See your optometrist if you have these symptoms.

the retina so images appear to be blurred. If you have nearsightedness the opposite is true—you cannot clearly see objects that are in the distance. Images are also blurred, but this is because the cornea and lens focuses the light rays in front of the retina.

WHAT NEXT?

If you have a problem with your eyesight, see an optometrist and ask for an eye test. The problem will probably get worse, so don't delay.

MY TREATMENT OPTIONS

Far- and nearsightedness can be easily corrected with glasses, contact lenses, or, sometimes, laser surgery.

HOW CAN I HELP MYSELF?

Make sure your vision is tested every two years.

Vision disorders

Farsightedness (hypermetropia) and nearsightedness (myopia) are very common vision disorders. Most of us will have some kind of visual problem in our lives. The older you get, the more likely you are to become farsighted, so it's perfectly normal to find that, in your 40s or 50s, threading a needle or reading the newspaper becomes more difficult. Sometimes one eye is more affected than the other.

WHAT IS IT?

If you have farsightedness you are unable to see clearly objects that are close to you. The cornea and lens focus the rays of light behind

Conjunctivitis

This common inflammation, known as "pink eye," affects the conjunctiva, which cover the whites of the eyes and the inside linings of the eyelids.

WHAT IS IT?

Conjunctivitis may be caused by a virus or a bacterium, in which case it is highly contagious. It can also be an allergic reaction to pollen or dust, and may be triggered by ultraviolet light, smoke, or pollution.

WHAT NEXT?

See your doctor who may take a swab from the lid of your affected eye to test for infection.

MY TREATMENT OPTIONS

Bacterial conjunctivitis is usually treated with antibiotic eyedrops or ointment. Viral conjunctivitis can't usually be treated, but should clear up in a couple of weeks.

HOW CAN I HELP MYSELF?

Bathe the affected eye with artificial tears, which you can buy. Wash your hands after touching the eye, and don't share towels or washcloths.

DO I HAVE THE SYMPTOMS?

You may have conjunctivitis if your eyes are:
- Red, itchy, and watery
- Producing a discharge.

See your doctor if you have these symptoms.

Cataracts

Nearly everyone over 65 will be affected by cataracts in their eyes at some time, but they can easily be rectified. Usually, one eye is more affected than the other.

WHAT IS IT?

Cataracts occur when the normally clear lens of one or both your eyes becomes opaque and slightly cloudy. This causes reduced vision, which usually comes on gradually and painlessly over months or years. Bright lights and sunlight may trouble you, and your color vision may be less than perfect. Cataracts are also more likely if you are diabetic, have low calcium levels, or are taking steroids.

WHAT NEXT?

Consult your doctor for advice if you develop a cataract. He or she will look at your eyes with a slit lamp and an ophthalmoscope.

MY TREATMENT OPTIONS

If your cataract affects your daily life, your doctor may recommend surgery to replace your defective lens with a plastic implant. After a short operation under a local anesthetic, your sight will be blurred for a few days but should improve greatly afterward. You may still need glasses to read.

HOW CAN I HELP MYSELF?

If you have a cataract in one or both eyes, make sure your glasses are correctly prescribed and that you read in good light.

DO I HAVE THE SYMPTOMS?

You may have a cataract if:
- Your sight is blurred
- Objects look yellow or reddish
- The pupil of an eye is cloudy

See your doctor if you have these symptoms.

EYE PROBLEMS THAT ARE MEDICAL EMERGENCIES

Some conditions affecting the eye can cause permanent damage to your eyesight—even blindness. Many of these can be treated successfully as long as you seek treatment early. If you have any of the following symptoms, you must see a doctor immediately:
- Seeing flashing lights
- Double vision
- Redness of the eye accompanied by severe pain
- Painful red eye if you have shingles affecting your face
- Sudden loss of vision or deterioration in your vision
- Loss of vision in one part of your visual fields.

Although not emergencies, conditions that mainly affect other parts of the body, such as diabetes (see pp320–5) and an overactive thyroid gland (see pp328–9), may also cause eye problems.

Glaucoma

Glaucoma is a potentially serious condition that can cause blindness. Although much less common than cataracts, glaucoma is more common in women than men and may also run in the family.

WHAT IS IT?

Glaucoma is due to abnormally high pressure of the fluid inside the eye. This pressure occurs when the fluid is prevented from draining away. It can permanently damage the retina and the optic nerve. It's age related: it is rare under the age of 40, but if you're over 80, you have a 1 in 10 chance of developing it.

In acute glaucoma, the symptoms will occur suddenly and you may also feel quite unwell. In chronic glaucoma, the pressure rises slowly and the symptoms appear later on.

WHAT NEXT?

See your doctor immediately if you think you have glaucoma symptoms. They will measure the pressure in both your eyes and, if necessary, will recommend immediate treatment.

DO I HAVE THE SYMPTOMS?

You may have acute glaucoma if you suddenly experience:
- Pain in the affected eye
- Aversion to light
- Loss of vision.

See your doctor or optician if you have these symptoms.

MY TREATMENT OPTIONS

If you have acute glaucoma, you'll be given eyedrops and medication to relieve the eye pressure, followed by surgery or laser treatment to encourage drainage of the fluid. Your sight may be saved if you are treated quickly. If you have chronic glaucoma, you'll be given eyedrops to use regularly to reduce fluid production. If needed, surgery or laser therapy is usually successful.

HOW CAN I HELP MYSELF?

Make sure you have regular eye tests, particularly if you have a close relative who has glaucoma.

Macular degeneration

Macular degeneration is the progressive deterioration of vision, usually in both eyes. It's age related, affects women more than men, and may run in the family.

WHAT IS IT?

Your vision is best at the macula, a yellowish spot in the retina near the optic nerve. In macular degeneration the cells supporting the macula are damaged, causing its light-sensitive cells to die.

In "dry" macular degeneration, which is the most common form of the disease, the loss of cells is patchy and very gradual. In the "wet" form of macular degeneration, blood vessels grow over the macula, which quickly causes a major loss of central vision.

WHAT NEXT?

Your doctor will look at your retina with an ophthalmoscope. If the wet form is suspected, an ophthalmologist may use fluorescein angiography to assess the blood vessels in your retina.

MY TREATMENT OPTIONS

No treatment can effectively restore your sight if you have the dry form of macular degeneration. The wet form can be treated with laser therapy to obliterate the new blood vessels. These vessels tend to grow again, so monitoring and repeated therapy may be needed. Keyhole surgery relocates the macula to a healthy area of supporting cells nearby. Drug therapy with antibodies, ranibizumab or bevacizumab, is also used.

HOW CAN I HELP MYSELF?

Preventative measures include reading in good light, use of magnifying glasses and other low-powered visual aids, and beta carotene, zinc oxide, and vitamins C and E. For the wet form, a diet rich in lutein and fish has shown benefits.

DO I HAVE THE SYMPTOMS?

You may have developed macular degeneration if you experience:
- Blurring or loss of the central portion of your vision
- Distorted vision that makes objects look bigger or smaller.

See your doctor if you have these symptoms.

Dizzy spells and falls

Dizziness usually passes quickly, but if you aren't careful, it can make you fall over unexpectedly, which can be dangerous and cause injury. It's common to feel dizzy or off balance if you change positions suddenly: this can happen, for example, if you stand up too quickly after bending over.

Dizziness

Dizziness is the feeling of being off balance and light-headed, as if you're about to faint.

WHAT IS IT?

Dizziness has many causes. Some are:
- Low blood sugar
- A disorder that causes low blood pressure, such as severe bleeding or overmedication with drugs for high blood pressure
- Episodes of very slow heart rate, known as "vasovagal attacks"
- Disease of the blood vessels in the neck
- Neurological diseases such as Parkinson's disease (see p197) and epilepsy (see pp194–5)
- Side effects of medications
- Excessive heat, or anything that causes blood vessels to dilate
- Panic attacks and hyperventilation.

DO I HAVE THE SYMPTOMS?

You may be suffering from dizziness if you feel:
- Off balance and light-headed
- Sweaty and pale.

See your doctor if you have the above symptoms.

WHAT NEXT?

Your doctor will diagnose the problem, recommend tests, and review your medications.

MY TREATMENT OPTIONS

Treatments depend on the cause. For example, low blood pressure may require elastic stockings and a drug such as fludrocortisone. Ask your doctor about side effects.

HOW CAN I HELP MYSELF?

Some simple self-help measures include the following:

Eat regular, balanced meals to combat bouts of low blood sugar (see also pp52–7, 325).

If you're elderly, hold on to something solid when you stand up from a chair. Use a sturdy cane when you're out and about.

Vertigo

Vertigo is the feeling that you or your surroundings are spinning.

WHAT IS IT?

Vertigo occurs when the brain fails to coordinate sensory information from your ears, eyes, and joints. It is often accompanied by nausea and vomiting. Vertigo can be caused by ear disease, Ménières disease (see box, below), migraines (see pp182–3), multiple sclerosis (see p198), head injury, viral infection, diabetes (see pp320–5), and strokes (see p196).

WHAT NEXT?

Your doctor will recommend tests to help with diagnosis.

MY TREATMENT OPTIONS

Your doctor will try to find and treat the cause. Meclizine may be prescribed. Ask about side effects. Physical therapy can help.

HOW CAN I HELP MYSELF

If you have an attack of vertigo, lie still and avoid sudden movements.

DO I HAVE THE SYMPTOMS?

Attacks of Ménières disease are sudden, and last minutes or days.
- Sudden dizziness and loss of balance
- Nausea and vomiting
- Jerky eye movements
- Buzzing or ringing in the ear
- Loss of hearing
- Pressure or pain in the ear.

See your doctor if you have any of the above symptoms.

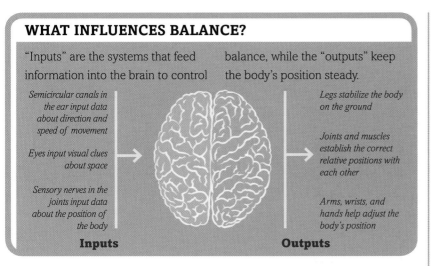

"Inputs" are the systems that feed information into the brain to control balance, while the "outputs" keep the body's position steady.

Semicircular canals in the ear input data about direction and speed of movement

Eyes input visual clues about space

Sensory nerves in the joints input data about the position of the body

Inputs

Legs stabilize the body on the ground

Joints and muscles establish the correct relative positions with each other

Arms, wrists, and hands help adjust the body's position

Outputs

DO I HAVE THE SYMPTOMS?

These symptoms of vestibular neuritis may be mild or severe:
- Vertigo, which may range from a subtle dizziness to a violent spinning sensation
- Nausea and vomiting
- Unsteadiness and imbalance
- Vision impairment
- Impaired concentration
- Inability to sit, stand, or walk.

See your doctor if you have any of the above symptoms.

Falls

Dizziness sometimes makes us fall, although of course not all falls are preceded by dizziness. The elderly are particularly vulnerable.

WHAT IS IT?

You might develop a tendency to have falls because you have:
- Dizziness or vertigo (see opposite)
- Faintness
- A lack of coordination; arthritis
- Weakness affecting a leg or ankle, or in the muscles, nerves, brain, or spinal cord
- Sensory nerve problems, such as numbness or tingling in the feet
- Poor vision
- Intoxication with drugs or alcohol.

WHAT NEXT?

Talk with your doctor if you are worried that you are prone to falls.

MY TREATMENT OPTIONS

Treatment is aimed at addressing the root cause of the problem.

HOW CAN I HELP MYSELF?

Improve your home lighting and turn lights on at night when going to the bathroom. Remove slippery mats and electrical cords from underfoot, fix uneven floors, wear sensible shoes, and use a cane. If you wear glasses check your prescription.

Vestibular neuritis and labyrinthitis

These are two disorders of the vestibulocochlear nerve, which connects the inner ear to the brain.

WHAT IS IT?

Vestibular neuritis and labyrinthitis result from infections that inflame the vestibulocochlear nerve. Symptoms of labyrinthitis are similar to vestibular neuritis, but may include tinnitus and/or hearing loss (see p188).

WHAT NEXT?

Discuss your symptoms with your doctor, who may prescribe medications to try to control the nausea and suppress the dizziness during the acute phase, after other illnesses have been ruled out.

MY TREATMENT OPTIONS

If a middle-ear infection is present, possible medications are steroids, an antiviral drug (e.g. aciclovir), or antibiotics (e.g. amoxicillin). Ask your doctor about the potential side effects. If you're treated immediately, there should be little or no permanent damage. If the dizziness or imbalance continues for several months, vestibular rehabilitation exercises can help to retrain your brain's ability to adjust. Full recovery may take several weeks.

HOW CAN I HELP MYSELF?

Keep moving around—only if you can—despite your natural inclination to remain still. Be aware of the risk of falls.

Epilepsy

Epilepsy is the most common serious brain disorder. About 3 in 100 people experience a seizure in their lifetime and 1 in 100 people experience at least two. Treatment with antiepileptic drugs is often extremely effective. Most people with epilepsy have no symptoms between seizures or long-term problems.

DO I HAVE THE SYMPTOMS?

If you think you have symptoms of either generalized or focal epilepsy, consult your doctor.

Generalized seizures

- Tonic-clonic seizures (formerly known as grand mal): you lose consciousness, become rigid, and collapse; then your limbs move in a jerking rhythm
- Absence seizures (sometimes known as petit mal): a type common in children; the child becomes vacant and appears to be daydreaming
- Myoclonic seizures: brief, sudden jerking of one or more limbs
- Status epilepticus: repeated tonic-clonic seizures with no regaining of consciousness in between.

Focal (partial) seizures

- Focal sensory seizures: abnormal sensations, such as seeing unexpected colors
- Focal motor seizures: limb twitches
- Temporal lobe epilepsy: starts with odd sensations or a feeling of déjà vu, then detachment from reality, and perhaps repetitive movements.

WHAT IS IT?

An epileptic seizure happens when there's sudden, abnormal, and excessive electrical activity in a group of nerve cells in the cortex (outer region) of the brain. Depending on how much of the brain is affected, seizures may be either generalized or focal (partial) in which you remain conscious (see box above).

Some seizures begin in one part of the brain (focally) and then spread and become generalized. Symptoms can range from a mild feeling of detachment to losing consciousness with jerking limbs. Most seizures last for a few minutes, but occasionally the seizure will not stop spontaneously and you'll need hospital treatment. Status epilepticus (see above) is a serious medical emergency that needs immediate attention.

Seizures can occur without any specific provoking factors, but they can also be triggered by external events. These include:

- Head injury
- Excessive fatigue
- Exposure to either flashing or flickering lights
- Low blood sugar levels
- Alcohol intoxication
- Alcohol withdrawal
- Some recreational drugs.

Sometimes epilepsy arises because there's an underlying structural abnormality in the brain, such as a brain tumor (see p181). Most often, however, the brain appears normal when it's viewed with a scanner, such as an MRI, and no specific structural cause can be found.

WHAT NEXT?

Descriptions of the symptoms, both from the sufferer and from an eyewitness, form a crucial part of the diagnosis. These will help to exclude other potential conditions such as simple fainting episodes and mini-strokes (known as transient ischemic attacks), in which the blood supply to a part of the brain is temporarily blocked. Even types of migraines can sometimes mimic epilepsy.

If your doctor suspects that you have epilepsy, you'll be referred to a neurologist. You'll need to have an electroencephalogram (EEG), in which electrodes are attached all over your scalp and the electrical activity of your brain is recorded. Usually, the EEG will be normal unless you're actually having a seizure, in which case abnormal activity will show up on the trace.

MY TREATMENT OPTIONS

Medication is the main treatment, and your doctor will discuss your options. How long you need to take it depends on the cause of your seizures. If you have an underlying brain abnormality, you may be advised to stay on treatment for life. If the seizures were caused by a specific episode—for example, a head injury—it may be possible to stop medication after a few years and subsequently remain seizure free.

Anti-epileptic drugs (AEDs)

There are many AEDs that act in different ways to reduce the excitability of the brain. Most people are seizure-free on one or two medications taken daily. Modern drugs can be very effective and produce fewer side effects than those used in the past, although many make the oral contraceptive pill less effective. Ask your doctor about potential side effects of your medication.

Surgery This is reserved for people who have severe, frequent seizures that don't respond to medication. The epileptic focus in the brain may be able to be completely removed, but the surgery may cause disability through loss of brain tissue.

HOW CAN I HELP MYSELF?

Maintain a healthy lifestyle

Minimize stress, eat regularly, and get enough sleep.. Avoid operating heavy machinery, climbing heights, or swimming unsupervised.

Avoid triggers like flashing lights if you have photosensitive epilepsy.

Take your AEDs as prescribed
Failure to take them correctly is one of the most common causes of uncontrolled seizures.

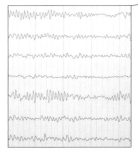

The screen shows different brain wave patterns arising from different areas of the cortex.

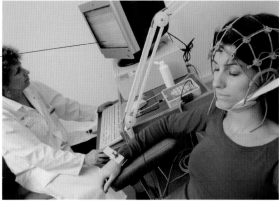

A woman suspected of having epilepsy undergoes an EEG
Electrodes on her scalp painlessly record brain waves. Some forms of epilepsy cause characteristic changes in the normal EEG, even when there is no seizure.

Stroke

Although the incidence of stroke in women and men is about the same, many women still think that stroke is a men's disease. Fortunately, maintaining a healthy lifestyle (see Chapter 3) and preventing or treating risk factors (see below) can help reduce your risk of stroke in later life.

DO I HAVE THE SYMPTOMS?

Stroke symptoms appear suddenly and vary greatly, depending on the specific blood vessels and brain regions involved. Strokes often occur at night so you may wake up with symptoms. Severe strokes can cause unconsciousness and may be fatal. **Contact your doctor urgently** if you experience any of the following symptoms:

- Weakness, numbness, and tingling in the hand, arm, and maybe the leg on one side of the body
- Drooping of one side of the face
- Slurring of speech, or difficulty finding the correct words
- Poor balance, marked clumsiness
- Impaired vision with inability to see objects in one half of the visual field in each eye.

AM I AT RISK?

Women should take note of these risk factors for stroke:

- High blood pressure
- Diabetes
- Smoking
- Obesity
- A diet high in fat
- Irregular heartbeat
- Oral contraceptive pills, particularly if you also get migraines
- Pregnancy. Strokes in pregnancy are rare. A few specific types, however, are unique to pregnancy
- Age. Strokes are more common in women over 65.

WHAT IS IT?

A stroke occurs when a part of the brain loses its function because its blood supply is disturbed by:

- A buildup of fatty tissue, or atheroma, in the blood vessels
- A blockage due to small particles (emboli) lodging in a vessel wall
- Bleeding into the brain tissue
- Reduced blood pressure.

WHAT NEXT?

A CT or MRI scan of the brain may show if you've suffered a stroke and may also reveal the cause. About half of all strokes are caused by blood clots that come from the heart, so you may need an electrocardiogram (EKG, see p168) and an echocardiograph (see p169).

MY TREATMENT OPTIONS

One dose of aspirin increases your chance of survival after a stroke and reduces the risk of another stroke in the following days. After that, a daily low dose of aspirin reduces the risk of future strokes.

Other treatments depend on the cause. For example, if your stroke was due to a blocked blood vessel, you may have an injection of a clot-busting drug, ideally within the first three hours. However, since the drug itself can cause excessive bleeding into the brain, the risk needs to be weighed carefully against any likely benefit.

Your long-term outcome depends on the cause of the stroke. Overall, one in three strokes are fatal, one in three cause some disability, and one in three leave no disability. With rehabilitation, people recover most functions in the first few months, but recovery can take a year.

HOW CAN I HELP MYSELF?

You will receive all kinds of care after suffering a stroke, including nursing, occupational therapy, and physical therapy, but you can also help yourself by establishing a routine of daily exercises and following a healthy diet.

Parkinson's disease

Parkinson's disease is the second most common neurological degenerative disease after Alzheimer's disease. This chronic disease usually affects older people, although in some cases it can occur in younger people. While there is no cure for Parkinson's disease, there are treatments to control symptoms.

DO I HAVE THE SYMPTOMS?

Symptoms may be attributed to old age, but the stance and gait of people with Parkinson's disease soon become obvious. Sufferers often don't swing their arms when walking, are unsteady when they turn, and have reduced facial movements, which makes them look depressed.

See your doctor if you have any of these early symptoms:

- Tremor—most marked in the hands (initially on one side). "Pill-rolling" tremor between thumb and index finger
- Stiffness of the limbs
- Rigidity of the body
- Slow, reduced movements—often hesitating when starting a movement, such as walking.

As the disease progresses more symptoms develop:

- Quiet, stumbling speech
- Coughing and choking
- Drooling due to excess saliva
- Disturbed sleep, vivid dreams
- Restless legs
- Depression
- Constipation
- Excessive sweating.

WHAT IS IT?

Nerve cells in the substantia nigra area of the brain secrete dopamine, which fine-tunes muscle control. In Parkinson's disease they degenerate and stop making dopamine.

WHAT NEXT?

A diagnosis can be made from any history of slowness, a tremor, and stiffness of the limbs. A CT or MRI scan may show brain areas where dopamine is made abnormally.

MY TREATMENT OPTIONS

Drugs to increase brain dopamine are the mainstay of treatment, but research may offer other options. Ask your doctor about side effects.
Drugs Your doctor will give you one or more drugs, such as levodopa, pramipexole, ropinirole, or selegiline.
Surgery Electrical stimulators in specific parts of the brain can reduce tremor and abnormal movements.

AM I AT RISK?

Most people develop symptoms during their 70s. Other risk factors include:

- Genetic predisposition
- Living in the country
- Exposure to some pesticides
- Exposure to some metals
- Repeated head trauma.

Associated treatment Drugs can help with sleep disturbances, mood disorders, and bladder and bowel problems. Physical therapy, speech therapy, occupational therapy, and specialized nurses can all help.

HOW CAN I HELP MYSELF?

Stay as active and positive as you can, and work with your doctor to get your medication just right. Join a support group and find out all you can about the disease.

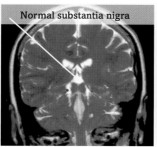
Normal substantia nigra

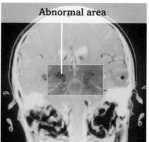
Abnormal area

Diagnosing Parkinson's
A comparison of the scans of a normal brain (far left) and a brain affected by Parkinson's disease (left) can help with diagnosis.

Multiple sclerosis

This complex disorder involves inflammation of the nerve fibers in the brain and spinal cord. Multiple sclerosis (MS) can affect young adults, and is twice as common in women as it is in men. Although there is no cure for MS, many people recover fully between episodes for a number of years.

WHAT IS IT?

MS is caused by inflammation of the myelin (insulating sheath) of nerves in the brain and spinal cord. This occurs when specific white blood cells that normally protect the body from infection become abnormal and attack the body's nervous system. Usually, the body's defenses heal the areas of nerve inflammation, but eventually, after many years, this is less effective. Some sufferers are left with permanent and increasingly severe disabilities although most are able to continue daily activities with minimal impairment. At first, the symptoms (see below) are vague, but real and worrying. Varying symptoms may occur at different times and may be more marked in hot weather or after a warm bath.

DO I HAVE THE SYMPTOMS?

Symptoms are variable in type and severity, occurring in "attacks" lasting from a day to a lifetime.

- Visual symptoms such as pain on moving your eyes, blurred vision, and altered color vision
- Weakness, clumsiness, or stiffness of the limbs
- Numbness, tingling, or tightness in an arm or leg
- Tingling in the face
- Unsteadiness in walking.

Persistent symptoms may include extreme fatigue, depression, cognitive difficulties, and bladder issues.

See your doctor on all issues.

WHAT NEXT?

If your doctor suspects MS, you'll be referred to a neurologist who may make the diagnosis based on a physical examination and your symptoms. MRI scans of the brain and spinal cord often show characteristic areas of inflammation. A lumbar puncture may reveal abnormal antibodies, which can contribute to making the diagnosis.

MY TREATMENT OPTIONS

Treatment is aimed at symptom relief and speeding recovery during relapses. Ask your doctor about the side effects of the following drugs:
Corticosteroids, intravenously or orally, may help shorten relapses. Because of the risks of long-term treatment, their use is restricted to severe flare-ups

AM I AT RISK?

No one yet knows what triggers mulitple sclerosis, but there are some pointers:

- The disease is much more common in temperate zones than in countries near the equator. This suggests that an environmental factor, such as a virus that thrives in temperate regions, may be involved
- You're more likely to get MS if one of your parents had the disease, which suggests a genetic link.

A selective serotonin reuptake inhibitor (SSRI) may be prescribed if fatigue and depression are troubling you.
A muscle-relaxant drug, such baclofen, may alleviate stiffness.
Injected interferon beta and copolymer 1 can suppress immune system oversensitivity, reducing the frequency and severity of relapses.

HOW CAN I HELP MYSELF?

Do regular gentle exercise to strengthen your muscles. Get plenty of support, and keep stress low.

Motor neurone disease

This rare degenerative disease affects the nerves that control muscles. Motor neurone disease (MND) usually begins in people over 50 and may progress rapidly. While the muscles become weaker, other brain functions such as memory, personality, and intellect remain unaffected.

WHAT IS IT?

MND is a rare but devastating disease of the motor nerves and pathways that control muscles. It results in muscle weakness in the limbs, difficulty in swallowing, and breathing problems.

This rapidly progressive disease is, understandably, very upsetting for those who have been diagnosed and for their close families and friends. Most people with MND die within a few years of diagnosis.

WHAT NEXT?

No tests specifically diagnose MND. specialist neurologist will need to perform a clinical examination involving MR imaging and blood tests to exclude other disorders. He or she will order electrical tests on your nerves and muscles.

MY TREATMENT OPTIONS

Treatment can't slow or reverse the muscle wasting, only help alleviate symptoms. Ask about the side effects of any medication you're prescribed.
Riluzole This drug can prolong survival on average by a few months.
Antibiotics These are used to treat chest infections.
Muscle relaxants These drugs help to ease stiff muscles.

AM I AT RISK?

The incidence of MND increases with age and is more common among smokers. In around 10 percent of cases, a parent has the disease and a genetic defect is sometimes found.

Artificial aids If swallowing and breathing are difficult, a feeding tube and ventilator can help.
Specialized support Experienced health-care professionals and palliative care physicians can help improve your quality of life as you become weaker.

HOW CAN I HELP MYSELF?

Keep your mind active, exercise gently if you can to maintain suppleness, and get plenty of support and counseling.

DO I HAVE THE SYMPTOMS?

Weakness and muscle wasting develop over a few months, with any of the following symptoms:
- Weakness in the hands or ankles
- Slurred speech or weak voice
- Stiff or floppy limbs
- Involuntary muscle twitching
- Worsening clumsiness affecting arms, legs, and neck.

Over one or two years, there is rapid deterioration leading to:
- Progressive weakness
- Shortness of breath
- Drowsiness
- Visible wasting of the muscles.

See your doctor if you have any of the symptoms described.

DEGENERATION OF MOTOR PATHWAYS

In MND, the motor nerves that make muscles move gradually degenerate, causing progressive wasting and weakness of the muscles.

Healthy neuron conducts impulses to the muscles

Muscle fibers are stimulated

Dead neuron no longer conducts impulses

Nerve ending relays impulses to muscle

Comparing healthy and dead neurons

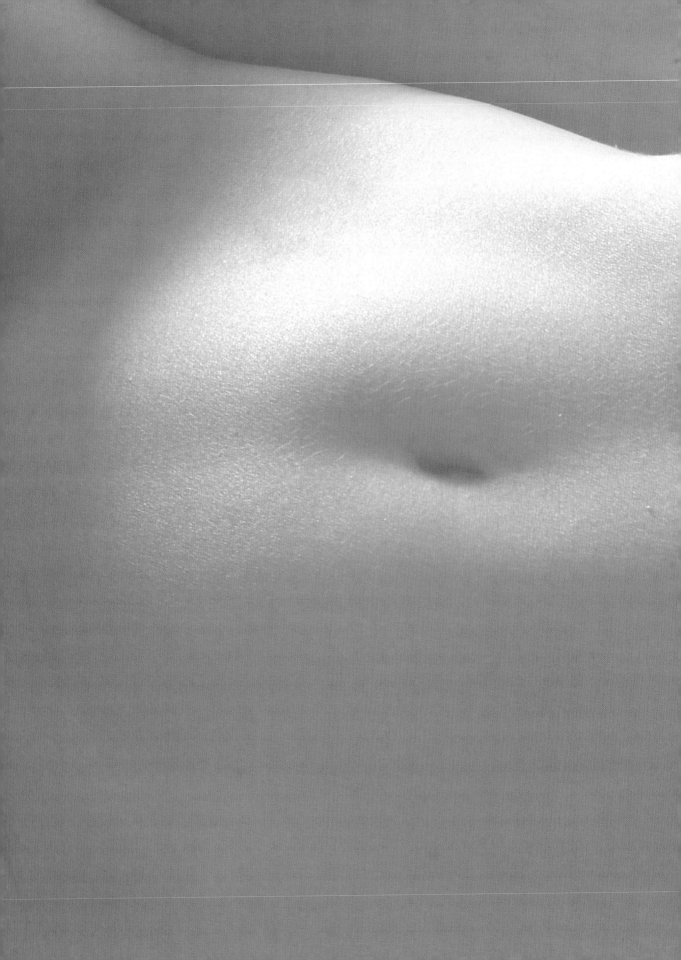

Mental Health

Catherine A. Birndorf MD
Alexandra C. Sacks MD

Mental health

In today's world, most women find themselves searching for balance in their lives. We work hard to integrate the demands of our relationships, families, and careers. We try, often at the very end of the day, to remember to care for ourselves and achieve mental and physical health. While some women are able to juggle these pressures and maintain wellness, there are many and complex reasons why others develop mental health problems. Fortunately, there are effective treatments for many of these problems; the first important step is to ask for help.

SUPERWOMEN

Many modern women feel an expectation from society to be perfect, and today's "superwomen" are expected to be accomplished in all areas, ranging from our beauty and physical wellness, to professional achievement, to happiness in our family and romantic lives. And we're supposed to pull it all off with a feeling of balance and expression of grace. In the post-equal-rights era, we have finally earned the right to do it all, but with these new freedoms have come the burden of new stresses.

MENTAL HEALTH PROBLEMS

All in all, we women tend to be caregivers and feel responsible for other people's needs. Yet many of us tend to overlook our mental wellness until a problem arises and we lose the balance in our lives. We know we can't always be happy and content, and that feelings of frustration, disappointment, sadness, and worry are part of the human condition. However, we can develop a mental health problem, or symptom, when these emotions become significantly distressing and impair our ability to function. Some psychological

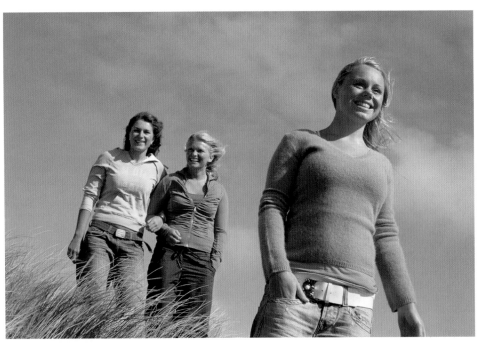

A good enough balance
What does achieving a healthy balance in life involve? Experts agree that a healthy approach is to find a *good enough* balance between work, play, and love. The balance doesn't have to be perfect – but it should be meaningful and satisfying to you.

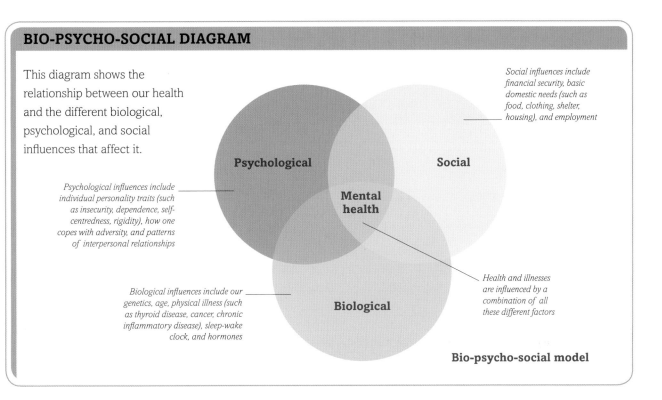

BIO-PSYCHO-SOCIAL DIAGRAM

This diagram shows the relationship between our health and the different biological, psychological, and social influences that affect it.

Social influences include financial security, basic domestic needs (such as food, clothing, shelter, housing), and employment

Psychological

Social

Mental health

Psychological influences include individual personality traits (such as insecurity, dependence, self-centredness, rigidity), how one copes with adversity, and patterns of interpersonal relationships

Health and illnesses are influenced by a combination of all these different factors

Biological influences include our genetics, age, physical illness (such as thyroid disease, cancer, chronic inflammatory disease), sleep-wake clock, and hormones

Biological

Bio-psycho-social model

symptoms may be expected for a given age group – many women experience a brief but manageable period of anxiety surrounding transitions, such as moving out of their childhood home, getting married, being pregnant or going through the menopause. Other emotions may be linked with hormonal changes as our bodies develop and change from menstruation through menopause.

This chapter addresses some of the mental health problems that women experience, from anxieties and depression to eating disorders and sexual dysfunction. Unfortunately, the history of psychiatric research has not always reflected gender differences, as women have frequently been excluded from studies. More recently, it has been recognized that women, due to their physiology, may have a different experience

> "Modern women have earned the right to do it all, but with these freedoms have come the burden of new stresses."

from men in their symptoms and treatment of mental health problems.

THE BIO-PSYCHO-SOCIAL MODEL

Despite significant progress identifying and treating mental health problems, their causes are still not fully understood. Many mental health problems, including depression, may be influenced by a number of different sources. In an attempt to explain these sources, and why some people develop psychological symptoms while others don't, scientists have developed a framework called the "bio-psycho-social" model. This combines the biological, psychological, and social influences (see box above), which all work together on the brain to alter the way neurotransmitters – chemicals in the brain – such as serotonin and dopamine, produce changes in our emotional states.

The following pages outline the mental illnesses that affect women the most. Specific treatments are mentioned in each article but refer to pp224–7 for a general discussion of treatment.

Anxiety disorders

Feelings of anxiety and panic, and the physical signs of sweating, palpitations, and breathlessness, can be a common response to stress. However, if you experience these reactions frequently and they disrupt your everyday activities, you may have an anxiety disorder.

Anxiety disorders, like other mental health disorders, are caused by a combination of biological, psychological, and social factors (see pp202–3). If you have a family history of an anxiety disorder, you may be more vulnerable to stress, and this may increase your risk of developing an anxiety disorder.

Sometimes there may be a medical factor that is responsible for your anxiety, such as thyroid disease or substance abuse, and any such possible medical causes must be ruled out before your doctor can diagnose anxiety as a mental health condition.

Generalized anxiety disorder

If you have generalized anxiety disorder (GAD), you worry excessively about anything and everything, although you might not know exactly why you feel so anxious. GAD affects more women than men and is most common during the early adult years.

WHAT IS IT?

Most people get nervous when they are stressed, but what makes someone with GAD different is that they are worried most or all of the time. Although to many people this may seem to be a minor problem, in fact it can seriously interfere with daily life.

If you have GAD, you may also have other mental health problems, such as major depressive disorder (see pp210–11), another anxiety disorder, or substance abuse (see pp220–1).

WHAT NEXT?

Your doctor will do a thorough evaluation and make a diagnosis based on your symptoms.

MY TREATMENT OPTIONS

Depending on your particular symptoms, your doctor may advise therapy, medication, or both.
Therapies Cognitive-behavioral therapy is effective for many people with GAD, although behavior therapy may also be recommended (see p225).
Medication The most common medication is either an SSRI or SNRI antidepressant (see p227), Ask your doctor about side effects.

HOW CAN I HELP MYSELF?

Symptoms may be alleviated by regular exercise, relaxation methods, avoiding caffeine, not drinking excessively, and not smoking,

DO I HAVE THE SYMPTOMS?

To be diagnosed with generalized anxiety disorder, you must be unrealistically anxious about two or more life circumstances for at least six months. You must also have at least three of the following symptoms:
- Problems sleeping
- Fatigue
- Muscle tension
- Restlessness
- Inability to concentrate
- Irritability.

See your doctor if you have symptoms that cause you distress in your daily life.

For your doctor to diagnose generalized anxiety disorder, your symptoms must not be caused by a medical condition or by another type of mental health disorder.

Panic disorder

Panic disorder is a condition in which a person experiences unexpected episodes of intense fear accompanied by physical symptoms. Panic disorder is roughly twice as common in women as in men and you can get it at any time in life, but women in their 20s–40s are at greatest risk.

WHAT IS IT?

If you have a panic attack, it doesn't necessarily mean that you have panic disorder. That diagnosis is only made if you also have anticipatory anxiety (anxiety about future panic attacks) on a regular basis for at least a month. Your attacks may be caused by specific triggers or situations, such as agoraphobia (the fear of being in crowds and public places) or you may get them more randomly.

Panic attacks also give you physical symptoms, and it's common for people to go to a hospital emergency room because they think they are having a heart attack.

Panic disorder rarely gets better on its own, and so it's important that you see your doctor if you think you may be suffering from it. In about 20 percent of the most severely affected people it can lead to attempted suicide, especially where it's coupled with major depressive disorder (see pp210–11).

WHAT NEXT?

Your doctor will do a thorough evaluation and make a diagnosis based on your symptoms.

MY TREATMENT OPTIONS

The two main treatment choices are therapy and medication.
Therapies Cognitive-behavioral therapy or behavior therapy (see p225) are often effective.
Medication Your doctor may prescribe antidepressants (see p227), including an SSRI, SNRI or tricyclic antidepressant. Benzodiazepines may also be used in some cases. Ask your doctor about any possible side effects.

HOW CAN I HELP MYSELF?

Creative visualization of a peaceful scene or situation, relaxation techniques, and regular exercise can all help to relieve symptoms.

DO I HAVE THE SYMPTOMS?

Panic attacks occur in discrete episodes peaking within 10 minutes. To be classed as panic disorder, you must have four or more symptoms featured in the box right, and accompanied by intense fear. You must also have:

● One month (or more) of worry about future panic attacks, worry about the implications of an attack, or changed behavior due to the attacks.

See your doctor if any of these features apply to you.

THE SIGNS OF A PANIC ATTACK

In addition to feelings of anxiety, panic attacks also produce physical symptoms, at least four of which must be present for an attack to be classed as a panic attack, together with a feeling of unreality, fear of losing control, and fear of dying.

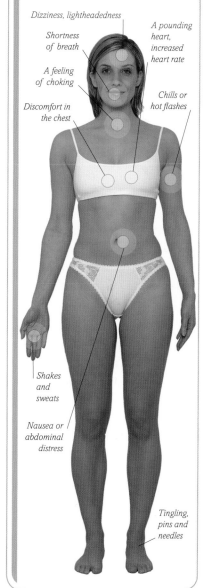

Dizziness, lightheadedness

Shortness of breath

A feeling of choking

Discomfort in the chest

A pounding heart, increased heart rate

Chills or hot flashes

Shakes and sweats

Nausea or abdominal distress

Tingling, pins and needles

Social anxiety disorder

At one time or another most of us have felt shy, lacking in confidence, or anxious in social situations, but these feelings are usually fairly mild and we manage to overcome them. However, if the distress is so severe that it affects your personal and work life, you may have social anxiety disorder.

WHAT IS IT?

Sometimes known as social phobia, social anxiety disorder makes you feel intensely anxious about being humiliated or embarrassed when you are in a social situation. You then become self-conscious and suffer from symptoms of anxiety, which may include blushing, a pounding heart, and sweating. As you become anxious, your symptoms cause more stress and this makes you even more anxious, so you find yourself in a vicious cycle. Eventually, these reactions may become your normal conditioned response to social situations. Such severe anxiety can have a negative impact on your personal life and your work life.

Common problems for people with social anxiety disorder are a fear of public speaking and other situations involving performance. Other symptoms may include fear of eating or drinking in public, and a fear of using public toilets. Associated personality features seen in people with social anxiety disorder include low self-esteem, oversensitivity to criticism, and difficulty being assertive.

Social anxiety disorder is a relatively common problem. About 7 percent of the population experience social anxiety in adulthood, and it is more common in women than men. The exact cause isn't known, but it probably has bio-psycho-social roots (see p203). It's likely that the chemistry of the brain and the functioning of the amygdala (a part of the brain concerned with emotions and feeling, including fear) are involved.

Many people with social anxiety disorder also suffer from depression (see pp210–11). Some also turn to substance abuse, possibly in an attempt to reduce their social anxiety by self medication.

WHAT NEXT?

Your doctor will do a thorough evaluation and make a diagnosis based on your symptoms.

MY TREATMENT OPTIONS

Your doctor may advise talk therapy, medication, or both.
Therapy Behavioral therapy and cognitive-behavioral therapy (CBT, see p225) may help. CBT, in particular, has proved to work for many women.
Medication Your doctor may prescribe an antidepressant (see p227), such as an SSRI (e.g. Prozac) or an SNRI (e.g. venlafaxine). Benzodiazepines may also be used in some cases.

HOW CAN I HELP MYSELF?

The most important thing is to persevere with treatment, even if it does not seem to be working at first. Both medication and therapy may take time to produce noticeable benefits.

DO I HAVE THE SYMPTOMS?

If you have social anxiety disorder, you will fear situations in which you may be exposed to scrutiny by others. This response must not be due to another medical or mental health condition and must last for at least six months. Symptoms of social anxiety disorder include:

- Fear of behaving in a way that is embarrassing
- Severe anxiety in social situations or situations in which you have to perform (e.g. speaking in public)
- A recognition that your anxiety is unreasonable
- Avoidance of stress-producing situations.

See your doctor if these symptoms interfere with your normal daily life.

"Although social anxiety disorder can feel overwhelming, it can often be treated effectively."

Obsessive compulsive disorder

In obsessive compulsive disorder (OCD), you are bothered by unwanted and intrusive thoughts and/or overwhelming urges—compulsions—to perform particular actions repeatedly. This obsessive-compulsive cycle may become so time consuming that it disrupts your daily life.

WHAT IS IT?

If you suffer from OCD, you have thoughts or worries that keep coming into your mind. Although you may realize these obsessions are irrational, they still make you anxious. For example, you may have such a powerful fear of germs that you can't go out because of your worry about contamination.

You may also feel compelled to perform specific rituals to reduce anxiety. Although these compulsions are intended to be reassuring, they may actually prevent you from functioning normally in everyday life. A classic example is repeatedly checking that a door is locked even though you know you've already locked it.

As with other mental disorders, OCD probably has bio-psycho-social causes (see p203).

About 1 percent of adults have OCD. In women it tends to appear in adolescence or early adulthood. Women may have a new onset of OCD symptoms when they are pregnant. Women with OCD may also find their symptoms are more severe before a period.

WHAT NEXT?

OCD is a long-term disorder that won't get completely better unless you have treatment, so if you're concerned that you have OCD, see your doctor. He or she will make a diagnosis based on your obsessions or your compulsions, although it's common to have both. For OCD to be diagnosed, your obsessions or compulsions must be distressing and disrupt daily activities.

MY TREATMENT OPTIONS

Your doctor will do a thorough evaluation and discuss the most appropriate therapies and medication with you.

Therapies Exposure and response prevention (ERP) is a specific behavioral therapy for OCD in which you are exposed to situations that make you fearful but are prevented from performing your usual rituals. This can be difficult at first but may be effective over time. Alternatively, cognitive-behavioral therapy (see p225) may be helpful.

Medication Your doctor may also prescribe an SSRI antidepressant (see p227) or the tricyclic antidepressant clomipramine.

HOW CAN I HELP MYSELF?

Treatment may take time to produce noticeable benefit, so the best way you can help yourself is to persist with it.

DO I HAVE THE SYMPTOMS?

You may have OCD if you have obsessions and/or compulsions that you recognize are unreasonable but that still interfere with daily life. Your symptoms must not be due to another medical or mental health condition. Symptoms include:

- Obsessions—recurrent thoughts, impulses, or images that you know are a product of your own mind but that still cause anxiety
- Compulsions—repetitive behaviors in response to obsessions that are aimed, unrealistically, at preventing distress.

See your doctor if any of these symptoms impair normal life.

Post-traumatic stress disorder

Any of us can witness or experience a distressing or life-threatening event and most of us recover without needing help. But for some people, with women being particularly at risk, such an event is experienced as a trauma that haunts them over time and, as a result, they suffer various symptoms that disrupt daily life.

DO I HAVE THE SYMPTOMS?

The symptoms of PTSD occur after a person has been exposed to a traumatic event. The symptoms must last for at least one month and must impair your daily functioning or cause distress. The memory of the event haunts you, recurring in flashbacks or nightmares that trigger the same intense fear that you originally felt. In addition, you will have three or more of the following:

- Emotional numbness
- Loss of pleasure in activities you usually enjoy
- Memory loss
- Active avoidance of reminders of the event.

You will also be constantly "on edge" (hyperaroused) with two or more of the following:

- Poor concentration
- Hypervigilance
- Insomnia
- Irritability
- Exaggerated startle response.

Consult your doctor if your symptoms are distressing and interfering with your daily life.

WHAT IS IT?

Post-traumatic stress disorder (PTSD) is a severe anxiety response that you can develop after you have been involved in or witnessed a psychologically stressful or life-threatening event. It can affect anybody, including children, and the symptoms (see Do I have the symptoms?) may develop immediately or may not appear until months after the traumatic event. Initially, it may be difficult to distinguish PTSD from acute stress disorder, which has the same features as PTSD. However, with acute stress disorder the symptoms always develop immediately after the traumatic event and usually get better within a month.

PTSD is about twice as common in women as in men; it's estimated that about 10 percent of women will suffer from PTSD at some time in their lives. More than half of rape victims are diagnosed with PTSD.

As well as causing unpleasant, life-disrupting symptoms, PTSD also puts you at increased risk for suicide and impulsive behaviors,

AM I AT RISK?

A number of factors make you more at risk of having PTSD:

- Directly experiencing or witnessing a violent personal assault, an accident, a violent terrorist incident, a natural or human-caused disaster, or war.
- Women are at higher risk of PTSD because they are more likely to be the victims of a sexual assault or of physical, sexual, or emotional abuse from their partner (known as intimate partner violence).

- Women who are pregnant, especially if the pregnancy was not planned, are at increased risk of being the victim of intimate partner violence and therefore of developing PTSD.
- People who have suffered from anxiety or depression in the past are at greater risk of suffering from PTSD.
- Children who have been exposed to a traumatic event are at greater risk of developing PTSD as adults.

especially if you have also been sexually assaulted. In addition to suffering from PTSD, victims of intimate partner violence may also experience anxiety and depression. They often have a diminished sense of self-worth and frequently feel socially isolated.

Although the various external factors that can result in PTSD are well known, the entire causative mechanisms and processes are unclear, and it is not known why some people who experience traumatic events develop PTSD while others don't.

Like many other psychiatric conditions, PTSD is thought to be due to a combination of biological, psychological, and social factors (see p203). On the biological side, it is thought that part of the brain called the amygdala may play a central role. The amygdala is part of the brain's limbic system (see box, right) and is considered by many scientists to be the place where we store our fears and the memories of our emotions. Other areas of the brain that play a part in the formation of memories and in the body's response to stress are also thought to be involved, notably the medial prefontal cortex, the hippocampus, the hypothalamus, and the thalamus (see Areas of the brain affected in PTSD, right).

WHAT NEXT?
Your doctor will do a thorough evaluation and will be able to diagnose PTSD from your description of the symptoms. He or she will probably refer you to a psychologist or psychiatrist.

MY TREATMENT OPTIONS
You may be offered therapy, medication, or a combination of the two, and the treatment will be tailored specifically for you.

Cognitive–behavioral therapy (CBT) This form of therapy is often used for PTSD and is usually very effective (see p225).

Eye movement desensitization and reprocessing (EMDR) This therapy involves you rhythmically moving your eyes to help you relax (see p225). Your therapist then asks you to talk about the trauma. The goal of this therapy is to break the link between your memories and your anxiety symptoms.

Supportive therapy This is an important part of treatment for victims of violence. It is particularly valuable for rape victims, since it can help them to regain their sense of self-worth.

Medications Antidepressants such as SSRIs (see p227) may also be helpful. Ask your doctor about side effects.

HOW CAN I HELP MYSELF?
You can best help yourself by seeing a doctor as soon as possible and then by following your treatment plan. It's never too late to seek treatment—PTSD can be treated even years after the trauma.

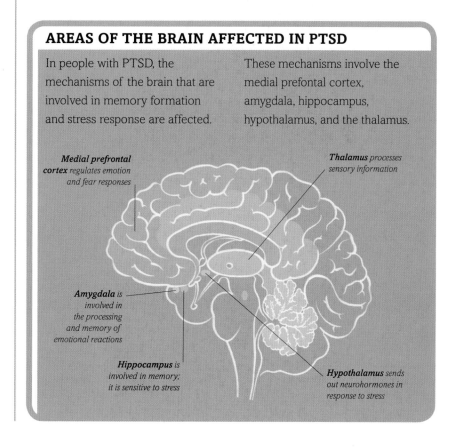

AREAS OF THE BRAIN AFFECTED IN PTSD

In people with PTSD, the mechanisms of the brain that are involved in memory formation and stress response are affected. These mechanisms involve the medial prefontal cortex, amygdala, hippocampus, hypothalamus, and the thalamus.

Medial prefrontal cortex regulates emotion and fear responses

Thalamus processes sensory information

Amygdala is involved in the processing and memory of emotional reactions

Hippocampus is involved in memory; it is sensitive to stress

Hypothalamus sends out neurohormones in response to stress

Depression

We all feel down or sad sometimes, but if "the blues" persists and becomes so bad that it interferes with daily life, this may be a sign of depression. Roughly 15 percent of people become clinically depressed at some point in their lives and, compared to men, women are twice as likely to develop depression.

WHAT IS IT?

In everyday life, when people say they are "depressed" they are often referring to feelings of sadness that will pass after a relatively short time. But in clinical depression, feelings of intense sadness, hopelessness, worthlessness, and loss of interest in life last for weeks or months and have a significant negative impact on your life. These feeling are deeper, more disruptive, and last longer than transient unhappiness. If you are depressed, you may also suffer from various physical symptoms, such as disrupted sleep, fatigue, aches and pains, and weight loss or gain. In the worst cases, people with untreated depression may even take their own lives. In addition, untreated depression can have secondhand effects on other family members and friends, and is a leading cause of disability. In the longer term, depression can also increase your risk of heart disease.

It is important to distinguish between depression, which is an illness, with grief, which is a natural reaction to loss. Both share many of the same features but, unlike depression, grief is a healing process that typically resolves itself in five stages and does not require treatment. The first stage is shock and denial. Then there is anger and guilt, followed by an urge to bargain to get back what you have lost. The fourth stage is deep sadness or despair. Finally there is acceptance, when you come to terms with the loss and are able to move forward. However, for some people the process does not resolve itself in acceptance; this is known as complicated grieving and requires professional help.

There are various types of depression and the causes are still unknown, but bio-psycho-social factors (see p203) may play a part. Women and men are different, and the anatomy and physiology of the female brain affect women in unique, specific ways.

Psychologically, we experience specific sources of stress, including worries about fertility, pregnancy, motherhood, and single parenthood. And socially, women have historically suffered more than men

DO I HAVE THE SYMPTOMS?

You may meet the criteria for a major depressive episode if you have at least five of the symptoms listed below (one of the first two symptoms must be present) during the same two-week period. These symptoms must be abnormal for you personally and must not be due to a physical illness, medications, or to substance use. They must also cause severe distress or impair your everyday life, and they must not be accompanied by symptoms of bipolar disorder (see p212) or be due to grief.

- Low mood
- Diminished interest or pleasure in activities you used to enjoy
- Significant weight loss or gain
- Inability to sleep or dramatically increased sleep
- Feeling as if your body is slowed down or feeling agitated
- Loss of energy
- Feelings of worthlessness or guilt
- Poor concentration
- Recurrent thoughts of death or suicide, or a suicide attempt.

See your doctor if you have a number of these symptoms. If you are suicidal, get help urgently.

from challenges such as juggling domestic and career duties, job discrimination, and abuse.

Each of the many different types of depression has different symptoms and different degrees of severity. The main types and their features are outlined below.

Major depressive disorder (MDD) Previously called unipolar depression, MDD is when episodes of depression are severe and involve a particular combination of features (see Do I have the symptoms?). For a diagnosis of MDD you must have one or more depressive episodes in the absence of manic, hypomanic, or mixed episodes. (Mania is a feeling of extreme elation; hypomania is similar to mania but milder; a mixed episode is when symptoms of both depression and mania are present at the same time.)

Minor depression This is diagnosed when you have some of the symptoms of depression but not all of the elements necessary for a major depressive episode (see Do I have the symptoms?).

Dysthymia This is characterized by symptoms that are relatively mild but long-lasting. If you have at least two of the symptoms of a major depressive episode but generally feel depressed in everyday life, then you may have this disorder.

Adjustment disorder with depressed mood This is diagnosed when you have the same symptoms as those of a major depressive episode (see Do I have the symptoms?), but

symptoms begin only after you've suffered a specific stressful event within the past three months.

Premenstrual dysphoric disorder (PMDD) A diagnosis of PMDD may be made when you have the same symptoms as those of a major depressive episode but the symptoms only occur during your premenstrual period and then clear up during the first few days of your period (see also pp92–3).

WHAT NEXT?

Your doctor will do a thorough evaluation and will be able to diagnose your specific type of depression from your symptoms.

MY TREATMENT OPTIONS

Modern treatments for depression are highly effective, so the sooner you seek help from your doctor, the sooner you'll be on the road to recovery. Your doctor may advise one or more of the following:

Talk therapies Commonly used talk therapies include cognitive–behavioral therapy, interpersonal therapy, and psychodynamic therapy (see pp224–5).

Medications There are several types of antidepressants but your doctor will probably prescribe an SSRI or an SNRI (see p227). Ask your doctor about any side effects.

Electroconvulsive therapy (ECT) This is usually reserved for severe depression that cannot be controlled by therapy and medications. It is done under carefully controlled conditions and involves passing an electric current

AM I AT RISK?

The following risk factors may increase your chance of developing the symptoms that may be diagnosed as one of the types of depression:

- Family history of depression
- Prior episodes of depression
- Having another mental health disorder
- Between 20 and 40 years old
- Recent stressful life events
- History of childhood abuse and/or sexual abuse
- Poor sleeping habits
- Smoking
- Alcohol or substance abuse
- Relationship stress
- Parenting stress.

through the brain to change the chemistry of the part of the brain that is causing the depression.

HOW CAN I HELP MYSELF?

The main way to help yourself is to follow your treatment plan. There are also self-help measures you can try, although you should discuss them with your doctor first.

Alternatives Many women have found that regular exercise (see pp56–7) and a healthy diet (see pp52–5) are helpful. Daily exposure to light, acupuncture, the herbal remedy St. John's Wort, and the dietary supplement SAMe (S-adenosylmethionine) might also be useful. A word of caution: these last two may react with medications, so it is vital to talk to your doctor first.

Bipolar disorder

Most of us have periods when our moods fluctuate but people with bipolar disorder experience extreme mood swings: they have episodes of depression followed by periods of feeling elated. These low and high phases are so extreme that they can have a major impact on every aspect of life.

WHAT IS IT?

A form of depression, bipolar disorder is probably caused by a chemical imbalance in the brain that is likely to be a genetic inheritance—having a parent with the disorder puts you at greater risk. It is categorized into two types.

Bipolar disorder I Once known as manic depression, this is characterized by alternating episodes of major depression (see pp210–11) and mania—a period in which you feel extremely high (see Do I have the symptoms?). These episodes last for a week or more. Most people with bipolar I spend more time in a state of depression than in a state of mania, although some people have only manic episodes. You must have at least one manic episode to be diagnosed with bipolar I.

Bipolar disorder II This is more common than bipolar I and is similar to it. The main difference is that the high periods (known as hypomanic episodes) are shorter—but still last for at least four days—and less extreme. Bipolar II may not adversely affect your social or work life and may not require hospitalization. If you suffer from bipolar II, you will have at least one hypomanic episode and at least one episode of major depression.

In both types, the occurrence of symptoms varies widely. Some people have only a few episodes while others have many.

WHAT NEXT?

Your doctor will do a thorough evaluation and make a diagnosis from your symptoms. If you have bipolar I or II, you will be closely monitored by your doctor because episodes of illness are likely to recur over the course of your life.

MY TREATMENT OPTIONS

If you have severe bipolar disorder, you probably need medication and treatment for the rest of your life.

Medication After a manic episode, you will require long-term medication. You will probably be treated with lithium or other mood-stabilizers (see pp226–7). Ask your doctor about side effects.

Monitoring Your doctor will make sure that you are monitored as an outpatient. You may have to be admitted to the hospital during a manic or depressive episode for safety and treatment.

HOW CAN I HELP MYSELF?

You should follow the treatment plan set out for you by your doctor.

DO I HAVE THE SYMPTOMS?

A manic episode is a period of abnormally elevated or irritable mood. It must impair daily life and must not be due to a medical condition, medications, or drugs. It must last for at least a week (but may be shorter if hospitalization is required) and include at least three of the following (at least four if your mood is irritable):

- Increased energy/activity
- Talking fast and emphatically
- Racing thoughts
- Poor concentration
- Decreased need for sleep
- Grandiosity/inflated self-esteem
- Distractability
- Excessive indulgence in pleasurable but dangerous activities (e.g. spending, sexual activity)
- Increased goal-directed activity or physical agitation.

See your doctor if you have these symptoms.

Seasonal Affective Disorder

During the dark winter months, many of us feel lethargic, less social, and generally a bit low. But for people with seasonal affective disorder, these symptoms are more severe; sometimes, they can be bad enough to cause significant problems with everyday activities.

WHAT IS IT?

Seasonal affective disorder (SAD) is a type of depression whose symptoms are linked to the changing patterns of sunlight during the year. The change in light levels causes alterations in brain chemistry that affect your mood, energy levels, and even sex drive. Most people suffer from SAD during the winter but some people experience symptoms during the summer. As with other mental health conditions, SAD is likely to be caused by bio-psycho-social factors (see p203). In some people, it may be inherited.

WHAT NEXT?

Your doctor will diagnose SAD only if you have had symptoms during the same season (usually fall–winter) in two consecutive years and are not suffering from major depressive illness (see pp210–11).

MY TREATMENT OPTIONS

SAD can usually be treated effectively with light therapy, antidepressants, or talk therapy.
Light therapy With this therapy, you sit in front of a special light box that produces bright light similar to outdoor light.

DO I HAVE THE SYMPTOMS?

Most people with SAD have symptoms of depression during the winter months. Symptoms of winter SAD may include:
- Lethargy and fatigue
- Food cravings for sugar, starch, and alcohol, and weight gain
- Irritability and anxiety
- Avoidance of social activities.

Symptoms of the less common summer SAD include:
- Insomnia
- Loss of appetite and weight loss
- Irritability and anxiety
- Increased sex drive
- Agitation.

See you doctor if you have any of these symptoms.

Therapy Psychotherapy or counseling (see pp224–5) may be helpful for some people.
Medication Your doctor may prescribe an antidepressant (see pp226–7). Ask your doctor about any side effects.

HOW CAN I HELP MYSELF?

The main way to help yourself is to increase your exposure to light, ideally by spending at least 30 minutes outside every day. It is also worthwhile making your home and workplace as light as possible.

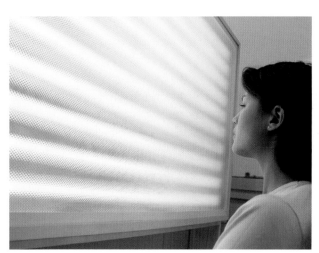

Light therapy for winter SAD
This involves sitting in front of a special light box every day (ideally in the morning) for between 30 minutes and two hours, depending on the strength of the light it gives out.

Depressions of pregnancy and childbirth

Pregnancy and childbirth are times of enormous biological, psychological, and social changes for women. Some women deal with these changes seamlessly but many others find that the challenges of pregnancy and childbirth cause old mental health problems to resurface or new ones to develop.

Prenatal depression

Depression during pregnancy has been historically underdiagnosed and undertreated; however, it may affect as many as 10–20 percent of pregnant women.

WHAT IS IT?

It's normal for women to have periods of feeling down during pregnancy but prenatal depression is more severe and causes significant distress. It is similar to a major depressive episode and causes the same symptoms (see Do I have the symptoms? below left). In addition, prenatal depression may result in you neglecting your own health, and this can be harmful for both you and your baby.

WHAT NEXT?

If you think you may have prenatal depression, you should see your doctor. He or she will perform a thorough evaluation and will make a diagnosis from your symptoms.

DO I HAVE THE SYMPTOMS?

To be diagnosed with prenatal depression:

- You must be pregnant and your symptoms must fulfill the various requirements necessary for a major depressive episode (see pp210–11)
- Your symptoms must cause significant distress in your daily life.

See your doctor if the features of your condition correspond to those listed above.

AM I AT RISK?

There are a variety of risk factors for developing depression during pregnancy. These include:

- A prior history of depression in yourself or your family
- A high-risk or complicated pregnancy
- Stress in your relationship
- Prior miscarriage or loss.

MY TREATMENT OPTIONS

In the past, doctors usually advised pregnant women to avoid medication at all costs because of potential effects on the baby. Today, however, it is thought that a woman's untreated illness may be more harmful than the effect of medication on the fetus. Your doctor will work with you to weigh the pros and cons of the therapy and medication choices.

Therapy This is usually the first choice and is highly effective for many women. Among the options that may be considered is short-term, symptom-focused therapy such as interpersonal psychotherapy (see p225), which may also help protect against postpartum depression (see opposite).

Medication If therapy alone does not work, you and your doctor should discuss which medication is the best choice.

HOW CAN I HELP MYSELF?

You should keep your doctor's appointments and follow your treatment plan. You should also take care of your physical health.

Postpartum depression (PPD)

The birth of a baby is a life-changing event and many new mothers find the period after the birth stressful. Feeling hypersensitive—the "baby blues" (see Other postpartum problems, below)—is common, but some mothers develop more serious, longer-lasting depression known as postpartum depression (PPD).

WHAT IS IT?

While most new mothers are concerned about how well they are able to care for their baby, if you have PPD you may be excessively anxious about your caretaking ability and your baby's well-being.

Paradoxically, you may also have negative feelings toward your baby—you may even have upsetting thoughts about harming him or her. Fortunately, mothers with PPD rarely act on such thoughts, but they can make it hard to bond with your baby.

The main symptoms of PPD are described on the left (see Do I have the symptoms?). They are similar to those of major depressive disorder (see pp210–11), but the distinctive feature of PPD is that it occurs specifically after you have given birth—usually within the first month but sometimes up to six months later—and is often characterized by severe anxiety.

WHAT NEXT?

If you think you may have PPD, you should see your doctor. He or she may ask you to fill out a short questionnaire called the Edinburgh Postpartum Depression Scale in order to diagnose PPD.

MY TREATMENT OPTIONS

PPD can be treated effectively with the same therapies and medications used for major depressive disorder (see p211). If you are breast-feeding, your doctor will take this into account when considering any medication.

HOW CAN I HELP MYSELF?

You should keep your doctor's appointments and also make sure you follow the treatment plan devised for you.

AM I AT RISK?

Women at highest risk are those with a personal or family history of a mood disorder, especially PPD or prenatal depression (see opposite).

DO I HAVE THE SYMPTOMS?

The symptoms of PPD are similar to those of major depressive disorder (see pp210–11). Other typical features of PPD include:

- Symptoms occur within four weeks of delivery, and during this period you have symptoms nearly every day for two weeks
- The symptoms are not typical for you personally and affect your daily life
- Anxiety about your baby that may disrupt your sleep.

See your doctor if you have any of these symptoms after having a baby.

OTHER POSTPARTUM PROBLEMS

As well as depression, other mental problems may occur in the postpartum period. The main ones are:

"Baby blues" This affects some 50–80 percent of women after they have had a baby. Milder than PPD, the most common symptoms are feeling low, tired, and emotionally hypersensitive. It clears up on its own within about two weeks.

Postpartum psychosis At the other end of the spectrum from "baby blues," postpartum psychosis is the most severe mental problem. Fortunately, it is rare and usually occurs only in women with bipolar disorder (see p212) or in women who have had postpartum psychosis before. Women with this problem lose touch with reality and behave in a confused way. There is also a high risk of infanticide and suicide.

Eating disorders

Ninety percent of people who have eating disorders are young and female, and most of them suffer from anorexia and/or bulimia. Although these eating disorders often begin with a focus on weight, they usually also involve complicated emotions, such as self-esteem.

Anorexia nervosa

People with anorexia are alarmingly thin, but most don't think there's anything wrong with their appearance or their health.

WHAT IS IT?

If you suffer from this body image disorder, you will be so worried about being fat that you will keep your intake of calories dangerously low. The constant worry about food and weight can cause serious emotional distress and can also distract you from all other areas of your life.

Because of the severe calorie restriction and weight loss involved, your body goes into starvation mode and you may start to experience physical symptoms. These may include constipation, loss of hair from your head, the growth of new lanugo (fine, downy hair) on your body, swelling of your limbs, feeling cold, and severe fatigue.

Malnutrition throws all your hormones out of balance, and you stop having periods. Over time, these hormone imbalances increase your risk for osteoporosis (see pp260–2) and infertility (see pp122–3). Finally, the starvation can make your heart beat abnormally, which can cause a fatal heart attack.

Unfortunately, about 5–18 percent of anorexics will die from the disease, either from cardiovascular problems, malnutrition, or suicide. However, roughly 50 percent will recover (with some relapse) with proper treatment.

DO I HAVE THE SYMPTOMS?

You may be anorexic if you meet the following four criteria:
- You refuse to maintain at least 85 percent of your normal weight (for your age and height)
- You constantly fear gaining weight or being fat, despite being underweight
- No matter how much weight you lose, you still think that you are fat or deny the severity of your weight loss
- You have missed three consecutive menstrual periods.

See your doctor if you have these symptoms.

AM I AT RISK?

You are at greater risk of anorexia if:
- You are still in adolescence and facing a stressful life event or have a poor body image
- You are involved in activities or professions that exert a pressure to be thin, such as ballet, gymnastics, and modeling
- You have anxiety disorders such as OCD (see p207) or depression (see pp210–11).

WHAT NEXT?

Your first priority is to return to a normal weight. Once you have started eating normally again, it's important to address the core psychological issues at the root of your problem to prevent a relapse. If you are medically and psychiatrically stable, agree to participate in a therapy program, and have the support of your friends and family to pull you through, you can be treated as an outpatient. Otherwise, you may need to be admitted to the hospital for medical monitoring and therapy.

MY TREATMENT OPTIONS

Treatment depends on your own individual circumstances and needs. Your doctor will assess your overall health and explore with you the medical care that will give you the best results with the fewest side effects. He or she will devise a specific treatment plan for you. It is very important to start your treatment as soon as possible, especially if you have lost a lot of weight.

Therapy Individual, group, and family-based therapies may work for anorexia (see pp224–6).

Medication Antidepressants, antianxiety, and antipsychotic medication (see pp226–7) may be used to address specific symptoms, but researchers are still investigating which medications may be effective in people with very low body weights. Ask your doctor about the possible side effects of medication.

HOW CAN I HELP MYSELF?

Once you have been to see your doctor and discussed the best treatment for you, you must make sure that you follow your treatment plan.

Bulimia nervosa

Bulimia is different than anorexia because bulimics often are a normal weight and often realize that their behavior is unhealthy.

WHAT IS IT?

Bulimia is a disease of bingeing (when you eat large amounts of food in a short time) and purging (when you try to prevent weight gain by fasting, exercise, and taking laxatives or diuretics).

If have bulimia, it's important to get treated because of the distress it can cause in your daily life. If you constantly make yourself vomit, you'll get dental cavities and dental erosion. You may also develop a life-threatening tear in your esophagus, and dangerous imbalances of electrolytes (salts).

Although all of this can severely damage your body, bulimia is less likely to cause death than anorexia; 75 percent of people who receive treatment recover, although up to 25 percent may experience a relapse.

WHAT NEXT?

Your doctor will do a thorough evaluation and make a diagnosis based on your symptoms.

MY TREATMENT OPTIONS

As with anorexia, safety comes first. If you are at risk of suicide or have severe medical complications, you may need to be hospitalized.

Therapy Individual, group, and family-based therapies may work (see pp224–6).

Medication As an outpatient, you may benefit from medications. Antidepressants (SSRIs) may be helpful in treatment (see p227). Ask you doctor about any side effects.

HOW CAN I HELP MYSELF?

Once you have been to see your doctor, you must make sure to follow your treatment plan.

DO I HAVE THE SYMPTOMS?

You may have bulimia if:
- At least twice a week for at least three months you have binged, eating excessive amounts in a two-hour period
- You repeatedly vomit, use laxatives or diuretics, or exercise excessively to prevent weight gain
- You overvalue your body shape and/or weight
- Symptoms occur separately from those of anorexia.

See your doctor if you have these symptoms.

AM I AT RISK?

You are at a greater risk of developing bulimia if:
- You are an adolescent
- You have begun dieting and are anxious about your weight
- You have a family history of eating disorders
- You suffer from anxiety disorders, substance dependency, or impulsive disorders (typically shopping disorders, sexual promiscuity, and self-harm).

Personality disorders

Our personality—the way we think, feel, and behave—makes us what we are. Sometimes a person behaves consistently in ways that produce recurrent problems in everyday life; such a person may have a personality disorder. The following are some of the personality disorders most common in women.

Borderline personality disorder

From time to time we all feel uncertain about our self-worth, or feel moody, isolated, impulsive, or fragile. People with borderline personality disorder (BPD) have these feelings—and others—in the extreme. BPD usually appears by late adolescence or early adulthood.

WHAT IS IT?

If you suffer from borderline personality disorder (BPD), as well as having the characteristic symptoms (see Do I have the symptoms?) you may also exhibit "splitting" behavior, in which you view the world in black and white—for example, seeing people as either perfect or evil—and this can make it difficult to establish and maintain relationships with friends, partners, and work colleagues.

People who suffer from BPD are at increased risk of also having major depressive disorder (see pp210–11) and/or a substance abuse problem (see pp220–1). They also have a high risk of self-harm, and about 9 percent take their own lives.

WHAT NEXT?

Your doctor will make a diagnosis based on your symptoms.

MY TREATMENT OPTIONS

The main options are therapy and medication, or both.

Therapy Dialectical behavior therapy (DBT, see p225) is a specific type of therapy helpful in the treatment of BPD.

Medication SSRI antidepressants and antipsychotic medications (see pp226–7) are the main types of medication used for BPD. Ask your doctor about any side effects.

HOW CAN I HELP MYSELF?

You should follow the treatment plan set out by your doctor. You may find that relaxation exercises (see pp62–3) and regular exercise (see pp56–7) help reduce stress.

DO I HAVE THE SYMPTOMS?

BPD manifests itself as a pervasive pattern of instability in several areas, with at least five of the following symptoms:

- Fear of being abandoned, and going out of your way to make sure that others don't leave you
- A pattern of unstable and intense relationships, both romantic and platonic. There is a tendency to idealize or dismiss people quickly, often the same individuals at different times
- Feelings of insecurity or uncertainty about who you are
- Impulsive behavior in at least two self-destructive areas, including spending, sexual activity, substance abuse, reckless driving, or binge eating
- Thoughts of, or attempts at, self-harm or suicide
- Intense moods that last for a few hours but less than a few days
- Chronic feelings of emptiness
- A strong temper and difficulty controlling yourself
- During times of stress, becoming paranoid (fearing things that are not in fact real) or feeling cut off from yourself.

See your doctor if you have had five or more of these experiences.

Dependent personality disorder

At some times in our lives we all need to be taken care of. But for people with dependent personality disorder (DPD) the reliance on others is so extreme they cannot function independently in daily life.

WHAT IS IT?

If you have DPD, you rely on others for every decision and tend to do what others want. You may also be anxious and depressed, abuse substances, and engage in abusive relationships.

WHAT NEXT?

Your doctor will make a diagnosis based on your symptoms.

MY TREATMENT OPTIONS

The main treatments for DPD are therapy, medication, or a combination of the two.

Therapy Commonly used therapies for DPD include psychodynamic, behavioral, and cognitive–behavioral therapy (see pp224–5).

Medication Specific symptoms may be treated with antidepressants or antianxiety medications (see p227). Ask your doctor about any side effects.

HOW CAN I HELP MYSELF?

You should make sure to follow your treatment plan.

DO I HAVE THE SYMPTOMS?

The following may indicate DPD:
- Fear of being left alone to care for yourself
- Difficulty doing things on your own due to low self-confidence
- Difficulty making everyday decisions without advice
- Needing someone else to assume responsibility for most major areas of your life
- Reluctance to disagree with others
- Actively seeking nurturing and support from other people

See your doctor if at least five of the above apply to you.

Histrionic personality disorder

We all overdramatize at times, but if this is your normal way of behaving and it causes you problems, you may have histrionic personality disorder. (HPD).

WHAT IS IT?

If you have HPD, you tend to have heightened emotions and react overdramatically to situations and relationships. It can affect all your relationships as well as how you react to losses or failures. You are also at increased risk of suffering from depression.

WHAT NEXT?

Your doctor will make a diagnosis based on your symptoms.

MY TREATMENT OPTIONS

The main treatments for HPD are therapy, medication, or both.

Therapy The goal of therapy is to target the problematic thoughts, behaviors, and feelings. Commonly used therapies include psychodynamic, behavioral, and cognitive–behavioral therapy (see pp224–5).

Medication The main medication options are antidepressants or antianxiety medications (see p227). Ask you doctor about any side effects.

HOW CAN I HELP MYSELF?

You should make sure to follow your treatment plan.

DO I HAVE THE SYMPTOMS?

The following may indicate HPD:
- You are moody, with rapid, shallow emotional shifts
- You are uncomfortable when not the center of attention
- You are often inappropriately sexually seductive/provocative
- You draw attention to yourself by your physical appearance
- You talk in an affected way
- You are overly dramatic
- You are easily influenced
- You consider relationships to be more intimate than they actually are.

See your doctor if at least five of the above apply to you.

Substance abuse and dependency

Drinking alcohol and taking recreational or prescription drugs are a part of the fabric of modern society, even though we know they can be harmful. Unfortunately, these habits can so easily lead to dependency and abuse, with potentially devastating consequences.

Alcohol abuse and dependency

An estimated 6 percent of adults worldwide will be diagnosed with alcoholism at some point. Most are men, but roughly a third are women.

WHAT IS IT?

Alcohol abuse occurs when drinking regularly creates problems in your daily life. Alcohol dependency is even more serious because you develop a tolerance. This means that you have to drink more and more to get the same effect, and when you don't drink, you have withdrawal symptoms.

Alcoholism is destructive to your well-being, makes you prone to a variety of illnesses (see p65), and can increase your risk of rape, unintended pregnancy, fetal alcohol syndrome, and breast cancer.

WHAT NEXT?

If you have problems, you need to seek professional help.

MY TREATMENT OPTIONS

Unsupervised withdrawal from alcohol can have deadly consequences, so should be done under professional care. Ask about the side effects of any medication.

Medical stabilization and detoxification Early on in withdrawal, you need medical and psychological support and care. Withdrawal symptoms are treated with benzodiazepines (see p227) to prevent seizures, shakes, hallucinations, and the DTs (delirium tremens). If you have any alcohol-related diseases or nutritional deficiencies, you will also have treatment for these.

Rehabilitation You may need a residential or outpatient program—for example AA's 12-step program.

HOW CAN I HELP MYSELF?

You must follow your treatment plan and go to your appointments.

DO I HAVE THE SYMPTOMS?

You may be abusing alcohol if, over 12 months, your drinking has led to one or more of the following:

- Inability to meet your major responsibilities at work, school, or home
- Drinking during dangerous activities (e.g. driving)
- Having legal problems
- Drinking despite knowing the problems it causes.

You may be dependent on alcohol if, over 12 months, you have three or more of the following:

- Increased tolerance to alcohol
- Withdrawal symptoms if you cut down or stop, or increased drinking to avoid withdrawal symptoms
- Drinking larger amounts over a longer period of time than you intended
- Inability to cut down on your drinking despite wanting to
- Drinking intrudes on the time you spend in social, recreational, or work activities
- Continuing to drink despite knowing the problems it causes.

See your doctor if you think you may have an alcohol problem.

Prescription drug abuse and dependency

Women are prescribed more prescription drugs, especially painkillers and antianxiety drugs, than men. This means women have more access to them and therefore may be at greater risk for abusing them.

WHAT IS IT?

Abuse of and dependence on prescription and recreational drugs is essentially the same as abuse of and dependence on alcohol, and the features that are used to diagnose drug abuse and dependence are the same as those for alcohol (see opposite).

Drug addiction is a brain disease and, over time, it will cause changes in the brain itself that will make it difficult for you to control yourself and will continue the chronic cycle of addiction.

WHAT NEXT?

If you have problems you need to seek professional help.

DO I HAVE THE SYMPTOMS?

The general symptoms of drug abuse and dependency are the same as those of alcohol abuse and dependency, as described opposite in Do I have the symptoms?
See your doctor if you think you may have a drug problem.

MY TREATMENT OPTIONS

You will be given a treatment plan based on your psychological, medical, and social profile, and the drug that is being abused. If you are taking prescription drugs and are concerned about the possibility of becoming addicted to them, talk to your doctor about when and how to take them, and about any possible side effects. If you take the following drugs as prescribed by your doctor, it is unlikely that you will have a problem.

Opioids These include painkillers such as codeine, morphine, oxycodone, and hydrocodone. They give you a sense of euphoria and make you feel sedated, but the risks are confusion, gastrointestinal symptoms, and coma.

Antianxiety medications These include sedatives and tranquilizers, such as benzodiazepines. They lower your inhibitions and decrease your anxiety, but the risks include poor concentration, passing out, coma, and, if breathing stops, death.

Stimulants These treat attention-deficit hyperactivity disorder (ADHD), the sleep disorder narcolepsy, and obesity. They include amphetamines that produce a high-energy state, but the risks are heart attack, weight loss, insomnia, paranoia, and panic.

HOW CAN I HELP MYSELF?

You must be sure to follow the treatment plan offered to you and go to all your appointments.

The following is a brief summary of some of the short-term effects and mental and physical health risks associated with some of the more commonly used recreational drugs.

Drug	Short-term effects	Health risks
Marijuana	Euphoria, sedation	Anxiety/panic attacks, confusion, paranoia, psychosis
Cocaine	Increased energy/mental alertness	Cardiovascular complications, stroke, seizures, heart attack
Ecstasy (MDMA)	Altered state of feeling/perception	Heart, kidney, and liver toxicity
Heroin	Pain relief, euphoria	Dangerous slowing of breathing, coma
PCP (phencyclidine)	Aggression	Memory impairment, cardiovascular problems
LSD	Altered state of feeling/perception	Persistent mental problems, cardiovascular risk

Sexual disorders

Modern society places great importance on having a good sex life, but many women experience sexual problems at some time. However, you should not focus on whether your sex life is "normal," but you should consider seeking help if it is a significant source of stress or negative feelings for you personally.

Hypoactive sexual desire disorder

Everyone lacks desire at some time, perhaps because of relationship problems or due to the stresses and strains of everyday life. However, for absence of interest in sex to qualify as a disorder, it must be something that is causing you significant problems and stress.

WHAT IS IT?

If you have this disorder you rarely, if ever, have any sexual fantasies or desire for sex, and this is a source of stress. It is the most common sexual disorder in women, and may be due to a drop in hormone levels through the onset of menopause, as well as some medications, such as drugs for high blood pressure (see p172) and a number of SSRI antidepressants (see p227). However, there may be psychological causes, perhaps if you have had a bad sexual experience in the past.

WHAT NEXT?

Your doctor will make a diagnosis based on a description of your symptoms and will refer you to a therapist if necessary.

MY TREATMENT OPTIONS

Therapy can help you work through any negative past sexual experiences that may be a factor.

DO I HAVE THE SYMPTOMS?

The following symptoms may indicate you have this condition:
- Lack of desire for sex
- Rarely having sexual fantasies.

See your doctor if you are distressed by your symptoms.

HOW CAN I HELP MYSELF?

Your therapist will guide you, but the following may be of help:

Fantasy and masturbation
These may help you achieve a good experience, which may make it more likely that you are able to desire such an experience with your partner.

Female sexual arousal disorder

DO I HAVE THE SYMPTOMS?

The following symptoms may indicate that you have this condition:
- Lack of arousal during sex

See your doctor if you are distressed by your symptoms.

There are times when we all find it difficult to become sexually aroused, due to interpersonal, psychological, or physical factors. It becomes a disorder if it causes you significant distress.

WHAT IS IT?

During sexual arousal your heart rate and breathing become faster, there is increased lubrication to your vagina and blood flow to the clitoris, and your nipples harden. If you suffer from female sexual arousal disorder, you can't experience this arousal phase and that will be the case long term.

This disorder often has an underlying physical cause, such as injury or surgery to the pelvis, hormonal changes, or side effects from medication. If you have hypoactive sexual desire disorder (see left) or dyspareunia (painful intercourse, see p109) you may be at a greater risk. There may be psychological factors, too.

WHAT NEXT?
Since the cause of sexual arousal disorder is often physical, your doctor will do an examination and workup, and will take a complete medical history. He or she will make a diagnosis based on the findings.

MY TREATMENT OPTIONS
Your doctor will help you find the best treatment. If necessary, he or she will refer you to a therapist. Even if your doctor can't find a physical or psychological cause, you may be offered medication. Ask about any possible side effects.

Medication You may be offered medication such as a vaginal lubricant or topical estrogen cream, especially if you are suffering from postmenopausal vaginal dryness, to help relieve any discomfort.

HOW CAN I HELP MYSELF?
Be aware of your sexual feelings and behavior, and talk to you doctor if they are a source of stress.

Female orgasmic disorder

Women's magazines are full of advice on "how to have an orgasm." And no wonder. It's something many women have a problem with at some time. However, for about five percent of women, it's always problematic and they have a chronic inability to reach orgasm.

WHAT IS IT?
If you cannot reach orgasm, even though your sexual desire is normal and you go through a normal sexual excitement phase, you may have female orgasmic disorder. Over the course of their lifetime, 16–30 percent of all women may experience it.

There are two types, but they are only considered to be disorders if they cause you significant distress:
- Total female orgasmic disorder means that you are unable to have an orgasm during any sexual experience.
- Partial female orgasmic disorder means you can orgasm from some sexual experiences (such as, clitoral stimulation or oral sex), but not during intercourse. Some antianxiety and antidepressant medications (see pp226–7) may have side effects that stop you from having an orgasm. Worrying about intimacy in your relationship, or being generally anxious may also be a factor. If you're less sexually experienced, you are more likely to have difficulty with orgasm and, of course, early ejaculation in your partner may be a factor.

WHAT NEXT?
Your doctor will make a diagnosis based on your symptoms.

MY TREATMENT OPTIONS
If your doctor thinks that the medication you are taking for some other condition is causing your problem, then he or she will discuss with you the risks and benefits of changing your medication. Ask about any other possible side effects.

HOW CAN I HELP MYSELF?
The following self-help measures may be useful:
Masturbation This will help you learn more about your body and what gives you pleasure.
Kegel exercises These exercises may help increase orgasm during intercourse (see p341).
Different sexual positions During sex, experiment with different positions and techniques to find those that help you to be more in control or free in your movement, or that incorporate manual clitoral stimulation (with hands or a vibrator).

DO I HAVE THE SYMPTOMS?

The following symptoms may indicate you have this condition:
- Inability to have an orgasm at any time
- Inability to have an orgasm during intercourse.

See your doctor if you are distressed by your symptoms.

Mental health treatment options

If you are suffering from a mental health problem you should first visit your doctor, who will try to find the right kind of treatment for you. There is a wide range of different therapies and medications available, and the main ones are summarized and explained in the next few pages.

After talking with you and listening to your troubles, your doctor will assess the kind of treatment you might need. He or she may be able to treat any of your symptoms that are mild or straightforward, but for more complicated problems, your doctor will refer you to a specialist in "talk therapies" (see opposite) or to someone who also specializes in prescribing medication (a psychiatrist). Throughout the process toward treatment, you will undergo the crucial steps of screening and diagnosis.

The next four pages explain the "menu" of treatment options that are available. The two main approaches to reducing symptoms are psychotherapies (when you talk to a professional about your thoughts and feelings) and medications (drugs that change the chemistry in your brain to regulate your mood and behavior). Your doctor will recommend if you need one or the other, choosing from the range of options outlined here. Most people do best with a combination of both.

Therapies

There are many different approaches to psychotherapy, and all of them involve some kind of talking, which is why they are often called "talk therapies." Ideally, you will meet face to face with a therapist, although some therapists offer the chance to talk things through over the phone or on the Internet. Therapy can be either one on one, with a whole family, as a couple, or with a group who shares the same symptoms or problem. Many different mental health professionals are trained as therapists (psychiatrists, social workers, nurse practitioners, psychologists, counselors, coaches), but only psychiatrists are licensed to prescribe medications.

PSYCHODYNAMIC THERAPY

This therapy is based on the idea that painful emotions and feelings buried in your unconscious need to come to the surface so you can experience and understand them. Often these hidden feelings stem from past experiences, so your therapist may want to explore your

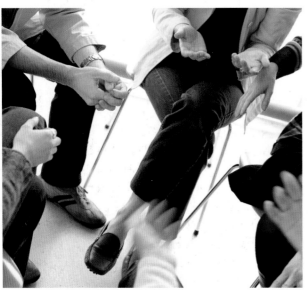

Talk therapies
Another term for psychotherapies, talk therapies come in many forms. They can involve anything from two people—the therapist and the person who is looking for help—talking together in a room, to a group of people who come together to work on a shared problem.

childhood memories; your dreams, which may give clues to your innermost fears, as well as your conflicts in daily life.

PSYCHOANALYSIS

This is an intensive "talk therapy" that is similar to, but more intense than, psychodynamic therapy. It is a long-term therapy, taking several years, and may involve 3–5 sessions a week. Usually you lie on a couch while your analyst helps you become more self-aware, often pointing out how patterns in your life are played out in your relationship with your therapist.

COGNITIVE-BEHAVIORAL THERAPY (CBT)

Consisting of a program that lasts for 16–20 weeks, CBT focuses on specific patterns of thinking or behavior that give you problems and shows you how you can change these irrational or unhelpful patterns. You are given homework assignments, such as keeping a diary of events that upset you, so you can explore your thoughts and feelings with your therapist.

BRIEF DYNAMIC THERAPY

This focused, short-term treatment, based on psychodynamic technique, is tailored to a specific problem in your life rather than looking into other larger issues.

BEHAVIORAL THERAPY

The goal of this therapy is to change your dysfunctional patterns of behavior by teaching you how to respond to things differently; the focus is on outward behavior, not internal states, with the emphasis on rewards and not punishments. Behavioral therapy often includes exercises such as relaxation training, stress management, and biofeedback (see right). The latter uses physical signs from your body, such as heart rate, to get information about and control your mental state in a stressful setting.

DIALECTICAL BEHAVIOR THERAPY (DBT)

This is a specific type of therapy that was originally designed for borderline personality disorder (see p218), although it may be useful for other problems, too. Its techniques are similar to those used in CBT. The goal of DBT is to teach you self-awareness, how to get along with other people, control of your emotions, how to avoid acting impulsively, and how to calm yourself down.

EXPOSURE THERAPY AND DESENSITIZATION (EDT)

Often known simply as EDT, this is a specific branch of behavioral therapy and CBT in which you must face your particular fear, either virtually, in the safety of the therapy room, or in reality. For example, if you have a fear of heights, your therapist will actually go with you to a bridge. This form of therapy may take you either gradually or suddenly through the process of exposure and desensitization.

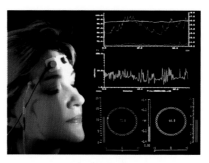

Biofeedback machine
This apparatus monitors the physical signs that accompany different moods.

SUPPORTIVE PSYCHOTHERAPY

This therapy is widely used to bolster self-esteem and coping mechanisms, and to help you become more successful in daily life. You may have a number of brief therapy sessions over a long period or a few extended sessions over a shorter period.

INTERPERSONAL THERAPY (IPT)

A short-term therapy often used to treat depression, IPT focuses on how the stresses of everyday life can trigger symptoms, and how emotional difficulties can lead to problematic behaviors. It is based on the theory that psychological problems may be caused by the way in which you relate to others.

GESTALT THERAPY

This therapy focuses on the here and now. It is based on the belief that the best way to understand yourself is to look at how you relate to others in a given context. Gestalt therapy emphasizes personal responsibility.

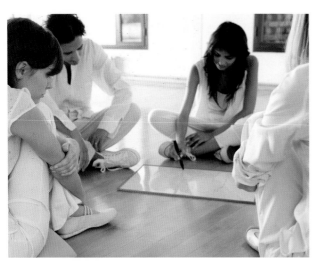

Art therapy
For people who struggle to express their thoughts and feelings, art therapy may be an effective way to communicate difficult emotions. Sessions may be one on one with the therapist or in a group situation.

SPIRITUAL AND EXISTENTIAL THERAPY

This focuses on the meaning of your behavior in the context of both your past and the human condition in general. It may use methods from other therapy types, as well as spiritual or religious readings to help you better find the meaning in your life.

INTEGRATIVE THERAPY (ECLECTIC)

Incorporating the various practices of psychotherapy, integrative therapy also includes aspects of other therapeutic approaches.

MOVEMENT/DANCE/ART/ MUSIC THERAPIES

These therapies use different arts to help you express your feelings. This practice is helpful for people who have difficulties putting their emotions into words.

FAMILY THERAPY

This therapy involves either part or all of a family coming together for therapy sessions. Some sessions may include only certain individuals to focus on specific issues. This is often useful when one family member has a problem that affects the others.

COUPLES THERAPY

This therapy involves a couple attending sessions together to address their relationship issues.

GROUP THERAPY

This is a process of sharing with others who have the same problem. It is facilitated by a group leader.

Medications

Drugs that treat mental health problems are known as psychotropic medications, and they are designed to have an effect on the chemistry of the brain. Many are good at controlling symptoms but they do not make the illness itself go away. A drug may be helpful or not; it all depends on the circumstances of

your body and illness. Sometimes, you may only need to take a medication for a few months; other people may take medications for their whole lives.

Psychiatrists have the most extensive training in psychotropic medications; they know the differences between the drugs and are trained in how to find the right match, dose, and timeline for you. Other types of doctors may also prescribe psychotropic medications for basic care. The following are general categories of medications, and you should refer to specific articles for the most commmonly prescribed medications for each illness.

ANTIPSYCHOTIC MEDICATIONS

Antipsychotic medications are designed to help people who suffer from diseases that confuse their understanding of reality. These drugs, also called neuroleptics, target brain chemicals, such as dopamine, that are thought to be out of balance. If you need to take these, your doctor will monitor you carefully for side effects such as changes in your blood count, weight gain, or diabetes.

MOOD STABILIZERS

These drugs help people feel on a more even keel, so they don't have any dangerous highs and lows. Mood stabilizers may be combined with antipsychotics or antidepressants. Many people need to stay on these medications for their whole lives to keep their mood stable and to reduce the kind of episodes that cause them problems. Some of these medications have significant side effects, so you may need monitoring with blood tests.

Mood stabilizers include lithium, valproic acid (Depakote, divalproex sodium), carbamazepine (Tegretol), and lamotrigine (Lamictal). You must not stop taking these medications suddenly, but follow the advice from your doctor who will gradually reduce your medication to avoid side effects.

ANTIANXIETY MEDICATIONS

Medications that relieve anxiety, called anxiolytics, include benzodiazepines. SSRI and SNRI antidepressants (see antidepressant medications) are also used to treat anxiety symptoms.

Benzodiazepines are drugs that work quickly to relieve anxiety, but they can make you feel drowsy and you can get addicted to them if you use them incorrectly. You can take benzodiazepines daily, several times daily, or only when you need to. If you drink alcohol while taking them, it can be dangerous and even life threatening.

These drugs are rarely used to treat anxiety long-term. If you decide to stop, you must consult with your doctor, because withdrawal can be difficult and dangerous. Benzodiazepines include clonazepam (Klonopin), alprazolam (Xanax), diazepam (Valium), and lorazepam (Ativan).

ANTIDEPRESSANT MEDICATIONS

Antidepressants are used to relieve the symptoms of depression and anxiety. Rather then being "uppers" or stimulants (which stimulate your central nervous system, increasing your heart rate and speeding up your mental alertness, for example, caffeine or cocaine), antidepressant medications simply make you feel like yourself again. They may help you fairly quickly, but it may take up to 8–12 weeks to feel the effects. It is important to work with your doctor to decide if a medication is working, and what to do next.

Most people stay on the drug for 6–12 months, even when they are feeling better. If you decide to stop, your doctor should reduce your dose gradually to avoid any withdrawal symptoms.

Selective serotonin reuptake inhibitors (SSRIs) These are one of the newest classes of antidepressants and they have the mildest side effects. They work by targeting the brain chemical serotonin. Some SSRIs may have some side effects, such as sexual problems, insomnia, and weight gain. SSRIs include fluoxetine (Prozac), sertraline (Zoloft), fluvoxamine (Luvox), paroxetine (Paxil), citalopram (Celexa), and escitalopram (Lexapro).

Tricyclic antidepressants (TCAs) These are among the oldest drugs for depression. They mostly target two brain chemicals—the neurotransmitters noradrenaline and serotonin. Although they are effective, they are not used so often because they can have unpleasant side effects, such as constipation, dry mouth, sexual problems, and dizziness. However, they may be a good option if the newer drugs don't work well for you. Tricyclics include amitriptyline, nortriptyline, imipramine, and desipramine.

Serotonergic noradrenergic reuptake inhibitors (SNRIs) These medications are used to combat depression and anxiety by acting on the same brain chemicals as the tricyclics: noradrenaline and serotonin. The SNRIs venlafaxine (Effexor) and duloxetine (Cymbalta) combine the features of SSRIs and TCAs.

Other antidepressants These are medications that don't fit into any of the other main groups of antidepressants, such as mirtazepine (Remeron), bupropion (Wellbutrin), and nefazadone (Serzone). These medications work in unique ways and have specific advantages. For example, Wellbutrin is one of the few drugs that rarely results in side effects such as weight gain or sexual problems.

Monoamine oxidase inhibitors (MAOIs) These are older drugs that are rarely used because they usually require you to be on a strict diet, since certain foods and drink cause dangerous side effects. MAOIs include phenelzine (Nardil), tranylcypromine (Parnate), isocarboxazid (Marplan), and selegiline (Zelapar).

Breathing and respiration

Cordelia T. Grimm MD MPH

Breathing and respiration

From the moment we emerge into this world, we breathe completely automatically and unconsciously. Breathing in is just the first step in a complex process that uses gas exchange to supply the oxygen we need to power our bodies; breathing out takes away the carbon dioxide waste product that is produced. Just like other body systems, such as your heart or muscles, your entire respiratory system is capable of responding to all the various demands you place on it—from running for a bus to doing a marathon.

WHAT IS THE RESPIRATORY SYSTEM?

You can think of your respiratory system as being made of two fundamental parts: an upper and a lower respiratory tract. The upper respiratory tract consists of your nose, sinuses, mouth, throat (pharynx), and voice box (larynx); the lower respiratory tract consists of the windpipe (trachea) and the tubes that branch from that in ever-decreasing sizes (bronchi and bronchioles), ending in millions of tiny balloon-like sacs called alveoli, within the lungs.

The main function of the respiratory system is to supply oxygen to the blood, which absorbs it and carries

WHAT HAPPENS WHEN YOU BREATHE

When you breathe, air flows down the trachea, into the bronchi and through smaller and smaller bronchioles until it reaches tiny, gas-permeable air sacs, the alveoli. In the alveoli, oxygen from the air diffuses into the blood stream, to be transported to all the cells of your body. At the same time, carbon dioxide waste produced by your body diffuses from the blood into the alveoli, to be breathed out.

Right lung

Larynx (voice box) contains the vocal cords

Pharynx (throat) links the back of the mouth and nose to the larynx and esophagus

Trachea is the main airway from the larynx to the lungs

Left lung

Bronchus branches from the trachea and divides into smaller airways

Heart

Alveoli

Diaphragm is the main muscle used for breathing in and out

Alveoli are tiny air sacs that pass oxygen into the blood

Bronchioles are tiny airways connected to the bronchus

it to all parts of the body, and to remove the waste-product carbon dioxide from it. Oxygen is required by every cell in the body and because it cannot be stored, we need a continuous supply from the outside air.

A healthy person breathes between 12 and 20 times per minute at rest. How fast and how deeply we breathe depends on our size and on how fit we are. Generally, an adult woman inhales about 16–18 fl oz (450–500 ml) of air—about the size of a pint of milk—in a normal breath, and can take in about 7 pints (4 litres) with a maximal breath. On average, lung capacity in men is 25 to 30 percent higher.

Breathing is one of the few automatic bodily functions that we can consciously control. Taking slow deep breaths can help us handle stress, as demonstrated by the techniques taught to women in labor through the Lamaze method.

BREATHING AND EXERCISE

As we get older, the amount of air we can breathe (lung capacity) and the amount of oxygen we can extract from each breath declines, but this doesn't mean an inevitable decline in fitness. Women of all ages should be able to exercise for 30 to 60 minutes and not get out of breath. If you are 35 years old, then you should be able to cycle at 15 mph (24 kph), play vigorous singles tennis, or jog 1 mile (1.6 km) in 10 minutes. If you are 50, then you should be able to jog 1 mile (1.6 km) in 12 minutes, and swim or walk vigorously. If you are 65 years old you should be able to cycle at 10 mph (16 kph), dance, or play doubles tennis. Even if you are 80, you should still be able to walk 1 mile (1.6 km) in less than 20 minutes, play golf (but no club carrying), or do water aerobics.

THE EFFECTS OF SMOKING

There is one huge threat to breathing (and health) that affects all parts of the respiratory system—cigarette

> "Breathing is one of the few bodily functions that can be controlled consciously and unconsciously."

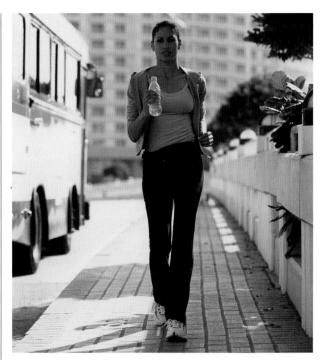

Benefits of exercise
Any vigorous exercise, such as power walking or jogging, will make you breathe harder and deeper, strengthening your lungs and delivering more oxygen to your body.

smoking. Smokers run a higher risk of developing each and every respiratory illness from coughs and colds (see p232) and laryngitis (see p236) to asthma (see pp238–9) and lung cancer (see pp242–3).

As a smoker you not only affect your own health but also the health of those around you, including your children and grandchildren. Living with a smoker puts children at a higher risk of developing asthma and allergies, and of missing school with colds and other respiratory infections. If the smoker in the family is the father, the risk rises by about one-third; but if mummy smokes, the risk goes up by a massive three-quarters.

People who grow up in a household with smokers are three times more likely to get lung cancer than people who grow up in non-smoking households, even if they don't smoke themselves. So, if you smoke, try to stop now (see p64); if you get enough support from family and friends as well as a smoking cessation clinic, you can make it the last time you quit. You want to be playing golf and swimming at 80, don't you?

Colds, flu, and chest infections

Colds and coughs are common infections and hard to avoid. As you grow older you may find it more difficult to shake off a cold and it might worsen into a chest infection, such as bronchitis, or, more seriously, pneumonia. Fortunately, these more severe conditions usually respond to antibiotic treatment.

Colds, flu, and acute bronchitis

DO I HAVE THE SYMPTOMS?

Colds, the flu, and acute bronchitis share many symptoms—it's their severity, location, and duration that defines them. Cold symptoms usually include:

- Sore throat
- Nasal congestion
- Sneezing
- Cough.

The flu can be dangerous, especially if you're over 65. Symptoms usually include:

- Fever over 102° F (39° C)
- Chills and sweats
- Muscle aches and fatigue
- Nasal congestion
- Sore throat
- Cough.

Acute bronchitis is inflammation of the airways and symptoms may include:

- Sore throat
- Nasal congestion
- Cough
- Shortness of breath
- Wheeziness.

See your doctor if symptoms persist for over a week.

If you're in good health, a cold is unlikely to be more than a nuisance. The flu, on the other hand, will probably keep you in bed for a few days. Acute bronchitis can also be debilitating.

WHAT ARE THEY?

A bad cold is often described as flu, but they're distinct respiratory infections. Acute bronchitis is characterized by chest symptoms, so confusion with colds and flu is less likely. However, a cold may develop into bronchitis.

You can pick up cold and flu viruses by touch or inhalation of particles that are released in a sneeze, so infection is more likely to occur in autumn and winter when people spend more time indoors together. There are more than 100 common cold viruses, and catching one gives you immunity against that virus only. There are fewer flu viruses and immunity lasts about 10 years.

WHAT NEXT?

If you have a cold, you won't get better faster by staying home, but at least you won't infect your work colleagues. If your symptoms don't improve or you develop a bacterial infection, then see a doctor.

MY TREATMENT OPTIONS

If you're in a high-risk group—for example, if you're elderly, suffer from respiratory problems, or have a compromised immune system—you must have an annual flu vaccine, since you're also more at risk of getting complications such as

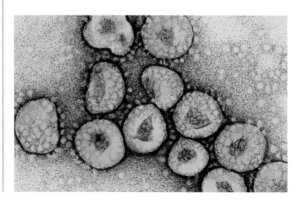

Coronavirus
About 10–30 percent of common colds are caused by a coronavirus.

pneumonia (see p234) or a bacterial infection. If you do have the flu, your doctor may prescribe antiviral medication such as olsetamivir (Tamiflu) or zanamivir (Relenza). You may be given antibiotics if you have acute bronchitis and you're in poor health generally or have a long-standing respiratory problem, such as asthma or emphysema. Your doctor may also prescribe bronchodilators for acute bronchitis.

HOW CAN I HELP MYSELF?

Rest—in bed if you're suffering from the flu or acute bronchitis— will help you recover more quickly.

To relieve symptoms, take:

- Plenty of hot liquids
- Analgesics such as ibuprofen and acetaminophen (but not aspirin)
- Decongestants
- Antihistamines
- Bronchodilators (for acute bronchitis).

To minimize infection:

- Wash your hands before eating or food preparation, particularly after touching an infected person
- Avoid touching your face, especially your nose
- Try not to remain near an infected person
- Don't share towels and wash-cloths with an infected person
- Keep surfaces clean
- Don't smoke.

Chronic cough

Coughing is a reflex action stimulated by specialized nerves in your respiratory system, designed to remove irritants such as dust or mucus from your airways. Most respiratory infections cause coughs, but they usually get better without treatment.

WHAT IS IT?

A chronic cough lasts for eight weeks or more. Because women have a more sensitive cough reflex than men, they are almost twice as likely to be susceptible.

One of the most common causes is chronic bronchitis. Often described as "smoker's cough," this is a phlegm-producing cough that is caused by narrowed, mucus-filled airways.

About one in two cases of a chronic dry cough is a result of postnasal drip (PND), in which excessive mucus is produced by the sinuses and accumulates in the throat, causing you to cough in

order to clear it. Other possible causes include asthma (see pp238–9), eosinophilic bronchitis, gastroesophageal reflux (see pp290–1), and sinusitis (see p235).

Women are more prone to a chronic cough around the time of menopause, if they smoke, and if they are overweight.

WHAT NEXT?

A careful history and physical examination can sometimes give your doctor clues about why you are coughing. Be sure to mention all your medications, since some can make you cough as a side effect. If a cause can be found, your cough will probably stop once the underlying problem is treated.

MY TREATMENT OPTIONS

Your treatment options depend on the underlying cause of your cough, but you may find that over-the-counter medications such as cough syrups and lozenges may give symptomatic relief, as well as drinking plenty of water.

DO I HAVE THE SYMPTOMS?

Symptoms may include:
- Persistent cough

See your doctor if symptoms persist for three weeks since it may indicate something serious.

HOW CAN I HELP MYSELF?

There are many self-help measures to ease a chronic cough including:

Don't smoke Over 50 percent of people with a chronic cough are smokers. If you need help with quitting smoking, ask your doctor for advice.

Avoid dust, chemicals, and indoor pollutants as far as possible since this may ease the problem. You may be particularly sensitive to aerosols such as hair spray or perfume, in which case try to find alternatives.

Lose weight if you're carrying extra pounds; you may discover that losing weight will help alleviate your symptoms.

Pneumonia

While pneumonia remains one of the top 10 causes of death in the US, vaccinations and antibiotics have lessened its devastating effects. It can affect otherwise healthy people, but is most common and most dangerous among the very young, the very old, and people who are seriously ill or have long-term ill health.

WHAT IS IT?

Pneumonia is inflammation of the lung, particularly of the alveoli (air sacs), making it difficult for oxygen to reach the blood. Infections from a virus or bacterium cause most cases of pneumonia, but sometimes a fungus, spirochete, or parasite is responsible. In the US, fungal pneumonia usually affects only people with a weakened immune system or a chronic respiratory problem, although it is more common in some other parts of the world including South and Central America and Africa.

WHAT NEXT?

Your doctor will order an X-ray of your chest, check the oxygen level in your blood with a pulse oximeter (a monitor that fits over your finger), and take blood for testing. If you're coughing up phlegm, your doctor will take a sample for laboratory analysis.

You can be treated at home if you have a mild form of the condition, if you are generally in good health, and you have a normal level of oxygen in your blood. However, many people suffering from pneumonia need to be treated in the hospital.

MY TREATMENT OPTIONS

Pneumonia is treated with drugs, and the medication you will be given will depend on the type of pneumonia you have.

Bacterial pneumonia will be treated with antibiotics. If you don't start to improve within two days of taking the antibiotics, tell your doctor, who may want to try a different type of antibiotic.

Viral pneumonia may be treated with antiviral medications. Viruses weaken your ability to fight off infection and temporarily damage your lungs, so you may also be given a course of antibiotics to prevent bacteria from causing a secondary infection.

DO I HAVE THE SYMPTOMS?

The more of these symptoms you have, the more likely you are to be suffering from pneumonia:
- Fever, or an abnormally low temperature
- Drenching sweats
- Cough, especially with phlegm
- Blood in the phlegm
- Shortness of breath
- Rapid breathing
- Chest tightness
- Fatigue
- Muscle aches
- Headache.

See your doctor if you have four or more of these symptoms.

AM I AT RISK?

You may be at higher risk for pneumonia if:
- You have asthma or another chronic respiratory illness
- You're a smoker
- You're over 65
- You are pregnant.

HOW CAN I HELP MYSELF?

A few basic precautions can help you avoid pneumonia, but if you do get it you can take steps to ease the symptoms.

To minimize your chance of catching pneumonia:
- Keep your distance from people with colds or other respiratory infections
- Wash your hands thoroughly after contact with people with respiratory infections
- If you are elderly, have a weakened immune system, or are prone to respiratory problems, ensure that you are vaccinated against the flu and pneumonia. It won't guarantee you avoid pneumonia, but it's likely to be less severe.

For relief of symptoms, try the following:
- Take analgesics such as acetaminophen to ease pain and reduce fever
- Drink plenty of fluids
- Soothe soreness from coughing with warm lemon and honey drinks. Avoid cough suppressants since coughing helps clear mucus from your lungs

Sinusitis

This condition can be very painful, but it's rarely serious and usually clears up on its own. Four pairs of sinuses behind your nose, eyes, cheeks, and forehead clean air before it enters your lungs by trapping small particles and bacteria in the mucus they produce. In sinusitis, they become inflamed and swollen.

DO I HAVE THE SYMPTOMS?

Symptoms vary depending on which sinuses are affected. The most common include:

- Headache that worsens when leaning forward
- Pain/pressure behind or between the eyes
- Pain in the upper teeth
- Postnasal drip (excessive mucus in the back of the nose and throat)
- Nasal congestion
- Sore throat
- Bad breath
- Loss of taste and/or smell
- Cough.

See your doctor if your symptoms are persistent.

WHAT IS IT?

Sinusitis is usually prompted by a cold, but may occasionally be caused by a bacterial or fungal infection. In some women, allergies can cause sinusitis. If you have small sinus drains or a deviated nasal septum (when the cartilage between the nostrils is out of place), you may also have sinus problems. Pregnant women are susceptible because their hormones can make the nose swell and may also increase mucus production.

WHAT NEXT?

Your doctor can usually diagnose sinusitis by your description and an examination. If your symptoms are very severe, or last longer than three months, your doctor may refer you to an ear, nose, and throat specialist (otolaryngologist) who may take a sample of mucus for laboratory analysis and a CT scan of your sinuses.

MY TREATMENT OPTIONS

Unless your symptoms are severe or long lasting, they will probably get better without treatment.
Medication You can take analgesics to reduce a headache, and decongestants to reduce pressure in your face. However, don't take antihistamines because they thicken mucus.

If your symptoms last for more than 10 days, you may need antibiotics. If you have chronic sinusitis, your doctor may prescribe a nasal steroid to reduce swelling that blocks the sinus drains.
Surgery In rare cases of chronic sinusitis, you may need surgery.

HOW CAN I HELP MYSELF?

If you are prone to sinusitis, you can try to avoid recurrences.
Don't smoke.
Protect yourself from chemicals, dust, and any other irritants.
Rinse your sinuses daily with a saline spray or wash.
Use a humidifier, but it must be cleaned regularly to avoid mold.

WHERE ARE MY SINUSES?

You have four pairs of sinuses—the sphenoid, the maxillary, the frontal, and the ethmoid sinuses. Your sinuses are closely connected, and the pain and discomfort of sinusitis may be pinpointed or felt in all areas.

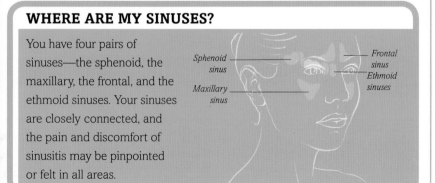

Sphenoid sinus

Maxillary sinus

Frontal sinus

Ethmoid sinuses

Disorders of the throat

When you develop a sore throat and can't swallow, or you lose your voice and can't speak, you soon realize the importance of your throat for eating and breathing. Your larynx and pharynx can become infected with viruses and bacteria, and the vocal cords can develop nodules.

Laryngitis

Laryngitis occurs when the larynx becomes inflamed. It can either be acute, when it comes on suddenly, or chronic, when it lasts for a long time. The symptoms are the same, but the time they have been present suggests the diagnosis.

WHAT IS IT?

Inflammation in acute laryngitis may be caused by an infection, such as the common cold, but also by irritants, such as dust, cigarette smoke, or stomach acid. It may develop if you overuse your voice, which may happen if you are a singer, actor, or teacher.

If the symptoms of laryngitis have lasted for more than three weeks, the condition has become chronic and you need to see your doctor. The chronic condition may be caused by one of a number of other conditions, such as gastro-esophageal reflux, (see pp290–1), nodules (see p237), polyps, or cancer of the larynx.

WHAT NEXT?

If self-help measures (see right) don't relieve your symptoms, or if the hoarseness persists beyond three weeks, get medical advice. Your doctor may refer you to a specialist who will examine your throat with a fiber-optic viewing tube called a laryngoscope. The specialist may take a biopsy (tissue sample) for laboratory analysis.

MY TREATMENT OPTIONS

Most cases of acute laryngitis can be successfully treated at home.

HOW CAN I HELP MYSELF?

If you have laryngitis, self-help measures may relieve the irritating inflammation in your throat.

Gargle with salt water (avoid mouthwashes that use alcohol).

Breathe through your nose.

Use humidifiers, such as baths, showers, and steam inhalation.

Drink warm liquids to soothe your throat.

Avoid talking, whispering, and clearing your throat.

Avoid exposure to irritants, such as dust and cigarette smoke.

DO I HAVE THE SYMPTOMS?

The symptoms may include:

- Sore throat
- Cough
- Hoarseness
- Voice loss.

See your doctor if your symptoms are persistent.

SIDE VIEW OF THE THROAT

The throat (pharynx) connects the back of the mouth and nose to the voice box (larynx) and esophagus. The voice box lies between the throat and windpipe (trachea). The adenoids are made of lymph tissue and help protect against infection. The epiglottis is a flap of cartilage that stops food or liquid from entering your lungs when you swallow.

Adenoids help fight infection

Pharynx, or throat, for swallowing

Epiglottis prevents food entering the lungs

Larynx (voice box) and vocal cords, for producing the sound of the voice

Trachea, or windpipe, for passage of air to the lungs

Pharyngitis

When your throat, or pharynx, becomes inflamed, your doctor may diagnose it as pharyngitis, which simply means a sore throat. You may have pharyngitis with a common cold, often before the nasal symptoms develop.

WHAT IS IT?

Pharyngitis is caused by viral or bacterial infections usually during winter. In most cases it isn't serious and usually clears up within a week without any medical attention.

WHAT NEXT?

If you develop any symptoms in the box (see right), your doctor may take a swab from your throat to see if you have an infection such as strep throat.

MY TREATMENT OPTIONS

Most sore throats can be treated at home, and antibiotics are only used for a bacterial infection.

HOW CAN I HELP MYSELF?

You can help yourself by avoiding using your voice and drinking plenty of liquids. Gargling with salt water may be helpful, too.

DO I HAVE THE SYMPTOMS?

A sore throat may be a symptom of something more serious. If you have any of the following symptoms, see your doctor:

- Fever above 101° F (38° C)
- Swollen glands in the neck
- Spots on the top of the mouth
- Pus from the throat
- Drooling
- Difficulty swallowing
- Rash
- Symptoms lasting more than two weeks.

Vocal cord nodules

Nodules on the vocal cords are small, gray-white growths that range in size from a pinhead to a split pea.

DO I HAVE THE SYMPTOMS?

You may have developed nodules on your vocal cords if you experience one or more of the following symptoms:

- Increasing hoarseness or some other change in the quality of your voice
- Increased effort required to talk or sing
- Painful swallowing (although this is rare).

See your doctor if your symptoms show no improvement after 2–3 weeks.

WHAT IS IT?

Vocal cord nodules usually result from overusing the voice, and are more common in women than men. Alcohol and inhaling cigarette smoke may make the symptoms worse. The people affected include singers, actors, and teachers. Untrained singers tend to be more prone to the problem than singers who have had a formal training.

WHAT NEXT?

Your doctor may refer you to a specialist who will look down your throat with a fiber-optic viewing device called an endoscope to confirm the diagnosis.

MY TREATMENT OPTIONS

The nodules may disappear if you avoid straining your voice. If they don't you may need:

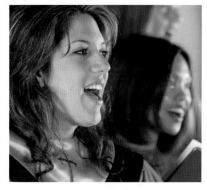

Straining the voice
Singers who put their voice under a great deal of strain may develop nodules.

Voice training or speech therapy to teach you how to avoid straining your voice.
Laser treatment or microsurgery to remove the nodules.

HOW CAN I HELP MYSELF?

Although vocal cord nodules are not a serious health problem, you can help yourself by resting your voice.

Asthma

Asthma has been on the increase over the past 20 years, and it is more common in women than in men. Fortunately, new methods of managing asthma and earlier recognition of symptoms have resulted in fewer hospital admissions. Healthier lifestyles have also contributed to a more positive outlook.

DO I HAVE THE SYMPTOMS?

The symptoms may be subtle in mild asthma, but debilitating in a full-blown attack and include:
- Wheezing
- Coughing—especially at night
- Shortness of breath
- Chest tightness
- Difficulty exercising.

See your doctor if one or more of the above asthma symptoms is very serious or persistent.

Despite the dramatic symptoms of a severe attack, people with asthma can lead normal, active lives. With advice from your doctor, you'll be able to manage or even eliminate your symptoms by making changes to your lifestyle and taking the right combination of medications. It's your responsibility to manage your condition—half of the asthma admissions to the hospital are people who aren't following a prevention plan. Asthma disproportionately affects women.
- 1 in 12 women have asthma compared with 1 in 16 men.
- Women with asthma have more attacks, are hospitalized more often, and are more likely than men to die from asthma.
- During pregnancy, one-third of women don't notice any change in their asthma symptoms, one-third experience an improvement, and one-third get worse.

WHAT IS IT?

Asthma symptoms are caused by inflammation in the airways: the bronchi and bronchioles. The inflamed airways swell, limiting space for air, and produce thick mucus that can plug the narrowed airways. The muscles in the walls also become hyper-responsive—they constrict readily and narrow airways even further.

There are a number of triggers that can cause symptoms. Although production of mucus and constriction of the airways are the lungs' normal responses to toxins, in asthmatics these responses can occur with normally harmless substances, such as:
- Dog or cat dander (skin flakes)
- Mold
- Pollens
- Exercise
- Cold weather
- Emotional upset.

WHAT NEXT?

Your doctor can usually diagnose asthma by your symptoms, and by examining you. You will be asked to breathe into a spirometer—equipment that measures how much air you can blow out after taking a deep breath. Your doctor may ask you to repeat the test after giving you medication to open up your airways. He or she may refer you to a specialist who may order more extensive lung function tests. However, such tests are rarely needed to make the diagnosis or determine the correct treatment.

MY TREATMENT OPTIONS

Your doctor will work with you to develop a plan to prevent attacks, monitor you, and adjust your medications if necessary. The first line of treatment is prevention.

AM I AT RISK?

You may be at risk of asthma if any of the following apply:
- You have a family history of asthma or eczema
- You have many allergies and/or hay fever
- You live in a city.

Medical management depends on how well symptoms are controlled. Your doctor will step up or step down the amount of medications you need based on how often you have breathing problems (see right).

Rescue medication The most familiar asthma medication is a beta-agonist, such as salbutamol or albuterol. When you start to wheeze, shake the inhaler and spray the medication into your mouth as you inhale sharply. Within minutes, the beta-agonist dilates the bronchi and bronchioles and relieves your wheezing.

Controller medication If you need to use your inhaler more than twice a week, your doctor will prescribe a longer-acting controller medication. The first-line controller treatment is an inhaler that contains corticosteroids, such as beclomethasone. You inhale the spray in regular doses over time to reduce airway inflammation.

If your symptoms continue, you will be given a steroid inhaler with a stronger dose, or additional controller medications such as long-acting B-agonists, leukotriene antagonists, or theophylline. People with severe asthma may need high dose corticosteroids in pill form.

Emergency medication For immediate treatment, you may need high-dose rescue beta-agonists delivered in nebulized form along with intravenous corticosteroids.

HOW CAN I HELP MYSELF?

Monitoring your ability to breathe and preventing attacks are key.

Monitor your condition Blow into a peak flow meter each day. If your ability to blow decreases, adjust your medications. If your symptoms are not controlled, you risk an attack that may require hospitalization. Be sure to call your doctor if your symptoms worsen.

Be aware of triggers (see left) and make sure you avoid them.

Get regular, manageable exercise (see pp56–7), which can help reduce your symptoms.

Asthma proof your house:
- Don't smoke or allow anyone else to smoke near you
- Wash all bedding every week to reduce dust mites
- Keep animals out of the house
- Use high-efficiency particulate air (HEPA) air filters
- Don't overhumidify the house since moisture encourages mold.

WHAT HAPPENS TO YOUR AIRWAYS?

During an asthma attack, the walls of your bronchioles contract and secrete more mucus, which narrows the internal space and restricts air flow to your lungs.

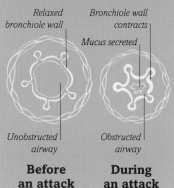

Relaxed bronchiole wall

Bronchiole wall contracts

Mucus secreted

Unobstructed airway

Obstructed airway

Before an attack

During an attack

STEP MANAGEMENT OF ASTHMA

Your doctor will help you monitor your symptoms, and together you can step up (increase) or step down (decrease) your medications according to your personal action plan. The goal is to use as few medications as possible while abolishing or at least minimizing your symptoms.

Step 1
Rescue inhaler.
Use inhaler as necessary

Step 2
Low-dose controller inhaler. Take daily as recommended

Step 3
Add long-acting bronchodilators. If no response, higher-dose preventer inhaler

Step 4
Addition of more drugs.
Add oral bronchodilators

Step 5
Addition of stronger drugs.
May need oral steroids

Step 6
Oral steroids

Chronic obstructive pulmonary disease

Although, historically, chronic obstructive pulmonary disease (COPD) was more common in men, the condition is now more common in women. The reason may be linked to the fact that more women smoke, and also because many industries that contributed to the disease in men are in decline in the developed world.

COPD is a combination of two lung diseases—chronic bronchitis and emphysema—where the airways and tissues of the lungs gradually become damaged over time, causing increasing shortness of breath. Although there is no cure, and the symptoms may worsen over time if they aren't treated, with an early diagnosis the decline can be slowed down.

WHAT IS IT?

In chronic bronchitis, the airways (bronchi and bronchioles) that carry air to the tiny air sacs (alveoli) embedded in the lung tissue become inflamed and blocked, making it harder for air to flow through them. In emphysema, the air sacs become damaged or destroyed, and the exchange of oxygen and carbon dioxide within the air sacs becomes more difficult. The main cause of both chronic bronchitis and emphysema, and therefore of COPD, is smoking.

COPD symptoms typically begin in people over 40 who have smoked for 20 years or more.

In the early stages, COPD may produce minimal or no symptoms, and as the disease progresses the symptoms in individual patients may vary (see opposite).

The prevention and early recognition of COPD in women is vital, as the following facts and figures show:

● COPD affects more women than men, and kills more women than men. The mortality rate in women has doubled since 1980.
● Chronic bronchitis afflicts twice as many women than men, and

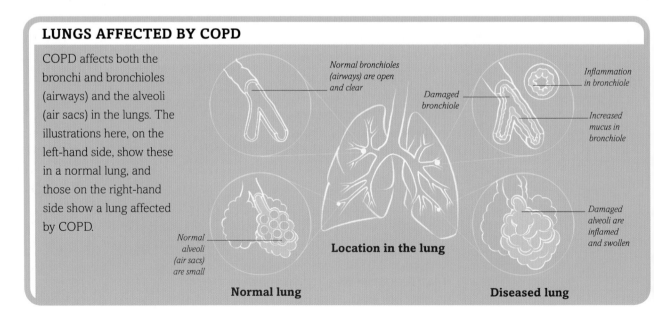

LUNGS AFFECTED BY COPD

COPD affects both the bronchi and bronchioles (airways) and the alveoli (air sacs) in the lungs. The illustrations here, on the left-hand side, show these in a normal lung, and those on the right-hand side show a lung affected by COPD.

Normal bronchioles (airways) are open and clear

Damaged bronchiole

Inflammation in bronchiole

Increased mucus in bronchiole

Normal alveoli (air sacs) are small

Location in the lung

Damaged alveoli are inflamed and swollen

Normal lung

Diseased lung

DO I HAVE THE SYMPTOMS?

As COPD progresses, your symptoms will gradually get worse:

- A cough is usually the first symptom to develop, and tends to come and go at first and then gradually become more persistent, with phlegm lasting for months
- Frequent coughs of any kind, especially in the morning
- Increased mucus
- Frequent clearing of your throat
- Shortness of breath when you exercise. Often the first sign is noticing that you need to rest more often while exercising
- More frequent colds, which last longer than in the past

See your doctor if you have two or more of the above symptoms.

emphysema is almost as common in women as men.

- Women with COPD are on the rise, while the number of men with the disease is decreasing.
- Women who smoke are more likely to get COPD, and die from COPD, than men who smoke.

WHAT NEXT?

Your doctor can diagnose whether you have COPD in much the same way as he or she would diagnose asthma (see p238). If your medical history and physical examination

AM I AT RISK?

There are a few definite risk factors for developing COPD:

- The disease is rare in women under 40, and most common in women over the age of 60
- It's usually seen in smokers
- Exposure to dust and/or chemicals at work may be responsible for 2% of cases of COPD in the US.

suggest that you might have COPD, your doctor will then refer you to a specialist to arrange lung function tests. One test is spirometry, in which you breathe hard into a tube that is attached to a monitor. The spirometer produces a graph showing how much air you can blow out.

Once you have a diagnosis, the first goal is to prevent any further damage to your lungs. If you smoke, you must stop (see p64). Infections can worsen your lung damage and to prevent them you should make sure that you receive these vaccinations:

- An annual flu vaccination at the beginning of the fall.
- A pneumonia vaccination, or "Pneumovax," every 10 years.

The next goal is to control the symptoms of COPD.

MY TREATMENT OPTIONS

COPD treatments aim to ease the symptoms rather than cure them. **Drug therapy** and preventive methods, such as those listed

below, are the main treatments:

- Inhaled bronchodilators
- Inhaled corticosteroids
- Vaccinations against flu and pneumonia.

Asthma medications such as bronchodilators, which relax the muscles of the airways, relieve shortness of breath, while anti-inflammatory drugs—mainly inhaled glucocorticosteroids—reduce inflammation within the airways (see p239). If you have severe COPD, you may need to take oral corticosteroid medicine also. When the disease is advanced, you may need oxygen therapy—pure oxygen delivered through tubes in your nostrils.

Pulmonary rehabilitation programs build up your exercise tolerance, and educate you about your condition and how to manage the symptoms better. This will include exercise training, disease management, and support. The goal is to increase your tolerance to exercise so you can get around without any shortness of breath, and encourage you to be more independent and less anxious.

HOW CAN I HELP MYSELF?

COPD develops very gradually. We all cough sometimes, and we get short of breath when we exercise more than usual. It's easy to dismiss early signs of COPD. **Pay attention to your body** and get help if you think you have COPD symptoms.

Don't smoke, if you do, get help to quit (see p64).

Lung cancer

Unfortunately, the rates of lung cancer among women are rising, and lung cancer is now the leading cause of cancer death in American women. Although this condition can be fatal, modern treatments can improve survival time—this is especially true for women—and in a few cases, even offer a complete cure.

Since the mid-1980s, men's lung cancer rates have been declining, while women's lung cancer rates continue to rise. This is likely due to smoking, although lung cancer can be found among non-smokers.

Women are less likely to quit smoking than men, and the rate of smoking among young women is increasing. Fortunately, data from 2008 shows that lung cancer rates in women are finally starting to plateau.

WHAT IS IT?

Lung cancer is either primary, where the initial growth occurs in the lungs, or it may be secondary, where the cancer has spread from another part of the body.

There are two basic groups of lung cancer:

Small cell lung cancer (or oat cell cancer). This type comprises about 20 percent of lung cancers and is the most closely associated with smoking.

Non-small cell lung cancer

About 75 percent of lung cancers are of this type. Several cell types are affected but are grouped together because they share some similarities in their causes and treatment. These types of cancers may or may not be linked to smoking.

WHAT NEXT?

If you have any of the symptoms (see left), seek help early from your doctor. The sooner lung cancer is diagnosed, the better the outlook.

One reason why lung cancer is so deadly is that there aren't any symptoms when the cancer is small and potentially treatable.

Once symptoms are evident, you'll be given a chest X-ray and sputum tests. However, chest X-rays usually only show lung cancer once it's large and difficult to treat. If lung cancer is diagnosed, your doctor will refer you to a cancer specialist, or oncologist. He or she will perform a number of tests, including CT scans, MRI scans, and occasionally PET scans, to determine the extent or stage of the cancer. These tests will help show whether you have lung cancer or not and if you do, what the best treatment will be.

MY TREATMENT OPTIONS

Cancer treatment has improved greatly over the years, and is now safer and more tolerable.

Non-small cell lung cancer has a better prognosis than small cell lung cancer. If it is caught early, about half the cases can be cured with a combination of surgery followed by chemotherapy. Women respond better to treatment than men, and have higher survival rates.

DO I HAVE THE SYMPTOMS?

Symptoms of lung cancer may include:
- Persistent cough
- Chest pain
- Shortness of breath
- Weight loss
- Loss of appetite
- Frequent colds that tend to last longer than usual.

See your doctor if you have a persistent cough whether or not it's accompanied by any of the additional symptoms listed above.

"Women respond better to treatments for lung cancer than men, and have higher survival rates."

Small cell lung cancer has usually spread by the time of diagnosis, but it responds to chemotherapy and radiation, and treatment can often improve survival time from a few months to over a year.

Despite the advances in therapy, the survival statistics for lung cancer are far from reassuring. Only about 50 percent of women with lung cancer will be alive a year after diagnosis, and only 15 percent after five years. Some people opt not to have treatment, particularly if the chance of curing the cancer is small. For those who decide against treatment, palliative care can alleviate symptoms and improve quality of life.

The treatment of lung cancer depends on what type of lung cancer it is and whether it has spread to other parts of the body. **Surgery** to remove the tumor is an option only if the cancer hasn't spread beyond the lungs. **Chemotherapy** involves taking medicine to combat the abnormal cells and is often recommended. **Radiation therapy**, in which X-rays are used to reduce the size of the tumor, is often effective. **Palliative care** can provide relief when other treatments are no longer an option.

HOW CAN I HELP MYSELF?

You can reduce your risk of lung cancer by avoiding these risk factors where possible:

Avoid inhaling smoke. Quit smoking, if you're a smoker (see p64), and avoid exposure to smoke in your home, car, and workplace.

Eat a healthy diet that is rich in fresh fruit and vegetables (see pp52–5); this may help your body to repair damaged cells, and reduce your risk of all types of cancer.

Cancerous lung
This colored X-ray shows the chest of a 73-year-old woman who is a heavy smoker. The lung cancer (red area) can clearly be seen in the right lung.

Exercising regularly (see pp56–7) decreases the risk of some cancers, including lung cancer.

Test your house for radon. This naturally occurring radioactive gas is present in some rocks and soil and can cause lung cancer. Radon is found in 1 out of 15 American homes. If the levels of radon in your home are elevated, you should have it treated immediately.

Avoid asbestos Asbestos exposure presents a high risk of lung cancer. Exposure can also lead to an unusual type of cancer called mesothelioma. Many old houses have asbestos insulation. There's no danger as long as it's sealed off, but it can be a problem if you do any renovations and the asbestos is disturbed.

AM I AT RISK?

You're at increased risk if you smoke, or if you live with someone who smokes. Smokers are at least 100 times more likely to develop lung cancer than nonsmokers.

- Cigarettes cause 90% of lung cancers in men, and 85% of lung cancer in women
- 10% of women who smoke will get lung cancer
- The more you smoke, the higher the risk; women who smoke two or more packs a day have a risk of lung cancer as high as 15%
- Smoking low-tar cigarettes offers absolutely no advantage
- Pipe and cigar smoking increases risk of lung cancer fivefold
- Marijuana smoking probably increases the risk of lung cancer
- Secondhand (passive) smoke increases the risk of lung cancer by 20–30%.

Less common risk factors include:
- Radon exposure
- Asbestos exposure
- Family history of lung cancer
- Air pollution.

Blood disorders

Judith C. Andersen MD
Director, Center for Bleeding Disorders and Thrombosis
Wayne State University School of Medicine
Karmanos Cancer Institute

Blood disorders

Although we're aware of blood as a life-sustaining substance, we're not always as familiar with its many functions. The blood circulating around your body in the arteries and veins is an extremely efficient transportation system, carrying substances essential for your survival such as oxygen, nutrients, and hormones to all your organs and tissues, and picking up waste products to process and eliminate from the body. In addition, your blood is vital to your body's defense system, containing cells that identify and fight invading organisms.

THE STRUCTURE AND FUNCTION OF BLOOD

Blood is made up of a fluid called plasma, which contains three different types of cell—red blood cells, white blood cells, and platelets. Plasma contains many essential substances, including glucose, proteins, fats, vitamins, and minerals, which it delivers to every tissue as it travels around the body. Plasma also collects waste products, such as urea and carbon dioxide, from the body's cells and carries them away for disposal—the carbon dioxide is removed from the body via the lungs, and other waste products are broken down and expelled via the liver and kidneys.

Red and white blood cells
Red blood cells have a distinctive biconcave disk shape and contain the red pigment hemoglobin. There are fewer white blood cells, but they play a vital role in defending the body against infection.

The red blood cells contain an important protein called hemoglobin, which has the crucial job of carrying oxygen from your lungs to every cell in the body's tissues and organs.

The white blood cells, of which there are various kinds, are part of the immune system (see p259). They fight infection, either by engulfing and destroying unwanted organisms, or by multiplying and producing antibodies that destroy invading bacteria.

The platelets are the smallest blood cells and are essential for clotting when a blood vessel is damaged or cut. They work together with various coagulation proteins (see p250) in the plasma to form a blood clot at the site of the damage. This quickly stems the bleeding.

HOW BLOOD CIRCULATES

Blood is transported around the body by a dense, branching network of arteries, veins, and capillaries. The blood absorbs oxygen in the lungs (see Breathing and Respiration, p230) and goes to the heart (see Your Heart, p160) via the pulmonary vein.

Arteries, which have thick muscular walls and carry blood under high pressure, carry the oxygenated blood around the body to the organs and tissues. Here, they branch into smaller and smaller vessels until they form tiny capillaries that release the oxygen and nutrients to individual cells. Tiny veins that gradually become large veins return the deoxygenated blood to the heart and to the lungs, where the carbon dioxide is exhaled and fresh oxygen is collected.

WHAT IS IN YOUR BLOOD

This cross section through a blood vessel shows the composition of the blood flowing through it. The plasma, which carries many essential substances (see opposite), accounts for about 55 percent of your total blood volume; 90 percent of that is water.

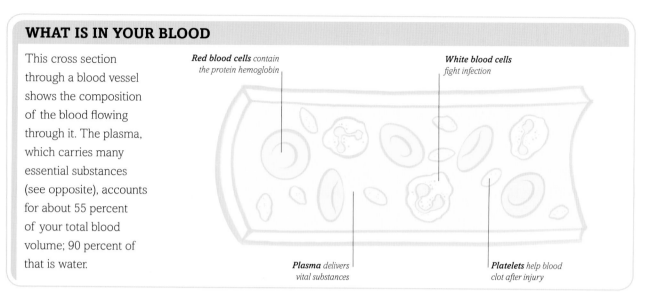

Red blood cells contain the protein hemoglobin

White blood cells fight infection

Plasma delivers vital substances

Platelets help blood clot after injury

HOW WOMEN ARE DIFFERENT

There are few differences between the blood of men and women, but a man, since he is normally larger than a woman, will have a greater volume of blood in his body. However, when a woman is pregnant, the volume of blood in her body increases, which ensures that the developing fetus will have all it needs in the way of blood, oxygen, and nutrients. Another difference is that men have more red blood cells than women, and they also have a higher concentration of hemoglobin.

Because they menstruate, women are more prone than men to iron-deficiency anemia (see p248). During menstruation they lose a small amount of blood (usually between 10 and 80 ml). Women who lose more than this over time without adequate dietary iron (or supplements) may become iron deficient, leading to anemia.

WHAT BLOOD REVEALS

When we talk about blood disorders we are referring to illnesses that affect blood cells rather than changes within the plasma component. Simple laboratory tests on blood samples provide a great deal of information about these disorders and illnesses.

If you are unwell or need an operation, you will probably have a routine test of your red and white blood cells and platelet counts in your blood. The analysis will also look at the size of your red blood cells and measure your total hemoglobin concentration. If your blood cells have an abnormal count, or if you have other symptoms, the blood cells' shape will be studied under a microscope to rule out conditions such as sickle cell anemia or hereditary spherocytosis.

BONE MARROW TEST

Red blood cells, white blood cells, and platelets are all produced in the bone marrow from cells known as precursor cells. In adults, bone marrow is located in the bones of the central skeleton, such as the pelvic bone, the sternum, and the long bones.

If there is no obvious explanation why your blood count is too high or too low, or your blood cells have an abnormal appearance, you may be given a bone marrow test. This might reveal some abnormalities in the precursor cells, or it may indicate the existence of another disease affecting the bone marrow, such as an infection, fibrosis, leukemia (see p254), or a cancer that is not related to the blood.

"Due to menstruation, women are more prone to iron-deficiency anemia than men."

Blood deficiency problems

Fatigue is the most common clinical complaint women have. Usually, it's a result of stress or inadequate sleep. If your fatigue persists, it's worth a visit to the doctor to be sure there isn't another medical explanation. Anemia, for example, commonly causes fatigue, and some types are particularly common in women.

WHAT IS IT?

Anemia occurs when the level of hemoglobin (see below) in the red blood cells falls and reduces the capacity of your blood to carry oxygen. You need enough iron, vitamin B_{12}, and folate (folic acid) to produce hemoglobin; if you are lacking any of these, you are likely to develop a type of anemia.

Anemia can also occur if your red blood cells are destroyed too quickly (hemolysis). This can be the result of an abnormal immune response—for example, to drugs such as penicillin. Sometimes, when we're unwell, our bodies can't use iron well. This is called "anemia of chronic disease." Rarely, anemia may indicate a bone marrow disorder, such as leukemia (see p254) or another type of cancer, which affects the way we produce hemoglobin.

Iron-deficiency anemia is usually caused by blood loss. It is fairly common in women of reproductive age, and is usually linked to menstruation and/or pregnancy. If you're older or only have light menstrual blood loss, it may be linked to something else, such as blood loss from the gastrointestinal (GI) tract.

Less commonly, you may have iron deficiency when there's no loss of blood. This may be due to a poor diet, or an inability to absorb iron efficiently during illnesses affecting the small intestine, such as celiac disease (see p301) or Crohn's disease (see pp310–11).

Pernicious anemia is more common in women than in men and can run in families. The vitamin B_{12} needed to produce red blood cells must bind with a protein called "intrinsic factor" before it can be

DO I HAVE THE SYMPTOMS?

If you experience the following, symptoms, you should have a blood test to check for iron-deficiency anemia:

- Fatigue
- Shortness of breath
- Inability to concentrate
- A craving for strange foods, known as "pica"
- Swollen ankles
- Brittle nails
- Painful cracks at the corner of the mouth.

The following extra symptoms are linked with a vitamin B_{12} deficiency:

- Tingling in fingers or toes
- Loss of balance
- Unsteady gait
- Memory impairment.

Low levels of B_{12} or folate can cause the following:

- Jaundice
- Glossitis (inflammation of the tongue).

See your doctor if you have one or more of these symptoms.

HEMOGLOBIN

Iron is a key component of hemoglobin, the oxygen-carrying molecules in your blood. A shortage of iron in the body means less hemoglobin, thus less oxygen reaching the tissues.

Hemoglobin molecule is made up of four protein chains

Four iron compounds are embedded in the protein chains

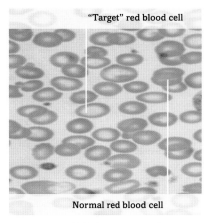

"Target" red blood cell

Normal red blood cell

Iron-deficiency anemia
These red blood cells have the typical irregular outlines caused by iron deficiency. Some lack their central pale area and look like the target for archery practice (so-called target cells).

absorbed via the small intestine. Some people make antibodies to intrinsic factor, which reduces their ability to produce the blood cells. This autoimmune response causes pernicious anemia.

Folate deficiency Folate, or folic acid, is another B vitamin needed to produce red blood cells. It is absorbed through the small intestine. Low levels in the blood indicate that our diet is lacking in it.

WHAT NEXT?

Your doctor will arrange for you to have a full blood count to confirm whether you have anemia and identify the type. He or she will ask you about symptoms, such as heavy periods or indigestion, and will review any medication you're taking, since some drugs such as aspirin can irritate the lining of the stomach and cause bleeding. If your doctor thinks your anemia is due to a lack of iron caused by heavy blood loss when you have your periods, then you may be referred to a gynecologist to help with this problem. Tell your doctor if you are having any gastrointestinal symptoms so that he or she can arrange extra tests, such as an upper GI endoscopy (see p290). B_{12} deficiency can mimic neurological disorders, so you may need to have additional tests.

MY TREATMENT OPTIONS

The treatment you are offered will be tailored to the type of anemia and its underlying cause.

Supplements Iron supplements can help iron-deficiency anemia, but if they cause diarrhea or constipation, you may need to lower the dose or choose an alternative. Some supplements contain very little iron and are easier to tolerate, but are less useful clinically. A folate deficiency usually responds to a course of folic acid supplements.

Injections Some people can't tolerate iron supplements and so need iron injections at the hospital.

Vitamin B_{12} deficiency can be treated with injections, which can be stopped once the cause is known, but if your body can't absorb vitamin B_{12}, you may need three-monthly injections for life.

HOW CAN I HELP MYSELF?

Iron- and folate-deficiency anemia may solved by adjusting your diet.

Nutrition You can increase iron intake by eating meat and fish. It's harder to absorb enough from vegetables, so some people may need supplements (see above). Good sources of folate include leafy green vegetables and whole grains.

"Iron-deficiency anemia is a common cause of fatigue and lethargy among women who suffer with heavy periods or who are pregnant."

Bleeding disorders

Having monthly periods means that women are used to bleeding. We often notice unusually heavier periods, but if that bleeding is heavy or prolonged, we may not consider that we have a clotting abnormality. Bleeding disorders are relatively common in women. While they are easy to diagnose, they are not always easy for women to detect.

WHAT IS IT?

When you damage a blood vessel, the clotting process in your blood immediately seals the wound. In this process, known as coagulation, the platelets in your blood (see p246) clump together and interact with proteins called clotting factors to stop the bleeding.

There are two types of clotting factor: "procoagulants" help the blood to clot and "anticoagulants" prevent it from clotting too readily. If your body's procoagulant and anticoagulant proteins aren't in balance, or if there's a problem with the number or the function of platelets, your blood can become either too runny or too sticky, and this can lead to a bleeding disorder.

Occasionally, a person has the normal numbers of platelets, but they don't work properly. This can result from an inherited condition or, more commonly, taking anti-inflammatory drugs such as aspirin or ibuprofen, which affect the way the platelets function.

Thrombocytopenia This is a reduction in the number of platelets. It can occur if they aren't being produced in sufficient numbers (for example with leukemia or after chemotherapy). It can also occur if the platelets are being destroyed too quickly, as when they are attacked by the body's immune system.

Hypercoagulability This occurs if there are too many platelets or coagulation factors. Some patients inherit extra-sticky clotting factors, and others, low levels of anticoagulant. These increase the tendency to form blood clots (or thrombus). If a thrombus starts to move freely in the circulation, it is called an embolism. If it gets stuck within the circulation of the lung, it can have potentially fatal consequences (see pp252–5).

(see pp252–5)

DO I HAVE THE SYMPTOMS?

The following symptoms may indicate a bleeding disorder:
- Easy or spontaneous bruising that is unexplained
- Recurrent severe nose bleeds
- Heavy periods from the menarche (the time that periods started)
- Prolonged or major bleeding after surgery/dentistry.

See your doctor if you suffer with any of the above.

AM I AT RISK?

The risk factors for a particular bleeding disorder depend on its cause. For example, you may have an increased risk of a bleeding if you:
- Have a family history of bleeding disorders
- Are taking drugs such as warfarin, aspirin, or ibuprofen.

Von Willebrand's disease is named after the Finnish doctor who discovered that some people lacked a key clotting factor, which then became known as von Willebrand's factor. This inherited disease is the most common bleeding disorder—between one and two percent of the population have it—and it affects men and women equally. Bleeding is excessive or prolonged.

Hemophilia is an inherited disease that involves excessive bleeding that can go on for hours or even days. Sometimes bleeding starts spontaneously. Hemophilia really only affects men (see p17), although some women can have mild symptoms. It is caused by a reduction in the level of a blood protein known as Factor VIII.

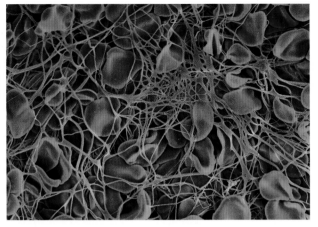

What happens when blood clots
When a blood vessel is damaged, a mesh of a protein called fibrin (colored green in this scan) develops to bind the blood cells together. The result is a blood clot, that prevents you from losing too much blood.

WHAT NEXT?

If your symptoms seem to suggest a bleeding disorder, your doctor will order a test to measure your full blood count, check the number of platelets, establish the presence of the clotting proteins, and measure your blood's clotting time. You may need further tests to measure the levels of specific proteins, such as Factor VIII and von Willebrand's factor. Platelet function tests may also be done in a specialized hematology center. Sometimes, test results are affected by stress, exercise, or medications, and the test may need to be repeated.

MY TREATMENT OPTIONS

There's no cure for bleeding disorders but treatment can enable women to lead normal, active lives. Treatment is either via medications or injection, and will depend on what causes the disorder. For mild disorders, medication is not really needed, other than after an injury, and before or after surgical or dental treatment. However, if the disorder is severe, you may need to take medication every day.

Desmopressin acetate helps to release clotting factors that are stored in the body. You can take it as an injection or via a nasal spray to combat heavy periods and stop nose bleeds.

Antifibrinolytic medications help prolong the life of a blood clot by preventing it from breaking down. They can be used before dental treatment, to stop nose bleeds, and to control mild bleeding in the intestine.

Intravenous injections of immunoglobulin or steroids can boost platelet numbers if your platelets are being broken down because you have an autoimmune disease. You can also have injections of plasma containing specific clotting factors, such as von Willebrand's factor or Factor VIII.

Changing medication If a bleeding disorder is caused by a medication, your doctor will suggest an alternative. If you are taking warfarin and need surgery, you may have to stop the warfarin

HOW CAN I HELP MYSELF?

Follow your doctor's advice with regard to your treatment and make sure your lifestyle is healthy (see Chapter 3, pp52–5).

EASILY BRUISED?

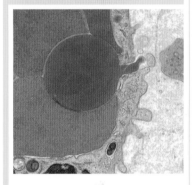

Damaged blood vessel
When the wall of a blood vessel (here shown in green) is damaged, red blood cells leak through into surrounding tissues, causing bruising.

Women seem to bruise more easily than men. Sometimes this bruising is unexplained and may indicate a bleeding disorder, particularly when it is accompanied by a bleeding nose or gums, and heavy or prolonged periods. If you have bruises that take a long time to disappear, consult your doctor.

> "Von Willebrand's disease is the most common inherited blood disorder in women, affecting about 1 in 100 women."

Venous thrombosis

We know that long, cramped flights and surgery can increase the risk of a venous thrombosis, but some women are at particular risk—for example, if you're pregnant, using the combined oral contraceptive pill or patch, or taking estrogen. Simple steps towards healthy circulation can reduce your risk of developing blood clots.

WHAT IS IT?

A thrombosis occurs when the flow of blood in a vein or artery is blocked for some reason. Fatty deposits on the inside of an artery—a condition called atherosclerosis (see p162)—are prime sites for thromboses. A venous thrombosis is a specific type of blood clot that occurs in a vein. In the case of the veins in your limbs, these are either near the surface (superficial) or deep. You can get a venous thrombosis in either of these. When a clot occurs in a deep vein, it is known as a deep vein thrombosis (DVT). Up to 50 percent of thromboses in veins may be linked to hormonal or biochemical changes in the composition of the blood. Veins may also develop thromboses after being immobile for prolonged periods—for example, being in a cramped airplane seat. A clot in a superficial vein may be painful, but it's unlikely to be dangerous.

Likewise, a DVT is not necessarily dangerous in itself, but it may break away from the place where it forms and become an embolus (abnormal blood clot) that travels in the blood to the lung. Once it reaches the lung, it can block a pulmonary blood vessel. This is known as a pulmonary embolism (PE), which can be fatal if an inability to oxygenate blood leads to shock and heart failure. It is important to note that venous thrombosis poses a long-term risk irrespective of the risk of embolism.

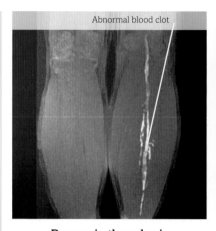
Abnormal blood clot

Deep vein thrombosis
This magnetic resonance imaging (MRI) scan shows a patient suffering from a DVT in a vein in the leg. The clot shows up as the white area.

WHAT NEXT?

It's important to diagnose and treat a DVT or a PE promptly. If your doctor suspects you have a DVT, he or she will first take a detailed medical history and order a blood test to identify whether you are at a high or low risk of a venous thrombosis. Depending on your symptoms, you may have an X-ray to establish whether a thrombosis has occurred. If a DVT is suspected, you may

DO I HAVE THE SYMPTOMS?

Venous thrombosis may be asymptomatic or you may have the following symptoms:
- Pain or tenderness in a limb
- A feeling of a cramp that doesn't go away
- Swelling of the affected limb.

In rare cases, when a clot travels to the lungs, the following symptoms can occur:
- Chest pain
- Shortness of breath
- A cough.

See your doctor as soon as possible if you suspect you have a DVT. If you have the symptoms of a pulmonary embolism, treat it as a medical emergency.

> "Although taking the pill or HRT has been linked to deep vein thrombosis (DVT), the actual risk of hormone-induced DVT is still very small."

AM I AT RISK?

The following factors can increase your risk of thrombosis:
- A family history of thrombosis
- The combined oral contraceptive pill
- Pregnancy
- Hormone replacement therapy (HRT)
- Recent hip or knee surgery
- Other major surgical procedures and a period of hospitalization
- Wearing a plaster cast
- Long-haul flights and prolonged road trips
- A prolonged period of immobility
- Cancer
- Inherited and acquired factors in the blood.

have a Doppler ultrasound scan to measure the blood flow within your veins and to establish whether a deep vein is blocked. If you have a suspected PE, you may have a scan to check the flow of blood and air in your lungs. Alternatively, you may have a computerized tomography (CT) scan, which involves taking a series of X-rays to build a detailed picture of your chest. If these tests don't give a clear diagnosis, you may need to repeat them a week or so later, or other tests may be done. If there is a wait of several hours or days for further tests, your doctor may decide to start treatment before the results are available.

MY TREATMENT OPTIONS

Venous thrombosis is commonly treated with anticoagulant drugs that thin the blood.

Anticoagulant drugs include warfarin. This takes a few days to beome effective so, during the first week, you may also have injections of the anticoagulant drug heparin (which works immediately). Increasingly used are low molecular weight heparins and newer agents such as fondaparinux, which are safer and can be used as an outpatient without laboratory monitoring.

Preventive measures "Post-thrombotic syndrome" can occur after a DVT and leads to pain, chronic leg swelling, vericose superficial veins, leg fatigue, and chronic leg ulcers. Wearing compression stockings for the two years immediately following the DVT can help reduce the risk of post-thrombotic syndrome in the future.

Blood tests can help find an underlying cause for an episode of thrombosis, but anticoagulants such as warfarin can affect the results. Repeat tests may be needed, or tests may be postponed until you stop taking warfarin.

HOW CAN I HELP MYSELF?

Several preventive measures can help you avoid DVT or a recurrence of the condition.

If you've had a thrombosis make sure that you tell your doctor if you become pregnant, require surgery, or are admitted to the hospital for any reason.

If you're high risk and due to have surgery, talk to the surgeon about the possibility of having heparin injections around the time of the surgery.

Keep your weight down You need to maintain a healthy weight to help you reduce your risk of developing a DVT.

When traveling, avoid alcohol and sleeping pills; try to walk around on long plane trips, and wear compression stockings and practice ankle exercises to help your circulation. Drinking plenty of water can help, too.

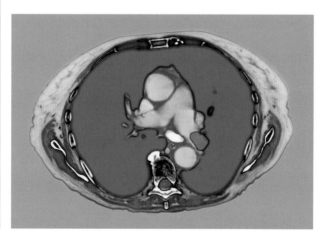

Pulmonary embolism
A computerized tomography (CT) scan of the lungs reveals a pulmonary embolism (green patch) in the left pulmonary artery.

Blood cancers

Cancers of the white cells in the blood and lymph system appear to affect men and women equally, and even though they are relatively common, they are poorly understood. However, many types of blood cancer (such as some types of leukemia) now have a good outcome and a decreasing incidence.

WHAT ARE THEY?

White blood cells are on the front line of our defenses, protecting us from illness by destroying invading organisms. The two main types of white blood cells, granulocytes and lymphocytes, work in different ways. Granulocytes engulf and destroy bacteria, while lymphocytes destroy organisms with antibodies. These two types of white cells are the ones affected when we talk about blood (hematological) cancers. There are several different types of blood cancer, each with its own characteristics.

Leukemia occurs when there is an increased number of abnormal white cells in the bone marrow. There are two main types: acute leukemia, which develops rapidly, and chronic leukemia, which can take years to develop and is more common among the middle-aged and elderly. There are two types of acute leukemia: acute lymphoid leukemia (ALL) is more common in childhood, while acute myeloid leukemia (AML) can occur at any age. There are also two types of chronic leukemia: chronic myeloid (CML) and chronic lymphocytic (CLL). Both types can cause bone marrow failure.

Lymphomas are cancers in which malignant lymphoid cells build up in the lymph nodes, liver, and spleen. There are two types of lymphoma: Hodgkins and non-Hodgkins lymphoma.

Myeloma occurs when plasma cells (see p246) become malignant, often in bone marrow. This impairs the production of normal blood cells, causing anemia (see p248). The malignant plasma cells also produce massive quantities of "paraprotein," an antibody that can lead to kidney failure. Myeloma most frequently results in skeletal disease with brittle bones and pathologic fractures.

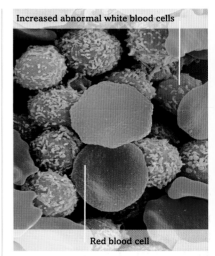

Increased abnormal white blood cells

Red blood cell

Leukemia
In chronic lymphocytic leukemia, there is an increased number of abnormal white blood cells in the bone marrow.

DO I HAVE THE SYMPTOMS?

The following are some of the general symptoms of chronic leukemia:

- Fatigue and shortness of breath, caused by anemia (see p248)
- Nose bleeds and bruising (see p250) caused by low platelet levels
- Fevers and infections, caused by low levels of white blood cells.

Chronic leukemia may initially have no symptoms, but in the later stages there may be:

- Anemia
- Easy bruising (see p251), bleeding
- A tendency to develop infections.

Symptoms of lymphomas include:

- Enlarged lymph glands in the neck, armpits, or groin
- Weight loss
- Raised temperature
- Drenching sweats at night
- Symptoms of anemia, such as fatigue and shortness of breath.

See your doctor if you have one or more of these symptoms.

"Many people with some types of blood cancers can be cured or can have the progress of their cancer halted for many years."

WHAT NEXT?

The diagnostic tests your doctor may recommend vary according to the type of blood cancer.

Acute leukemia needs to be diagnosed and dealt with quickly. Your doctor will order an immediate full blood count, which may reveal low numbers of red and white cells and/or platelets. If your blood count is abnormal, the laboratory will look for leukemia cells in a blood sample. If there are only a few circulating abnormal cells, you may be given a bone marrow test.

Chronic leukemia is identified by blood tests and confirmed by further specialized tests. In CML, an abnormal chromosome, known as the Philadelphia chromosome, is usually present.

Lymphoma requires special scans to assess the extent of the condition. You may also have a gland removed for examination.

Myeloma requires tests to identify two or more of the following: a significant number of plasma cells in the bone marrow; bone problems identified through a skeletal X-ray; and the presence of "paraprotein" antibodies in the blood or urine.

MY TREATMENT OPTIONS

Chemotherapy, radiation therapy, medications, and stem cell transplants are used in the treatment of blood cancers.

Chemotherapy/radiation Acute leukemia is potentially curable, particularly in children and young adults. Chemotherapy is usually given in the hospital; you will probably go into isolation to reduce your exposure to infection.

Chemotherapy can reduce the number of malignant cells in CLL but it doesn't cure. Treatment is only started if you have particular symptoms or signs of bone marrow failure, such as anemia, a low platelet count, or too few neutrophils (a type of white blood cell).

Some lymphomas, such as Hodgkins lymphoma, are curable with chemotherapy and/or radiation. In younger myeloma patients, chemotherapy can lead to remission but not to a cure. However, high doses can improve the length and quality of survival. Older patients are usually treated with chemotherapy in pill form and/or radiation therapy to help symptoms.

Other medications A drug called imatinib and its widely used successor, dasatinib, are designed to reverse the process of leukemia in CML without affecting other tissues.

HOW CAN I HELP MYSELF?

It is essential to follow your doctor's advice carefully and to lead a healthy lifestyle (see Chapter 3, pp52–5).

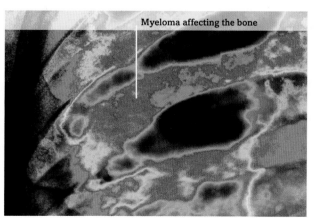

Myeloma affecting the bone

Myeloma
This color X-ray of a patient's ribs shows myeloma affecting the bones on one side of their chest. An X-ray will help in the diagnosis of the condition.

Bones and joints

Robin K Dore MD FACR
Clinical Professor of Medicine,
David Geffen School of Medicine,
Division of Rheumatology, University of California
Chronic fatigue syndrome Donnica Moore MD

Your bones and joints

Your skeleton is the bony, rigid framework that supports your body, gives it shape, protects some of the delicate internal organs, and allows you to move around. A complex system of overlying muscles, tendons, ligaments, cartilage, and other connective tissues works alongside your bones, allowing you to perform almost any movement you want. Your joints are the meeting points between two bones and are designed to help you make smooth, fluid movements, as well as cushion sudden jumps or falls.

HOW JOINTS WORK

In a healthy joint that is mobile, the end of each bone is covered with smooth cartilage, which allows movement at the joint, reduces friction, and acts as a cushion. A membrane called the synovium lines the joint and produces synovial fluid to lubricate the joint. The outer layer of the synovium is called the capsule. Tough bands called ligaments help hold the joint together by attaching one bone to another. Fibrous tendons attach muscles to the bones.

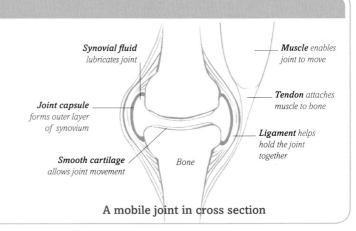

Synovial fluid lubricates joint

Muscle enables joint to move

Tendon attaches muscle to bone

Joint capsule forms outer layer of synovium

Ligament helps hold the joint together

Smooth cartilage allows joint movement

Bone

A mobile joint in cross section

BONE REMODELING

Throughout your life your bones are continuously broken down (bone resorption) and rebuilt (bone formation). This so-called bone remodeling is essential for the growth and maintenance of healthy bones. During childhood, bone is built up more rapidly than it is broken down—which is how you grow to be an adult—and so your bones become denser. Your bone density (also called bone mineral density or BMD) continues to increase until young adulthood (25–30 years), when it peaks. Bone resorption and bone formation are tightly coupled so that bone density remains pretty constant during this period.

After the age of 30, though, your bone density gradually declines year after year—between her 30s and 50s, the average woman loses 0.5 percent of bone density each year—so regular weight-bearing exercise (which promotes bone formation) is needed in order to

maintain bone density. If the processes of resorption and formation become uncoupled, as with the condition osteoporosis (see p260), there's an increase in bone resorption without a matching rise in formation. The result of this disparity is lighter, less

BONE DENSITY OVER A LIFETIME

Bone mineral density (BMD) peaks between the ages of 25 and 30. After 31, BMD gradually declines as more bone is lost than is made.

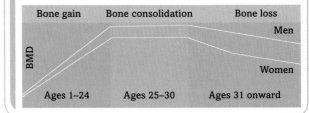

Bone gain | Bone consolidation | Bone loss

Men

BMD

Women

Ages 1–24 | Ages 25–30 | Ages 31 onward

dense, and more fragile bones. Estrogen provides women with added protection against bone resorption, but because estrogen levels decline after menopause, the rate of bone loss accelerates.

HOW ARE WOMEN DIFFERENT?

In addition to the anatomical differences between women and men (women have a flatter, more rounded pelvis; they are normally shorter than men; and they have narrower rib cages, to name but a few), women suffer much more from autoimmune diseases, such as rheumatoid arthritis (see pp266–8).

The hormones our bodies produce may actually put us at risk of developing autoimmune diseases. Doctors think that female hormones influence the immune system, which is backed up by the fact that at times of hormonal flux, such as pregnancy or menopause, some autoimmune diseases can flare up or subside.

JOINTS, MUSCLES, AND CONNECTIVE TISSUES AND YOUR IMMUNE SYSTEM

Discomfort you experience in your joints, muscles, and connective tissues can be linked to problems in your immune system. Inflammation is the way in which your body defends itself against infection or injury and fights off bacteria and viruses. If there is a breach of your body's defenses, your body increases blood supply to the affected site, which brings in elements of your immune system and raises your temperature (giving you a fever). Blood vessels become leaky, allowing other cells to join the assault. These cells make chemicals and antibodies to attack the foreign substances. This response is how your body staves off disease and keeps healthy.

If you have an autoimmune disease, your body's immune system triggers such a response when there are no foreign invaders. Instead, it produces an immune response against itself, damaging its own tissues in the process. If you have an autoimmune disease, it is highly likely that your blood contains autoantibodies— antibodies made against yourself. The damage such a disease can do can be wide ranging: on the joints in rheumatoid arthritis (see pp266–8); and on joints, skin, heart, lungs, kidneys, and nerves in lupus (see p269).

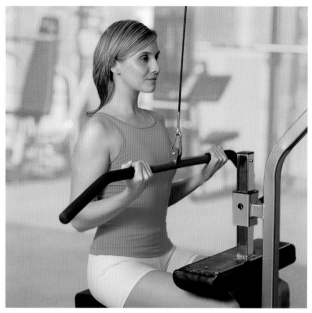

Exercise to build bones
Lifting weights not only boosts muscle strength but the action of the tendons pulling on bones promotes bone density, too.

THE INFLAMMATORY RESPONSE

When invaders such as bacteria get into your body (in this example into your skin), your body triggers an inflammatory response that helps fight them off.

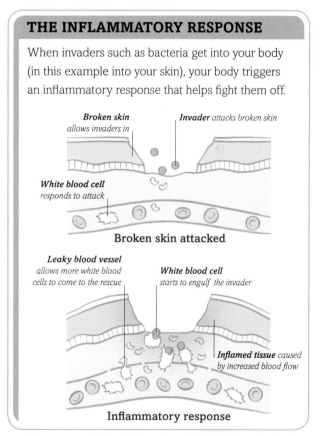

Broken skin allows invaders in

Invader attacks broken skin

White blood cell responds to attack

Broken skin attacked

Leaky blood vessel allows more white blood cells to come to the rescue

White blood cell starts to engulf the invader

Inflamed tissue caused by increased blood flow

Inflammatory response

Osteoporosis

Your bones are strongest in your late 20s, but as you age they become thinner and lighter. Estrogen helps keep bones strong, so after menopause (when estrogen levels fall) your built-in protection subsides and it's more important than ever to have a bone-conscious lifestyle to prevent osteoporosis.

WHAT IS IT?

Osteoporosis, which literally means "porous bones," results in weaker bones that are more brittle and so can break more easily. In fact, bones can be so brittle that even mild exertions, such as coughing or lifting a heavy bag of groceries, can cause a fracture.

Anyone can develop this condition as they get older, although some people have a higher than normal risk of osteoporosis (see Am I at risk?, opposite).

With age, we gradually lose some height as our backs become

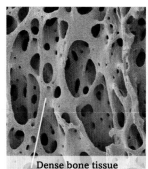

Dense bone tissue

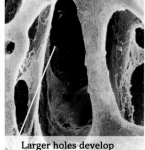

Larger holes develop

Normal and osteoporotic bone
Younger bones have a strong, dense structure with a small "honeycomb" effect (far left). With age the bone becomes less dense and larger holes appear as bone material is lost (left).

more curved than in our youth. These physical changes may well be related to the effects of osteoporosis on the spine. Amazingly, you can have a spinal fracture without any symptoms at all, but some fractures may cause persistent back pain and restrict what you can comfortably do.

WHAT NEXT?

Osteoporosis is often first diagnosed when you break a bone after a minor bump or fall. If your doctor suspects that you have osteoporosis, he or she may ask you questions to see how many of the risk factors (see box, opposite) might apply to you.

Then, it's likely you'll be sent for a bone density scan (dual-energy X-ray absorptiometry scan or DEXA scan for short). This procedure is quick, simple, and accurate. It

measures the density of bones in your spine, hip, and wrist (those areas most likely to be affected by osteoporosis).

You may also have to give a blood sample for tests to detect or rule out any underlying conditions.

MY TREATMENT OPTIONS

Obviously, you need to prevent any future fractures and also reduce the symptoms related to any existing fractures. The medications listed below are long-term treatments, and work by reducing bone loss and/or by helping to build new bone. Ask about side effects when discussing these with your doctor.

Calcium and vitamin D dietary supplements You may benefit from taking daily calcium and vitamin D supplements. Premenopausal women should consume 1,000 mg calcium per day

DO I HAVE THE SYMPTOMS?

Osteoporosis does not have any symptoms, but you may have the condition if:

- You suffer any hip, wrist, or spine fracture
- You are between 45 and 65 and you fracture your wrist in a fall
- You are over 70 years old and frail, and you fracture your hip in a fall.

Your doctor may then decide you have this condition.

while postmenopausal women (who don't take estrogen) should increase their intake to 1,500 mg. Everyone should take 800 IU of vitamin D. The body requires plenty of calcium and vitamin D to make bone.

Bisphosphonates These drugs slow bone loss. Your doctor is likely to prescribe alendronate or risedronate, which are taken daily or weekly, to reduce the risk of further hip and spine fractures (although these drugs can irritate your esophagus).

Hormone replacement therapy If you have had an early menopause, your doctor may prescribe hormone replacement therapy (HRT, see pp137–8). Although HRT contains estrogen, which is good for bones, it does come with side effects.

Selective estrogen-receptor modulators You may be prescribed raloxifene, which has a similar effect to estrogen and reduces spine fractures. It may give you hot flashes, however, and it can increase your risk of blood clots.

Strontium This newer treatment slows bone loss, helps build new bone, and reduces the incidence of spine and hip fractures.

Calcitonin is a hormone that is naturally produced in your body to help keep your bones strong. Doctors can give calcitonin as an injection or as a nasal spray.

Teriparatide This drug helps build new bone as well as reduce your risk of fractures. You'll need daily injections for up to 18 months. Currently, it's mainly given to people who continue to have fractures despite using other treatments or to those who can't tolerate other treatments.

HOW CAN I HELP MYSELF?

Did you know that one in two women over the age of 50 in the US will break a bone mainly because of osteoporosis? Well, that statistic may be enough to spur you on to do something about your bone density—it's never too early or too late to start. You can help prevent osteoporosis by leading an active life and eating a diet rich in calcium and vitamin D (see p262).

Reduce the risk of falling Make sure that there's nothing you can trip over at home, wear sturdy shoes, and be careful when you go outdoors during the winter. Use a cane if you have problems or need some extra assistance. If you're prone to falling, it may be worth looking into getting some hip protectors (specially padded underwear that cushions the hips). If your osteoporosis is severe, you need to be careful when carrying or lifting things, as sudden stresses can easily cause a spine fracture.

Eat foods that build bones It's easy to get enough dietary calcium by eating bone-building foods (see p262) or taking supplements.

Exercise for strong bones Weight-bearing exercise like walking and running helps keep your bones strong. Lifting weights can also promote bone density but should be avoided in those with osteoporosis. Women with osteoporosis should walk briskly for 30 minutes three to four days a week. Keeping physically active may reduce your risk of falls and improve your nerve and muscle responses if you do fall.

Stop smoking Chemicals from tobacco worsen bone loss and interfere in calcium absorption.

AM I AT RISK?

Bone loss affects everyone to some degree as they age, but your risk of osteoporosis increases if:

- You have had an early menopause (before the age of 45)
- You took corticosteroid drugs for a long period of time
- You have a family history of osteoporosis (especially if your mother broke a hip)
- You eat a diet that's low in both calcium and vitamin D
- You live, or have lived (particularly in your teenage years), a sedentary lifestyle, or you can't exercise for some reason
- You smoke
- You drink too much alcohol (see p65)
- You have certain conditions, such as celiac disease (see p301) or hyperthyroidism (see pp327–9)
- You're underweight, or have suffered from an eating disorder (see pp216–17) in the past.

How to get your daily calcium

For healthy, strong bones you need plenty of calcium, and you need vitamin D to be able to absorb the calcium from your food. Your skin makes vitamin D from sunshine—10–15 minutes outside without sunscreen at the hottest time of every day in summer (not enough to burn your skin) will usually give you enough vitamin D to last you all year round.

Recommended daily allowance (RDA) of calcium

Under 60 years old: 1,000mg RDA of calcium   **Over 60 years old: 1,000–1,500mg** RDA of calcium

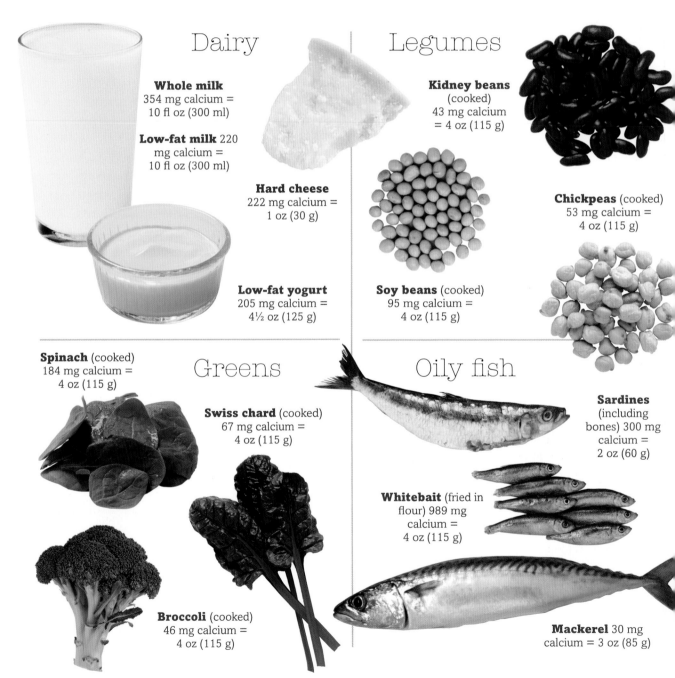

Dairy

Whole milk
354 mg calcium =
10 fl oz (300 ml)

Low-fat milk 220
mg calcium =
10 fl oz (300 ml)

Hard cheese
222 mg calcium =
1 oz (30 g)

Low-fat yogurt
205 mg calcium =
4½ oz (125 g)

Legumes

Kidney beans
(cooked)
43 mg calcium
= 4 oz (115 g)

Chickpeas (cooked)
53 mg calcium =
4 oz (115 g)

Soy beans (cooked)
95 mg calcium =
4 oz (115 g)

Greens

Spinach (cooked)
184 mg calcium =
4 oz (115 g)

Swiss chard (cooked)
67 mg calcium =
4 oz (115 g)

Broccoli (cooked)
46 mg calcium =
4 oz (115 g)

Oily fish

Sardines
(including
bones) 300 mg
calcium =
2 oz (60 g)

Whitebait (fried in
flour) 989 mg
calcium =
4 oz (115 g)

Mackerel 30 mg
calcium = 3 oz (85 g)

Osteoarthritis

It's normal to have the occasional creaky or stiff joint as you get older; none of us is the bionic woman. But if you notice a hip or knee, for example, that is becoming troublesome, it might be suffering the effects of osteoarthritis—a "wear and tear arthritis"—that develops slowly over many years.

WHAT IS IT?

In a joint affected by osteoarthritis, the surface of the cartilage on the end of the bones becomes rougher and thinner, and the bone beneath thickens and grows outward, forming bony spurs. Movements are no longer smooth and fluid; joints become swollen, painful, and creaky as you try to move.

It's unclear why osteoarthritis can affect one joint but not another, and why, for example, one hip is affected more than the other.

Osteoarthritis is most common in the weight-bearing joints of the knees and hips, and in the spine (see Back and neck pain, pp272–5). In women, it also affects the hands (especially the fingers and the base of the thumb) and the big toes (see Bunions, p265).

WHAT NEXT?

After going through your medical history your doctor will want to know about your symptoms. Tell him or her about any joints that are tender, swollen, or unstable. Before you visit your doctor, try to pin down the times when your pain or stiffness is worst and what, if anything, makes it better or worse.

Your doctor will then want to examine you. He or she may be able to feel bony swellings and any creaking of an affected joint, as well as discover if there is any restricted movement at that joint.

You will probably have to give some blood, which will be sent for laboratory testing. Blood tests are

DO I HAVE THE SYMPTOMS?

Symptoms of osteoarthritis can come and go, but they gradually worsen over time. You may find that there is:

- Pain after moving the joint
- Stiffness in the joint after rest; this improves when you start moving the joint
- A creaking sound when moving the affected joint
- A smaller range of movement in the joint, or it may even give way suddenly.

See your doctor if symptoms persist or cause you distress.

AN ARTHRITIC MOBILE JOINT IN CROSS SECTION

Osteoarthritis is more common in women than in men, especially in the knees and the hands; what's more, we tend to suffer with more severe symptoms. Compare the normal knee with the arthritic one and you will see how the cartilage at the bones' ends has roughened and thinned, and the bones have developed the tiny spurs typical of osteoarthritis. The capsule around the joint also thickens and stretches.

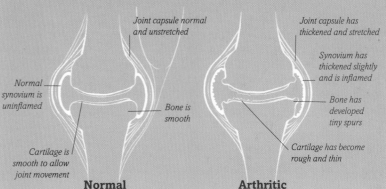

Joint capsule normal and unstretched

Joint capsule has thickened and stretched

Synovium has thickened slightly and is inflamed

Normal synovium is uninflamed

Bone is smooth

Bone has developed tiny spurs

Cartilage is smooth to allow joint movement

Cartilage has become rough and thin

Normal   **Arthritic**

normally done to exclude other types of arthritis (such as rheumatoid arthritis, see pp266–8) since there are no specific tests that can detect osteoarthritis. You may also need an X-ray to see if there is any narrowing within a joint or if there are bony spurs. Be aware that X-rays may be normal in the early stages of osteoarthritis.

MY TREATMENT OPTIONS

Unfortunately there is no cure for osteoarthritis—our joints just don't seem to be designed to work perfectly for a lifetime. But there are plenty of medicines to relieve any associated pain and stiffness. However, as with any drug, these can come with side effects.

Analgesics Acetaminophen is the safest analgesic to take for short-term relief. It can also be used in combination with other analgesics, such as codeine-like drugs. Medicines known as nonsteroidal

anti-inflammatory drugs (NSAIDs), such as ibuprofen and naproxen, can also reduce your pain, swelling, and stiffness.

Injections Steroids or hyaluronic acid (which is similar to the thick, viscous component of normal synovial fluid, see p258) can be given as injections into an affected joint. These injections may provide longer relief and ease your pain for several weeks at a time.

Physical therapy In sessions with a physical therapist, you can learn exercises that will help to stabilize and protect your joints. You may also have some hydrotherapy, which involves hot and cold water treatments, to increase your range of mobility in an affected joint, especially a knee.

Joint replacement If, despite taking medication, your pain continues to be severe and your joints become so badly swollen or damaged that they restrict your mobility, your doctor may refer you to an orthopedic surgeon. Depending on your particular problem, the surgeon may recommend that you have surgery to replace the affected joint with a prosthesis. As with any surgery, there are risks that your doctor will talk to you about.

Replacing an osteoarthritic hip

This X-ray image shows a hip joint after joint replacement surgery. Osteoarthritis had damaged the cartilage around the ball-and-socket joint where the thigh bone meets the pelvis at the pelvic socket.

AM I AT RISK?

Osteoarthritis becomes more common as you get older; it is rare before the age of 40. It's not known why one woman and not another will develop osteoarthritis, but there are some known risk factors.

- Being overweight or obese. The heavier you, are the more weight your knees and hips have to bear; being overweight or obese also increases the chances of osteoarthritis worsening
- Doing hard and repetitive exercise, such as seen in ballet dancers or gymnasts
- Having a history of osteoarthritis in the family
- Having a joint abnormality at birth
- Having had an injury or operation on a joint.

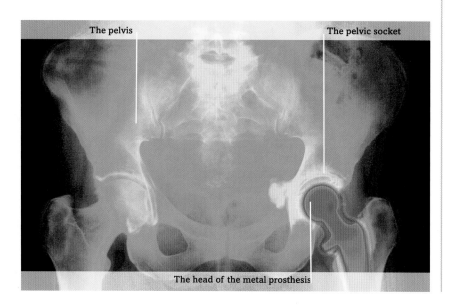

The pelvis

The pelvic socket

The head of the metal prosthesis

Advances in surgical techniques and materials technology mean that artificial joints may last 10–25 years. The implants can provide you with mobility that is both stable and pain-free.

Hips and knees are the most commonly replaced joints, and surgery for these is generally very successful. However, other joints, such as the shoulder, ankle, elbow, and knuckles, can also be replaced with varying amounts of success.

Depending on the procedure you have, you can expect to stay in the hospital between two and five days. Afterward, your recovery is likely to be slow and steady; many people feel much better three to six months after joint replacement surgery, but it can take up to a year to feel totally back to normal.

HOW CAN I HELP MYSELF?

There are several measures you can take to help you relieve the symptoms of osteoarthritis.

"There are plenty of osteoarthritis treatments so that you can still enjoy life to the fullest."

Lose excess weight First and foremost, losing weight if you are overweight will be a great help; you'll be significantly reducing everyday stress on your hips, knees, and feet. Try to keep active, and pace your activities throughout the day with regular breaks (see Eat a healthy diet, pp52–5; Exercise to stay healthy, pp56–7; Weight issues, pp58–9).

Wear comfortable shoes You might find that certain footwear helps: shock-absorbing sneakers with thick soft soles or flat shoes may be much more comfortable and help lessen any aches and pains. If you suffer with bunions or the beginnings of one, then steer clear of pointed toes or high heels, or at least restrict your wearing of them to short periods.

You may take a supplement Many people take glucosamine and/or chondroitin supplements, which are available from health food stores, to "help with their joints." Such substances may have a modest effect on cartilage loss, and some people find that they provide pain relief. There is no evidence, however, that cod liver oil has any noticeable impact on osteoarthritis.

Use a walking aid If you find that a joint simply gives way from time to time, try using a cane (you can get collapsible ones that are easy to store and transport). Wearing a joint brace to support a knee, for example, can also help.

Modify your home and work Occupational therapists can give you advice on modifications to both your home and your work environment, as well as useful gadgets, such as jar and bottle openers, to help with daily life.

BUNIONS

Osteoarthritis at the base of the big toe may result in stiffness of the joint and a bony deformity—one of the causes of painful bunions. The big toe leans toward the other toes and the joint at the base sticks out (see right). The tissues overlying the bunion can become inflamed, causing pain and swelling. Bunions are more likely to cause symptoms when you wear shoes with a tight toe box or high heels. Standing for a long time may also aggravate symptoms. Your doctor may recommend that you wear pads over the bunion or wear a custom-made device inside your shoes. Alternatively, you may want to visit a podiatrist for exercise recommendations and orthotics (special devices inserted into shoes). In severe cases, surgical treatment may be necessary.

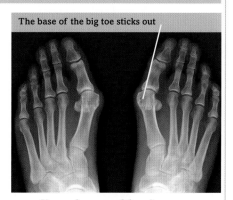

The base of the big toe sticks out

X-ray image of bunions

Autoimmune diseases

In this section, we look at rheumatoid arthritis, lupus, Raynaud's phenomenon, and Sjögren's syndrome. These diseases, in which your body attacks itself, are more common in women. As with so many conditions, it is not yet known what causes the body to prompt such an attack, or how this assault will affect the body.

Rheumatoid arthritis

This autoimmune disease can affect people of any age, although it most often occurs in people in their early 40s and is three times more common in women than in men.

WHAT IS IT?

Arthritis means inflammation of joints, and rheumatoid arthritis is a common form of arthritis. In rheumatoid arthritis (RA), the body's own immune system attacks the lining (synovium, see p258) of joints, in particular those of the hands, wrists, and feet, or other joints in the body. This results in inflammation, swelling, stiffness, warm joints, and pain. The joint can become painful when the cells in the synovium are irritated by inflammatory mediators called cytokines, resulting in a thickened, inflamed synovium and joint.

It is not known exactly what triggers this joint inflammation (see p259), which over time can also damage the cartilage, the ligaments, and the bone near a joint. Rheumatoid arthritis may also affect tendons and sometimes other body parts, such as the lungs, eyes, and blood vessels, and lumps called rheumatoid nodules may occur in elbows, hands, and feet. Patients with rheumatoid arthritis are also more at risk of cardiovascular disease and heart attacks. Treatment with steroids and some NSAIDS may also increase the risk.

In most cases, RA symptoms develop gradually over several weeks or so. The disease is usually characterized by recurrent moderate attacks. The frequency of attacks, the number of affected joints, and the severity of symptoms are variable. Some people have a mild form of the disease, with very few symptoms. Most people have periods of flare-ups when their joints become more painful and inflamed. Such flare-ups may last for weeks or months. For some people, their rheumatoid arthritis becomes progressively worse quite quickly.

WHAT NEXT?

There is no single test to diagnose rheumatoid arthritis, and because there are many other possible conditions that may cause your joints to be painful, it may initially be difficult to diagnose RA. Your doctor will make a diagnosis based on a discussion with you about your symptoms, your medical history, the findings of a physical examination, and the

DO I HAVE THE SYMPTOMS?

There are several main and "extra-articular" ("outside of the joints") symptoms to look for:

- Pain and swelling in the fingers, wrists, or balls of feet
- Morning stiffness
- A general feeling of being unwell
- Fatigue
- Feeling hot and sweaty
- Feeling depressed or irritable
- Unexplained weight loss
- Dry, irritable eyes

See your doctor if you have one or more symptoms in addition to stiff, aching joints.

"You can reduce your risk of developing RA by adopting a healthy lifestyle."

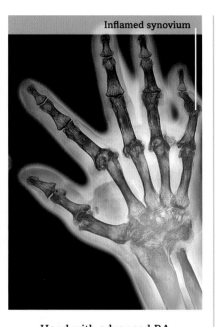

Inflamed synovium

Hand with advanced RA

This X-ray shows the swelling of the joint caused by the collection of fluid and cells in the synovium.

results of any blood tests and X-rays that might be appropriate. Blood tests can check for:

- Inflammation—erythrocyte sedimentation rate (ESR) and C-reactive protein (CRP)
- Rheumatoid factor (80 percent of people with RA have this protein in their blood)
- Anti-cyclic citrillinated peptide (CCP) antibodies (these antibodies are highly specific to rheumatoid arthritis).

X-rays may show damage caused by the disease process. There are also newer techniques, such as ultrasound scanning and magnetic resonance imaging (MRI), which may pick up earlier changes due to the disease.

AM I AT RISK?

Rheumatoid arthritis exists all over the world, and approximately 1 person in every 100 of the population is affected by it. Rheumatoid arthritis can begin at any age, but it most commonly starts between the ages of 30 and 50 and symptoms typically appear when people are in their early 40s.

As with many diseases, rheumatoid arthritis can run in families, but genes are only part of the picture. Certain lifestyle factors may increase your risk of contracting rheumatoid arthritis, so the best way to help reduce this risk is by adopting a healthy lifestyle. Cigarette smoking is

thought to increase the risk of rheumatoid arthritis, so if you are still a smoker, turn to p64 for tips on how to quit.

It's also important to eat a balanced, varied diet, because a diet that is typically high in caffeine and low in antioxidants, may increase the risk of this condition.

Rheumatoid arthritis has also been found to be slightly less common in people who drink alcohol in moderation.

If you are overweight or obese, the excess weight that your body carries can put extra pressure on joints, so losing any excess weight can make a positive difference to your health.

JOINTS AFFECTED BY RHEUMATOID ARTHRITIS

Rheumatoid arthritis is likely to affect the joints highlighted *(below)*, and tends to affect the body symmetrically. The degree of damage, and the number of joints affected, will vary from person to person, since RA seems to affect everyone differently.

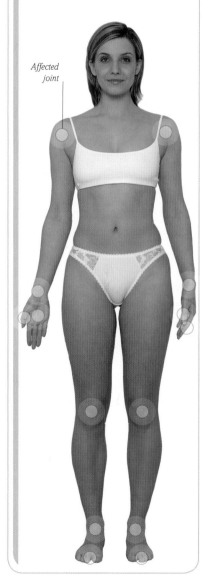

Affected joint

MY TREATMENT OPTIONS

The main goal of RA treatment is to suppress the inflammation in the joints as early as possible in order to prevent any more damage; once the joints have been damaged by inflammation, they do not heal very well. Key treatments for rheumatoid arthritis include:

Analgesics, such as acetaminophen, will help reduce pain, and can be given in combination with stronger codeine-like drugs. However, simple analgesics are not enough, and are usually prescribed together with NSAIDS.

Nonsteroidal anti-inflammatory drugs (NSAIDS) reduce both the pain and the swelling of joints.

Disease-modifying antirheumatic drugs (DMARDs) can treat more than just the symptoms of rheumatoid arthritis—they also slow down the course of the disease itself. These drugs may take many weeks or months to become effective, and tend to be taken for many years.

Since they can all potentially cause side effects, these drugs require regular monitoring by doctors. There are a number of drugs in this group:

- Methotrexate, sulfasalazine, leflunamide, azathioprine, and hydroxychloroquine.
- Newer biological therapies, such as antiTNF drugs, abatacept, and rituximab, are very effective and may work more quickly

Steroids, which can cause a number of side effects if used long term.

HOW CAN I HELP MYSELF?

There are several ways to take care of yourself to minimize the disability of rheumatoid arthritis as much as possible:

Take an omega-3 fatty acid supplement, which may have a modest beneficial effect on the symptoms of RA.

Keep your weight within healthy levels. Eating a good, healthy diet may also help, and lose weight if you are overweight.

RHEUMATOID ARTHRITIS AND PREGNANCY

Most women with rheumatoid arthritis feel better during pregnancy. Unfortunately, the disease can flare up again after the baby is born. Also, some medicines cannot be taken during pregnancy, so if you are thinking of becoming pregnant (or if you are already pregnant), discuss this condition with your doctor.

Try to be as active as possible, because the muscles around the joints will become weak if they aren't used. Regular exercise to increase muscle strength may also help reduce pain and improve joint function. However, you should work within your limits; you don't want to harm your muscles and joints.

Vary your level of activity from day to day, depending on how you feel. Swimming, cycling, and walking with supportive shoes are all very beneficial. Physical and occupational therapists can also advise on particular exercises to keep the joints mobile and the muscles around the joints as strong as possible, and also on joint protection, adaptations to your home to make daily tasks easier, and useful aids.

Beneficial treatment
Swimming is a good way to exercise many major muscles in the body without straining the joints too much.

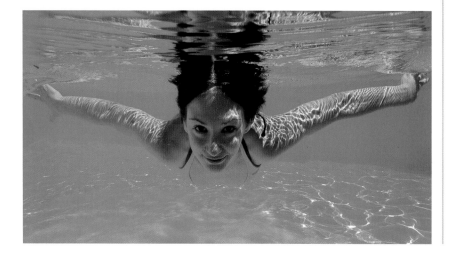

Lupus

Systemic lupus erythematosus (its full name) is usually called lupus or SLE for short. This autoimmune disease is nine times more common in women than in men, and it affects about 1 in every 1,000 people.

WHAT IS IT?

Lupus is an unpredictable, persistent disease that causes inflammation in various parts of the body. It can be mild or severe; it can flare up and then simply subside; and it can present in many ways and mimic many diseases.

DO I HAVE THE SYMPTOMS?

Lupus can cause a variety of symptoms, of which these are the most common:
- Joint pain
- Fatigue
- Skin rashes
- Increased sensitivity to light
- Fever
- Weight loss
- Swollen lymph glands
- Hair loss
- Mouth ulcers
- Poor circulation to the fingers and toes (Raynaud's phenomenon, see p270).

Every individual who has lupus may have a different selection of these symptoms from another person with the condition. **See your doctor** if you have a selection of these symptoms.

Lupus most typically develops in women of childbearing age, although people at any age can be affected, and it has been found to be more prevalent among women of African-American and Asian origin.

It's not known why lupus and other autoimmune diseases occur. Some factors may trigger the immune system to make abnormal antibodies, which cause the inflammation and damage to various body tissues. Possible triggers may include viruses, environmental factors such as sunlight and infections, hormones, and genetic factors, although lupus is not a simple hereditary disease. Some women also have specific antiphospholipid antibodies that can result in a miscarriage during pregnancy, or in blood clots.

Lupus has wide-ranging effects on various body organs and systems, including:
- The kidneys: inflammation here leads to high blood pressure and kidney failure
- The brain and nervous system: causing anything from a simple headache to anxiety and depression, epilepsy, strokes, and even mental health problems
- The heart and lungs: resulting in breathlessness and chest pain
- The digestive tract and liver: leading to loss of appetite, sickness, vomiting, and diarrhea
- The spleen: an enlarged spleen can be found when a patient is examined
- The eyes: causing dry eyes and a dry mouth.

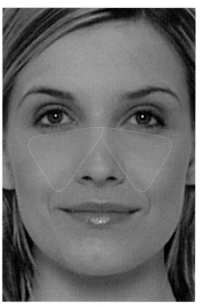

Butterfly rash
A red raised rash across the nose and cheeks in the shape of a butterfly is a common characteristic of lupus.

WHAT NEXT?

Your doctor will make a diagnosis based on your symptoms (see Do I Have the Symptoms?, left), medical history, a physical examination, as necessary, and the results of a range of specific blood tests. The tests can detect certain types of antibodies (ANA, antiDNA, and other antibodies) or signs of disease activity in your blood. The blood tests may also show evidence of anemia and abnormalities of other blood cells, and assess kidney and liver function.

MY TREATMENT OPTIONS

Although there is currently no cure, much progress has been made in the treatment and management of the disease, and the outlook for patients with lupus has improved dramatically. Most people with lupus are seen by a specialist who will advise on the right treatments.

Medication can ease symptoms in most cases. Depending on how many of the symptoms you are suffering from, your doctor may prescribe one or more of the following effective medications:

- Painkillers and NSAIDs: to provide relief from joint pain
- Hydroxychloroquine pills and steroid cream: both medications are used for the treatment of skin rashes; hydroxychloroquine pills also treat joint pains and fatigue
- Steroids: to treat inflammation in other parts of the body, such as the heart or the lungs
- High-dose steroids and immunosuppressants: for severe forms of the disease.

HOW CAN I HELP MYSELF?

There are some simple measures you can take to look after yourself if you suffer from lupus:

Avoid the sun Strong sunlight can aggravate the symptoms of lupus (and not just the skin symptoms). Cover up and apply sunscreen of SPF 25 or above on exposed skin.

Quit smoking because smoking can increase the risk of lupus.

Try to avoid infections, since you are more prone to infection— particularly if you take steroids or immunosuppressant medication.

Avoid using certain drugs, if possible, that are known to cause drug-induced lupus or lupus flare-ups.

Take an omega-3 fatty acid supplement, which may be helpful.

Raynaud's phenomenon

This common disease affects the extremities of the body (usually the fingers), which change color and become painful. Approximately 1 in 20 people develop the symptoms and it can affect all ages, but its symptoms are usually mild. Fewer than 1 in 10 people affected by this condition have an underlying disease (such as an autoimmune disease), but it can also be a side effect of drugs, such as beta blockers.

WHAT IS IT?

Raynaud's phenomenon is due to constriction of the small blood vessels when exposed to the cold, or to a change in temperature. The skin on your fingers, for example, changes color, first becoming pale and cool, then a bluish color, and finally pink (muscle spasm in the arteries restricts the blood supply briefly). Along with this color change comes pain, numbness, and tingling. It can affect your feet and even your nose, earlobes, or tongue, but it's your hands that are usually the problem.

WHAT NEXT?

If you're unable to control the condition on your own, your doctor may prescribe medication to dilate the blood vessels.

MY TREATMENT OPTIONS

Discuss your symptoms with your doctor and see what kind of treatment is appropriate for you.

HOW CAN I HELP MYSELF?

There are several ways to self-treat:
Keep your hands warm with hand warmers and heated gloves.
Avoid sudden exposure to cold.
Quit smoking, as it constricts the blood vessels in your hands.
Reduce stress in your everyday life and and learn to relax as much as you can (see pp62-3).

DO I HAVE THE SYMPTOMS?

Typically, these symptoms develop when you become cool, for instance in cold weather:

- Pain, numbness, throbbing, and tingling in fingers
- Skin on fingers changes color when cold due to the constriction and dilation of blood vessels in the fingers
- Occasional problems with your feet.

See your doctor if these symptoms develop when you experience cold weather.

Sjögren's syndrome

Sjögren's (pronounced "show-grins") syndrome is a serious and common autoimmune disease. Although this disease can strike at any age, women between the ages of 40 and 60 are most likely to get it.

WHAT IS IT?

In this autoimmune condition, your immune system attacks and damages the tissues of the salivary glands and the tear glands. The resulting symptoms (see Do I Have the Symptoms?, right), may prove to be uncomfortable but can be trseated. In addition to the attack on your salivary and tear glands, your body's immune system may also cause inflammation of your joints, kidneys, and lungs. If you have Sjögren's syndrome and become pregnant, there is a risk that some of the autoantibodies your body has created may pass across the placenta to your growing baby and cause a disturbed heart rhythm. The babies of patients who carry these antibodies need to be monitored carefully during pregnancy, and may also need to have steroid treatment.

WHAT NEXT?

After taking your medical history and examining you, if necessary, your doctor will measure your tear and saliva production, arrange for blood tests to detect any autoantibodies, and perhaps ask for a lip biopsy (when tiny salivary glands are removed from the lower lip for close examination under a microscope). To determine your tear production, your doctor will gently insert a small piece of paper under your lower eyelid for several minutes and ask you to keep your eyes closed. How much saliva you can produce is measured simply by how much you can spit into a cup.

MY TREATMENT OPTIONS

Although there is as yet no cure for Sjögren's syndrome, doctors can prescribe a variety of treatments:
Artificial tears can help to lubricate dry eyes.
Special eyeglasses keep in moisture and reduce eye dryness.
Artificial saliva, given as a mouth spray or as lozenges.
Painkillers (including NSAIDs) can be helpful.
Hydroxychloroquine, the antimalarial drug, helps with joint pain and fatigue.
Steroid drugs can be used for arthritis and swollen glands or other organs, such as the lungs.
Minor surgery is offered for particular cases.

HOW CAN I HELP MYSELF?

There are several general measures to take to help your condition:
To treat dry eyes, avoid wind, air conditioning, dust, and smoke.
To treat a dry mouth, drink lots of water, chew sugarless gum, keep your teeth, gums, and mouth clean, and visit your dentist regularly.

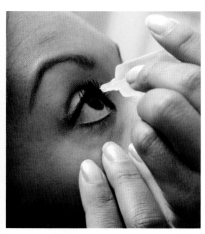

Artificial tears
Eye drops provide lubrication. Tilt your head back and pull the lower lid down to apply drops inside the lower lid.

> ### DO I HAVE THE SYMPTOMS?
>
> The symptoms to look for are:
> - Aching in the joints
> - Dry eyes
> - Dry mouth and dental problems
> - Fatigue
> - Swollen salivary glands and lymph nodes.
>
> Other organs of the body can also be affected by this condition.
> **See your doctor** if you think that you have more than one of these symptoms.

> "Some people may only notice mild symptoms, such as dry eyes and a dry mouth."

Back and neck pain

In the US, more working days are lost to back pain than any other condition—back pain accounts for 100 million lost work days per year. Neck pain is also common and occurs more often in women. The good news is that most pain resolves itself within a few weeks. But see your doctor if the pain persists.

DO I HAVE THE SYMPTOMS?

Symptoms may come on over weeks or appear suddenly.
- Pain, which could be referred to arms or legs
- Stiffness, clicking, or cracking felt with movement (neck pain).

See your doctor urgently if you have weakness, numbness, or tingling in your arms or legs; numbness in your bottom; bowel problems or with passing urine; dizziness when looking up.

WHAT IS IT?

Pain due to bad posture or straining muscles or ligaments—so-called mechanical pain—is very common. Largely worse after movement and relieved by rest, the pain doesn't usually radiate (called "referred pain") to your arms or legs and tends to resolve fairly quickly. However, the painful muscle spasm that's sometimes associated with it may last for several weeks.

"Referred" pain in your limbs may also be accompanied by numbness or tingling. Conversely, a painful shoulder (see p282) may

result in pain felt in the neck.

Common causes of neck and back pain are:
- Bad posture
- Abnormal exertion
- Osteoarthritis of the spine
- Injury, such as whiplash
- A "slipped disc"
- Narrowing of the spinal canal (spinal stenosis)
- Abnormal curvature of the spine.

Bad posture whether hunching over a steering wheel or slumping at a desk can wreak havoc on your muscles, often triggering painful muscle strains.

Abnormal exertion can happen when overreaching or lifting something too heavy or at an awkward angle. The resulting pain is a symptom of stress or damage to any of your spine's ligaments, muscles, tendons, or disks.

Whiplash injuries, where a person's head is thrown forward and then backward violently (as in a car accident when a car is hit from behind) is a common cause of neck pain.

A "slipped disk" is more accurately described as a "prolapsed" (bulging) or "herniated" (ruptured) disk. The cause of this serious back pain is the jellylike

material held within the cushioning intervertebral disks. This prolapsed or ruptured disc can squash a nearby nerve root or the spinal cord. Pressure causes pain as well as symptoms in other parts of the body, such as numbness or tingling in your arms or legs, and can even affect bladder and bowel control.

Osteoarthritis of the spine is also referred to by doctors as spondylosis: cervical spondylosis if the osteoarthritis is in the neck or lumbar regions, spondylosis, if

space between vertebrae has narrowed

roughened vertebra

Cervical spondylosis
This X-ray shows the vertebrae of the cervical spine. The osteoarthritic vertebrae are close together and have roughened edges.

in the lower back. Osteoarthritis (see p263) is a "wear and tear" arthritis. In the spine it affects both the facet joints and the intervertebral disks (see below). As we age, these disks become thinner and the spaces between the vertebrae become narrower. Bony outgrowths or spurs, called osteophytes, form at the edges of the vertebrae and the facet joints. These bony growths may cause localized pain or referred pain in an arm or leg, for example, if they pinch a nerve.

Spinal stenosis Narrowing of the spinal canal by a disk or a bony growth is known as spinal stenosis. This narrowing puts pressure on the spinal cord and can be associated with numbness, weakness in the legs, or bladder or bowel problems.

Abnormal curvature of the spine If your spine curves in an abnormal way or if the curve is exaggerated, it may result in pain. Scoliosis, where the spine curves to the side, may also cause pain.

Other causes of back and/or neck pain include: rheumatoid arthritis (see p266), ankylosing spondylitis, fibromyalgia (see p276), polymyalgia rheumatica, fractures associated with osteoporosis (see p260), infection (such as tuberculosis), certain cancers that may have spread to the vertebrae, and trauma and/or injury.

WHAT NEXT?

Normally, your doctor will make a diagnosis based on your medical history and a physical examination.

Your doctor will want to find out where the pain is coming from,

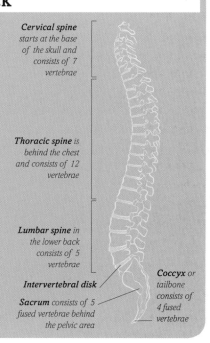

prolapsed disc

spinal cord

Lumbar disk prolapse
In this MRI scan, a prolapsed disk between the lumbar spine and the sacrum is putting pressure on the spinal cord.

how much you can move before the pain kicks in, and whether any muscles are in spasm. To this end, he or she may want to examine your back and assess your ability to sit, stand, bend over, walk, and lift your legs.

If it's your neck that's painful, your doctor will want to see your range of movement and the exact location of the pain as well as determine the kinds of activities that bring it on. Your reflexes may also be tested.

Further tests, such as X-rays, CT, or MRI scans, are often done to rule out a herniated disk, trapped nerve, spinal stenosis, spinal fracture, inflammation, infection, or a tumor.

You may have to give a sample of blood for laboratory testing to help determine the diagnosis.

THE BONES OF YOUR BACK

Your back consists of stacked vertebrae forming the spinal column from skull to pelvis. It is divided into three main sections: the cervical spine (7 vertebrae); the thoracic spine (12 vertebrae); and the lumbar vertebrae (5 vertebrae). The sacrum is 5 fused vertebrae; the coccyx is 4. Cushioning disks sit between the vertebrae, while facet joints connect them at the back. The vertebrae are held together by ligaments, allowing flexibility. Your spinal cord lies within the spinal column. Nerves run from your brain through your spinal cord to the rest of your body.

Cervical spine *starts at the base of the skull and consists of 7 vertebrae*

Thoracic spine is behind the chest and consists of 12 vertebrae

Lumbar spine in the lower back consists of 5 vertebrae

Intervertebral disk

Sacrum consists of 5 fused vertebrae behind the pelvic area

Coccyx or tailbone consists of 4 fused vertebrae

LOWER-BACK PAIN

Because of the complex and interconnected nature of your lower back, any small amount of damage to a muscle, ligament, tendon, or disk can result in a lot of discomfort. The location of the pain—be it high up in the middle of the back or radiating down one leg, as shown below—will give your doctor clues as to the cause of your pain.

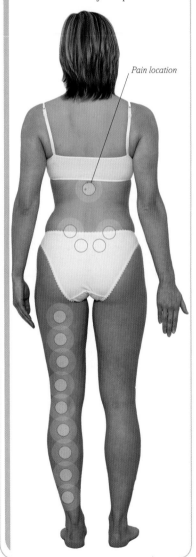

Pain location

MY TREATMENT OPTIONS

Most instances of back or neck pain resolve within weeks and need little or no treatment, except for some pain relief. But if your pain is severe or your doctor has identified the cause of your pain, then other options, which may have potential side effects, are available.

Pain relief While your pain resolves you may get enough relief from regular doses of acetaminophen or ibuprofen. If these drugs are not quite enough, your doctor can prescribe stronger nonsteroidal anti-inflammatory drugs (NSAIDs), such as diclofenac or naproxen.

Steroid and local anesthetic injections These can help with pain from a prolapsed or herniated disk or facet joint arthritis.

Other drugs Many people get relief from sciatic pain (pain in the buttocks and down the back of the thigh caused by pressure on the sciatic nerve) from the antidepressant drug amitriptyline and the anticonvulsant drugs gabapentin and pregabalin.

Manipulative therapies Your doctor may refer you to a physical therapist, who can use various treatments to lessen the pain, such as heat, ice, ultrasound, TENS (transcutaneous electrical nerve stimulation), and muscle-release techniques. What's more, he or she will be able to teach you exercises and stretches to restore muscle function and strengthen your neck and/or back muscles.

Surgery If all forms of pain relief and/or manipulative therapies fail, then surgery may be necessary. In cases of spinal stenosis or a prolapsed or herniated disk, a surgeon can remove the cause of the pain. After such surgery, it's usual to spend a few days in the hospital. It may take a few weeks afterward for the pain to resolve.

A pain-management program If, despite all treatments, the pain persists, your doctor may refer you to a pain-management program. Usually run as outpatient sessions, these involve a multidisciplinary team (doctors, nurses, physical therapists, and psychologists) to give advice and information about exercise, coping strategies, pacing of activities, and the use of medications.

HOW CAN I HELP MYSELF?

In addition to following your doctor's advice, there are some things you can try to help relieve the pain. Then, it's a good idea to learn how to prevent future occurrences by strengthening your muscles and keeping healthy (see opposite).

Rest It may help to spend a few days resting, but it's not a good idea to spend a long time in bed.

"Walking, swimming, and cycling
are all excellent to strengthen
your back muscles."

Try to get back to normal activities and work as soon as possible. Resting for too long may hinder your progress and weaken muscles, and significant time off work may also dent your confidence.

Gentle stretches For neck pain, gently move your head to one side and hold for 30 seconds. Then, repeat on the other side. Stretch your neck in as many directions as your pain allows. Stretching, strengthening, and stabilizing exercises can help relieve back pain. Such exercises are designed to restore the strength of your back muscles and the flexibility of your spinal column.

Sleep right You spend a third of your life sleeping and if you sleep in an awkward position—hugging a pillow, for instance, or even just lying on your front—you can be putting extra stress and strain on your back and neck muscles every single day. Try to train yourself to sleep lying on one side rather than on your front. Choose a supportive mattress and change it if you wake up first thing in the morning with backache; experts recommend that you change your mattress every 10 years.

Osteopathy, physical therapy, and chiropractic Many women seek the services of an osteopath, physical therapist, or chiropractor. Each professional has a different approach to problems relating to the spine. Normally, a short course is all that's needed, along with paying attention to your posture in your day-to-day life.

KEEP YOUR BACK HEALTHY

By following these few simple guidelines you can build a strong, healthy back and lead a full and pain-free life.

- Exercise your back regularly—walking, swimming, and using exercise bikes are all excellent to strengthen your back muscles
- Always bend your knees and your hips, never your back, when lifting an object
- Exercises, such as Pilates, that build "core strength" work your pelvic and abdominal muscles to support your back by working like a natural "corset"
- Never twist and bend at the same time
- Always lift and carry objects close to your body
- Try to carry loads in a backpack, and avoid shoulder bags
- Always maintain a good posture—avoid slumping in your chair or walking around with your hands in your pockets
- When working at a desk, always use a chair with a back rest and sit with your feet flat on the floor or on a footrest under the table
- Choose a firm mattress and ensure you sleep in a comfortable position.

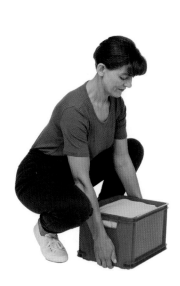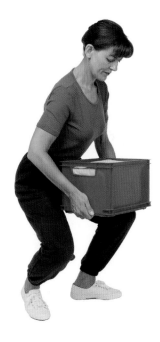

Good lifting technique
Step 1 To prevent back problems, learn how to lift correctly—using the power of your legs. Squat down in front of the object you need to lift.

Step 2 Then, while keeping your body straight and the object in front of you, straighten your legs and stand up.

Fibromyalgia

You may well know someone who has this common condition since it affects 1 person in 20, and 9 out of 10 sufferers are women. Fibromyalgia causes widespread and unremitting muscle pain, along with specific tender points. This discomfort is often accompanied by sleep disturbance and severe fatigue.

WHAT IS IT?

As with many conditions, the cause of fibromyalgia is unknown. It may be that chemical changes in the brain and nervous system lead to an increased sensitivity to pressure, so that what's normally felt as pressure becomes acutely painful. Recent research has suggested that fibromyalgia sufferers have lower than normal levels of a chemical called serotonin in the brain. Serotonin is involved in pain control and also in the regulation of sleep. Fibromyalgia may run in families; you're most likely to be affected if you have a relative who also suffers from it.

No one knows exactly what triggers fibromyalgia, but it often comes on after you've had a period of emotional stress or illness, or following surgery or an accident. Fibromyalgia often occurs together with other conditions, including irritable bladder, premenstrual syndrome (see pp92–3), painful periods (see p91), and irritable bowel syndrome (see pp304–5).

WHAT NEXT?

Your doctor may suspect you have fibromyalgia if you've had widespread pain for at least three months and you have tenderness in 11 out of the 18 characteristic locations (see opposite). If, after reviewing your medical history and carrying out a physical examination, your doctor thinks that fibromyalgia may be the cause of your symptoms, he or she will order X-rays and blood tests to rule out other conditions that may cause similar symptoms, such as overactivity of the thyroid gland (see pp328–9). There's no specific test that will positively confirm the diagnosis of fibromyalgia.

MY TREATMENT OPTIONS

Fibromyalgia can be treated in a combination of ways and, in addition to appropriate medication (which may have side effects), treatment includes learning about the condition and looking at how your behavior could be contributing to your symptoms. A carefully planned program of exercise is often integral to treatment.

Pain relief Acetaminophen is recommended for the relief of pain. If this doesn't provide adequate relief, you might also be given NSAIDS, and lastly, opioid painkillers, such as tramadol. Low doses of antidepressants, including amitriptyline, fluoxetine, duloxetine, and milnacipran (sometimes used in combination), can be used for relieving pain and can also help with sleep problems. For some, the anticonvulsant drugs pregabalin and

DO I HAVE THE SYMPTOMS?

Fibromyalgia is likely to cause a combination of any of the following symptoms:
- Pain at many sites
- Tender points (see opposite)
- Stiffness, which is often worse in the morning
- Feeling exhausted, even when you've just woken up
- Frequently waking at night and having trouble getting back to sleep
- Joints that feel swollen, although they look normal
- Tingling
- Poor concentration
- Memory problems
- Headaches
- Light-headedness, anxiety, and/or depression.

See your doctor if you have been suffering from a number of these symptoms.

gabapentin are effective both for relieving pain and for helping to counteract any sleep disturbances, though pregabalin is the only FDA-approved medication to treat fibromyalgia.

Cognitive behavioral therapy This form of talking therapy aims to help you understand that your thoughts, beliefs, and expectations can all have an impact on your symptoms. Changing the way you think about your symptoms can sometimes lessen their severity.

Exercise plan By getting some exercise you'll be able to continue your everyday activities. Regular exercise also has a beneficial effect on sleep patterns. Your doctor may refer you to a physical therapist, who will be able to help design an exercise program that will increase your strength, provide aerobic conditioning, and improve your flexibility and balance. Some of the best forms of exercise for fibromyalgia sufferers include low-impact aerobic exercise, such as swimming and walking, and activities such as yoga that involve stretching.

HOW CAN I HELP MYSELF?

Together with any medical treatment your doctor may prescribe for you, making a few simple changes to your lifestyle can reap big rewards in terms of a reduction in the severity of your symptoms and improving the frequency and length of your pain-free interludes.

Try to get a good night's sleep, training yourself to do so if necessary (see pp60–1).

Eat a healthy, balanced diet; Although there are no special foods that will help the condition, it can make a difference (see pp52–5).

Learn how to relax and handle stress (see pp62–3).

Physical therapies such as massage can sometimes relieve pain and eliminate stiffness as well as help you relax.

Join a fibromyalgia support group. The opportunity to share your experiences with others who are going through the same thing can be a great source of comfort and self-help ideas.

CLASSIC TENDER SPOTS

Your doctor will test each of the highlighted areas for tenderness. If 11 out of 18 sites are tender, then it's likely you have fibromyalgia.

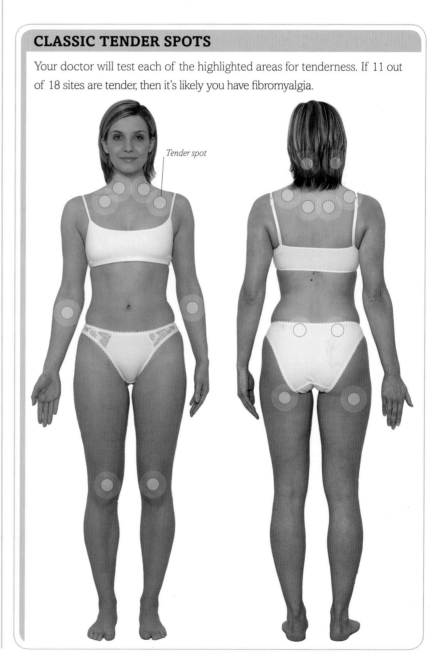

Tender spot

Chronic fatigue syndrome

Many of us in today's busy world complain of being "tired all the time," but if you have chronic fatigue syndrome (CFS), you literally *are* tired all the time. This long-term, often disabling, exhaustion persists even if you've had a good night's sleep. However, there are treatments to try, and ways to help yourself.

DO I HAVE THE SYMPTOMS?

CFS causes persistent physical and mental fatigue for at least six months, and any four primary symptoms:

- Weakness and extreme exhaustion, lasting more than 24 hours, after any mental or physical activity
- Unrefreshing sleep, insomnia, or excessive daytime sleepiness
- Substantial impairment of short-term memory or concentration
- Unexplained muscle soreness

- Pain that moves from joint to joint without swelling or redness
- Headaches of a new type, pattern, or severity
- Tender lymph nodes in your armpit and/or neck
- Persistent or frequent sore throat. In addition, there are some common secondary symptoms:
- Unexplained abdominal pain
- Hypersensitivity to light, noise, and to emotional overload

- Dizziness, fainting, lack of balance
- Palpitations, irregular heartbeat
- A need to urinate often
- Shortness of breath
- IBS (see pp304–5)
- Chills and inappropriate sweating, often at night
- A new allergy or sensitivity to a food, medication, or chemical.

See your doctor if you have any four primary symptoms and any secondary symptoms.

WHAT IS IT?

Also known as ME (myalgic encephalomyelitis or myalgic encephalopathy), CFS is recognized as a serious illness marked by prolonged exhaustion and wide-ranging symptoms (see box, above). CFS is a complex, mysterious condition and research is still ongoing into the exact cause; it is discussed in this chapter because of its close relationship with fibromyalgia (see pp276–7). CFS can affect people at any age, mostly 20s to 40s, and can either develop suddenly or appear gradually over a period of years. Three to five times more women than men have CFS.

WHAT NEXT?

Currently, there's no diagnostic test for CFS, so your doctor will make a diagnosis based on your medical history and a physical examination, as well as tests to rule out all other possible causes of your symptoms. To be given a diagnosis of CFS, you have to meet some of the criteria set out in the Do I have the symptoms? box (see above). Since fatigue can have other causes, your doctor may take a blood sample to exclude autoimmune diseases (see

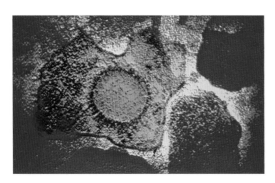

Cytomegalovirus
Although the cause of CFS is not yet known, one theory centers on a viral infection, such as might be caused by cytomegalovirus (left). It is also believed that a head trauma can trigger CFS.

pp259, 266–71), iron-deficiency anemia (see pp248–9), underactive thyroid gland (see p327), depression (see pp210–11), or viral infection.

Doctors generally find it hard to diagnose CFS because its signs and symptoms are similar to many other diseases. There are, however, a small number of self-designated chronic fatigue syndrome specialists in the US, mostly in teaching hospitals in major cities. If you want a referral to see one of these doctors, discuss this option with your doctor.

MY TREATMENT OPTIONS

Although a cycle of relapses and remissions—triggered by overexertion, infectious illnesses, or seasonal changes—is a common pattern of CFS, many people gradually improve over time after trying these treatments:

Medications to ease the various symptoms can be prescribed by your doctor. Although there are no specific medications to treat CFS, analgesics, such as acetaminophen, or NSAIDs, such as ibuprofen or diclofenac, may relieve existing muscle or joint pain, or headaches. Some antidepressants may help regulate your sleep, promote appetite, and relieve pain; types commonly used are tricyclics (see p227) and selective serotonin reuptake inhibitors (SSRIs) (see p227). Blood pressure drugs, such as fludrocortisone, may help to stop you from feeling dizzy and faint. Low-dose antidepressants, such as amitriptyline, may help you

> ### THE CFS SPECTRUM
>
> Chronic fatigue syndrome is often organized into four categories: mild, moderate, severe, or very severe.
>
> **Mild CFS** You can take care of yourself, but you may need to take days off work to rest.
>
> **Moderate CFS** You may only be able to do a little, although symptoms vary. You may have disturbed sleep patterns and doze in the afternoons.
>
> **Severe CFS** You can perform daily tasks like brushing your teeth, but may need a wheelchair for bigger chores. Concentrating may be hard.
>
> **Very severe CFS** You can't perform any daily tasks, and spend most of your day in bed. You may be highly sensitive to noise and bright lights.

get a good night's sleep. Antihistamines and decongestants, such as pseudoephedrine and fexofenadine, may help alleviate any allergy-related symptoms.

Pace yourself to strike the right balance: you need adequate rest, but too much rest can make you weaker. Your doctor may also encourage you to slow down and eliminate any unnecessary or excessively stressful activities. Ideally, you should follow a gentle, graduated exercise program, such as walking, under your doctor's supervision, to increase your activity by no more than one minute a day.

Cognitive behavioral therapy helps identify negative beliefs and behaviors that may be making your condition worse or delaying recovery, and replaces them with healthy, positive ones.

Nutritional counseling and lifestyle counseling can be very beneficial. Many patients benefit

from dietary supplements, such as daily multivitamins, omega-3 DHA, and probiotics for those with gastrointestinal symptoms.

HOW CAN I HELP MYSELF?

You can make simple changes to your lifestyle to help your recovery.
Complementary therapies, such as acupuncture, massage, t'ai chi, and biofeedback therapies, may prove helpful.

Develop good sleep habits, such as going to bed and getting up at the same time, and napping if necessary (see pp60–1).

Avoid caffeine so it can't affect your sleep patterns.

Don't smoke For advice, see p64.

Learn to relax by avoiding stressful situations and knowing when to take "time out." If you feel like doing certain activities, that's fine, just make sure that you relax regularly. Even people who feel they've recovered from CFS find they need more rest than their peers.

Localized problems

All of us have had nagging aches and pains in joints at one time or another. It's when a pain in a knee or a wrist, for example, turns into a persistent ache or sudden intense pain that you know there's a problem. With the appropriate treatment and then some preventive measures, you'll soon be as good as new.

Repetitive strain injury

WHAT IS IT?

Better known as RSI, repetitive strain injury is not one condition but a term used for various disorders that develop as a result of repetitive movements, awkward postures, and sustained force. RSI is common in adults of working age and is more common in women. It mainly affects soft tissues in the upper parts of the body: the shoulder, forearm, elbow, wrist, hands, and neck.

Initially, symptoms may be felt when doing a particular activity and subside when you finish that

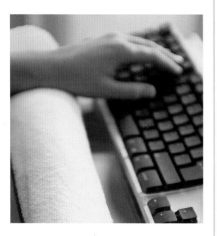

Wrist support
An occupational therapist may advise that a wrist support could alleviate your RSI when you are working at the computer.

work and rest. If such symptoms remain untreated, however, they can worsen so that you feel pain all the time.

Certain occupations put you at risk of developing RSI, including:
- Working in any manufacturing industry
- Typists and those working in computer data entry
- Dressmakers and tailors
- Musicians
- Hairdressers
- Professional athletes.

Even activities performed as part of your favorite hobby or sport can put you at risk of strain, so you must always be careful.

WHAT NEXT?

Your doctor will be able to make a diagnosis based on your medical history and a thorough physical examination. If your pain is in your wrist and forearm, he or she may tap gently in different areas to elicit a response that will indicate one condition over another.

MY TREATMENT OPTIONS

Some people get better without any treatment but many need a

DO I HAVE THE SYMPTOMS?

Symptoms of RSI can vary with the person and most commonly affect the neck, shoulder, elbow, hand and wrist, or carpal tunnel (see p283). They include:
- Pain
- Stiffness
- Tenderness
- Swelling or tingling (pins and needles)
- Loss of strength or sensation.

See your doctor if you experience any of the symptoms listed above.

combination of the following. When discussing potential treatments with your doctor, ask about any side effects.

Rest If you can, you should stop doing the activity that has caused your RSI. If this is impossible since it involves your job, talk to your employer so that adjustments can be made to your work.

Firm splints can be used to support the injured soft tissues during the healing process. Your doctor may be able to prescribe you one but you can buy them, too.

A course of nonsteroidal anti-inflammatory drugs, such as ibuprofen and diclofenac, may be prescribed by your doctor for effective pain relief and to address any inflammation or swelling.
Physical therapy can help to improve strength in targeted muscles to speed recovery and prevent future episodes.
Occupational therapy can address any ergonomic issues in your workplace.

HOW CAN I HELP MYSELF?
To relieve your symptoms and to prevent any more episodes in the future, you may need to take a long, hard look at your lifestyle. If you're an athletic person, you need to be conscientious about warming up and cooling down before and after your chosen activity.

A lot of cases of RSI result from our highly computerized world. But a few simple steps can limit the impact of typing.

Adjust your screen, seat, keyboard, and mouse if you sit at a desk all or most of the day so that they cause the least amount of strain on your back, wrists, hands, and fingers.
Try to be aware of your posture (see p67). Sit tall and ensure your eyes are level with the top of your screen.
Take frequent breaks.
Stop and stretch out your neck, hands, and fingers regularly.

Golfer's elbow and tennis elbow

WHAT ARE THEY?
Such soft-tissue problems occur when the tendons attaching the muscles that straighten or bend your fingers and wrist to the upper arm bone (humerus) become inflamed where they attach to the elbow. It's normally a short-lived complaint, although some people suffer repeat episodes. Any strain on the tendons can cause golfer's elbow and tennis elbow, as can any repetitive activity that involves gripping and twisting, such as using a screwdriver. Pain normally lasts for 6 to 12 weeks, or longer.

WHAT NEXT?
Consult your doctor or physical therapist on the best course of action for you.

MY TREATMENT OPTIONS
Rest your arm. Ask your doctor about potential side effects of drugs prescribed.
A course of nonsteroidal anti-inflammatory drugs (NSAIDs), such as ibuprofen, can help to relieve pain as well as reduce inflammation.
Cold treatment Ice packs can help counter any pain.
Steroid injections can reduce inflammation around the tendon if the pain doesn't resolve with a course of NSAIDs.

DO I HAVE THE SYMPTOMS?

Symptoms are worse when you use or twist your elbow.
- Pain on the outside, just by the bony lump of your elbow
- Pain on the inside, just by the bony lump of your elbow
- Pain that radiates down the arm toward the wrist.
See your doctor if you have any of these symptoms.

HOW CAN I HELP MYSELF?
Physical therapy can be helpful in restoring the strength and the tone of the muscles.
Rest from the sport or repetitive action that caused the injury in the first place.

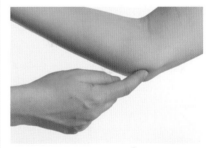
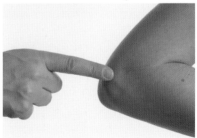

Location of the pain
In golfer's elbow (top), it's the tendons on the inner side of your elbow that are painful. In tennis elbow (below), it's those on the outer side of your elbow.

Painful shoulder

WHAT IS IT?

Your painful shoulder may be caused by a process within the shoulder joint itself; the pain can be over the front of your shoulder, in your upper arm, or at the tip of your shoulder. Often shoulder pain produces secondary pain in the neck muscles. Conversely, neck problems (see p272) can also result in shoulder pain. Osteoarthritis (see p263–5) and rheumatoid arthritis (see p266–8) can also cause shoulder pain, as can calcific tendinitis (calcium deposits in the rotator cuff tendons) or tears in the rotator cuff tendons, and subacromial bursitis (inflammation of the subacromial bursa).

WHAT NEXT?

Your doctor will be able to make a diagnosis based on your medical history and a physical examination. A diagnosis can be made in most cases without an X-ray. In complicated cases an MRI scan may be needed.

MY TREATMENT OPTIONS

Ask your doctor whether your treatment has any potential side effects.

Nonsteroidal anti-inflammatory drugs may relieve pain and reduce inflammation.

Physical therapy can help alleviate any stiffness and improve your range of movement.

Steroid injections can reduce inflammation within the joint itself if the pain is severe.

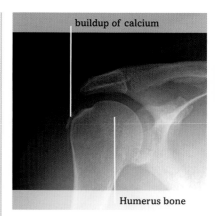
buildup of calcium

Humerus bone

Calcific tendinitis
This X-ray of a shoulder joint shows a crescent-shaped buildup of calcium in the rotator cuff, causing pain and stiffness.

HOW CAN I HELP MYSELF?

Follow the treatment plan recommended by your doctor.

DO I HAVE THE SYMPTOMS?

- Pain and tenderness in your shoulder, especially when reaching, lifting, pulling, or sleeping on the painful side
- Shoulder weakness, especially when trying to lift your arm straight out to the side
- Any loss in the range of motion of your shoulder.

See your doctor if you have any of these symptoms.

WHAT'S GOING ON INSIDE YOUR SHOULDER JOINT?

Inflammation of the tendons within the shoulder joint, known as the rotator cuff, often causes shoulder joint pain. The rotator cuff actually comprises four tendons: supraspinatus, subscapularis, teres minor, and infraspinatus. If you injure one of these, your doctor will probably refer you for physical therapy.

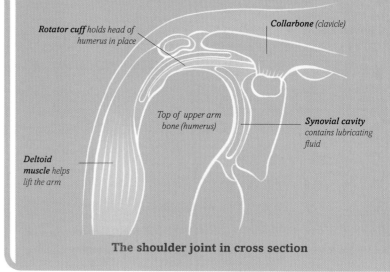

Rotator cuff holds head of humerus in place

Collarbone (clavicle)

Top of upper arm bone (humerus)

Synovial cavity contains lubricating fluid

Deltoid muscle helps lift the arm

The shoulder joint in cross section

Carpal tunnel syndrome

WHAT IS IT?

Women are far more likely to have carpal tunnel syndrome than men, and it's a condition that can strike at any age. It is due to entrapment of the median nerve at the carpal tunnel, which lies in the wrist. Tendons in the forearm that help move the fingers and the median nerve all pass through it.

The main nerve to your hand is called the median nerve. Before it branches into smaller nerve bundles in the palm of your hand, it passes through the carpal tunnel at your wrist. Space in the carpal tunnel is tight. So if a tendon is injured and inflamed, there is no room for it to expand. Swelling puts pressure on the median nerve, resulting in pain, tingling, or a pins-and-needles sensation.

In addition to tendon injuries from repetitive movements, for example, the nerve may be squeezed if there is arthritis of the wrist joint or a wrist fracture. Furthermore, any fluid retention, for example during pregnancy, or accumulation of fat, for instance in weight gain or in an underactive thyroid gland (see p327) may also result in carpal tunnel syndrome.

WHAT NEXT?

After doing a thorough examination, your doctor may arrange a nerve conduction test. Such tests will indicate to the doctor if the problem is related to the median nerve or the nerves originating from the neck.

MY TREATMENT OPTIONS

Your doctor will advise you as to which of the following treatment options is best suited to your case. He or she should also let you know about any potential side effects.

Rest your wrist when you can.

Nonsteroidal anti-inflammatory drugs may relieve pain and reduce inflammation.

Support your wrist by wearing a splint (your doctor will prescribe one) in the short term.

Steroid injections can cure it.

Surgery may be necessary in severe cases and can be done as an inpatient case in the hospital.

HOW CAN I HELP MYSELF?

Follow the treatment plan recommended by your doctor.

DO I HAVE THE SYMPTOMS?

Symptoms are usually worse in the thumb, index, and middle fingers (and in one half of your ring finger). They are also often worse at nighttime.

- Pain or aching in your hand; sometimes this pain radiates into your forearm
- Numbness
- Tingling and weakness in one or both hands.

See your doctor if you have any of these symptoms.

WHERE IS THE CARPAL TUNNEL?

The carpal tunnel is formed by the bones of the wrist (the carpal bones) and a strong ligament that lies over them. The median nerve, which both controls movement in the thumb, index, middle, and half of the ring fingers and relays sensations from them, runs through this tunnel, alongside the tendons. Everything fits just so within the carpal tunnel, so any injury that results in inflammation will have an impact on the function of the median nerve, and cause pain.

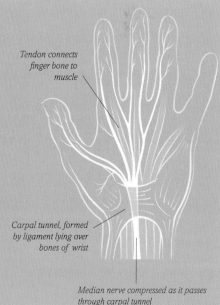

Tendon connects finger bone to muscle

Carpal tunnel, formed by ligament lying over bones of wrist

Median nerve compressed as it passes through carpal tunnel

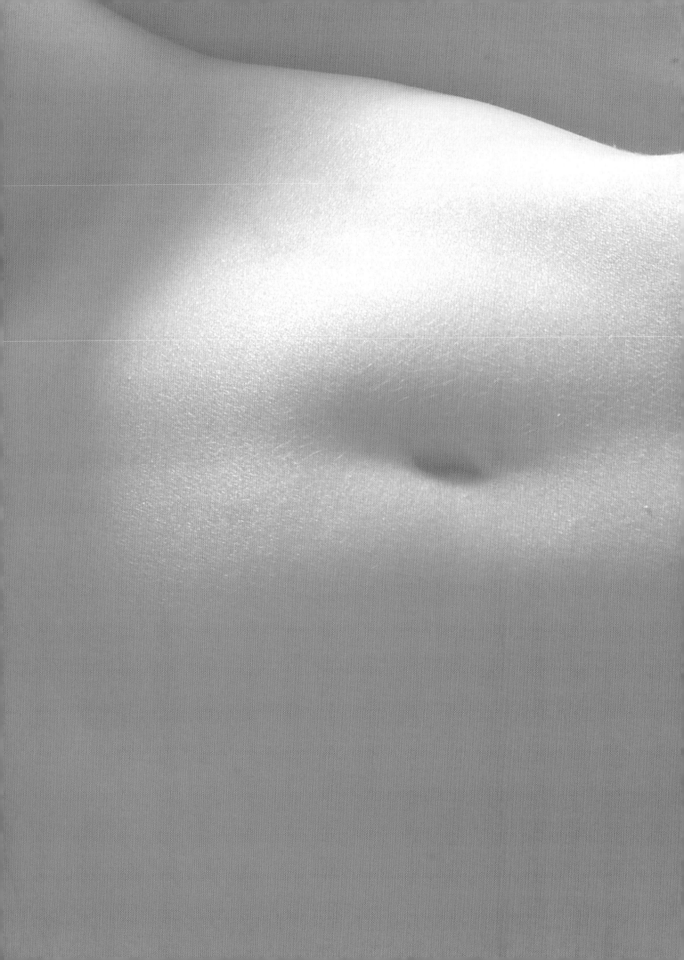

Digestive system

Lauren B Gerson MD MSc
Associate Professor of Medicine

Your digestive system

The gastrointestinal system is a remarkable piece of machinery, most of which is contained within the chest and abdomen. Its main function is to process the food we eat so that the body can absorb and use nutrients in the diet for energy and as building blocks for the growth and repair of muscles, bones, and other tissues in the body. The various parts of digestive system are subject to a variety of disorders, the most common of which are minor and easily treated by simple measures.

THE DIGESTIVE SYSTEM

The entrance to the digestive tract is the mouth (below), which is connected to the esophagus. The organs of the digestive system are shown in cross section (right). The tract itself is a long tube to which a number of organs are connected. These send digestive juices into the tract to help break down the food you eat. One of those organs is the liver, which produces bile, a digestive juice that helps the breakdown of fats. Bile drains from the liver into the gallbladder, where it is stored, to be released next time you eat.

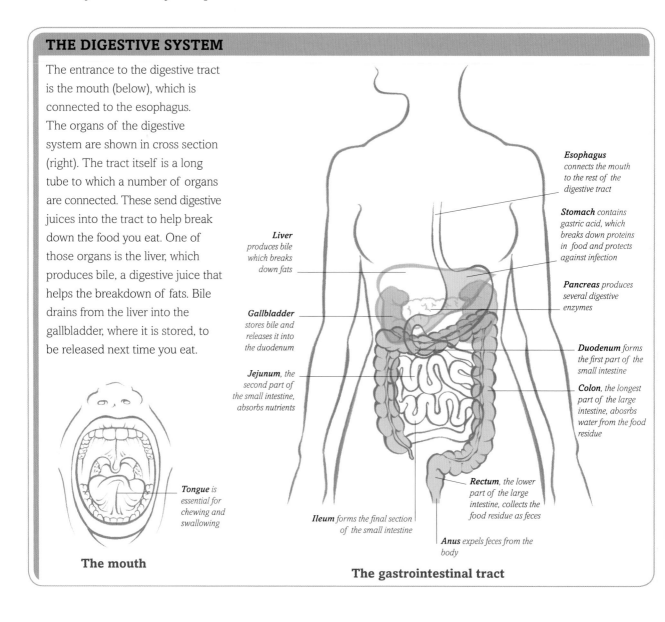

Liver *produces bile which breaks down fats*

Gallbladder *stores bile and releases it into the duodenum*

Jejunum, *the second part of the small intestine, absorbs nutrients*

Tongue *is essential for chewing and swallowing*

The mouth

Esophagus *connects the mouth to the rest of the digestive tract*

Stomach *contains gastric acid, which breaks down proteins in food and protects against infection*

Pancreas *produces several digestive enzymes*

Duodenum *forms the first part of the small intestine*

Colon, *the longest part of the large intestine, abosrbs water from the food residue*

Rectum, *the lower part of the large intestine, collects the food residue as feces*

Ileum *forms the final section of the small intestine*

Anus *expels feces from the body*

The gastrointestinal tract

The gastrointestinal system is essential for life, but we are able to survive and function quite well even if large parts are damaged or removed. Gastrointestinal diseases are common and, not surprisingly, diet plays a part in the cause or treatment of many of them. For instance, heavy alcohol drinking not only damages the liver but also causes pancreatic disease and is a risk factor in the development of mouth and esophageal cancers and polyps in the colon, while a low-fiber, high-fat diet increases the risk of colon cancer. Although the structure of the digestive system is the same in both sexes, the effects of female sex hormones, particularly in pregnancy, on muscle contraction mean that women may be more likely to suffer from certain digestive-tract problems, such as constipation. Moreover, women are more likely to suffer from liver damage as a result of drinking alcohol.

THE PROCESS OF DIGESTION

During the digestive process, the proteins, fats, and carbohydrates in the food you eat are broken down into amino acids (from dietary proteins), fatty acids (from dietary fat), and simple sugars (from dietary carbohydrates). These small molecules are all produced by a combination of mechanical churning of your food and the work of the digestive juices on it. These juices contain acid and digestive enzymes produced by the pancreas gland and bile from the gallbladder.

The small molecules that are the result of these actions are then absorbed via the wall of your small intestine and are carried in the lymph ducts and in the bloodstream, via the liver, to all parts of your body ready for use as needed.

The starting point of the whole digestive process is your mouth, which is the entry point for the food that you eat and the liquids that you drink. The first part of the process takes place here—the initial breakdown of food by chewing and by the action of the digestive enzymes found in your saliva.

From your mouth, the chewed-up food moves into the esophagus. This is a long muscular tube that pushes food and liquid on and into your stomach. The stomach behaves like a mixer; it churns the food around and mixes it with acid that it secretes. This acid

HOW WE ABSORB NUTRIENTS

Semiliquid food passes from the stomach into the small intestine. Here the nutrients are absorbed through the inner lining of the small intestine. In order for them to be absorbed as quickly as possible, this inner lining is covered in millions of tiny fingerlike projections called villi, which in turn are covered in brushlike structures called microvilli. These give the small intestine a huge surface area—the equivalent in size to a tennis court—through which the nutrients can rapidly be absorbed.

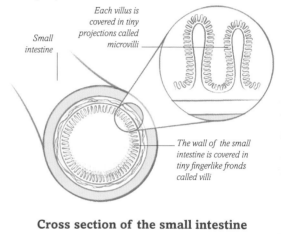

Small intestine

Each villus is covered in tiny projections called microvilli

The wall of the small intestine is covered in tiny fingerlike fronds called villi

Cross section of the small intestine

helps continue the process of digestion.

The semi-liquid food then leaves the stomach and enters the small intestine. This can be anything from 13–23 ft (4–7 meters) long and is made up of three parts—the duodenum, jejunum, and ileum. It is where the food is broken down even further and the small molecules are produced, ready to be absorbed.

The mainly digested food residue then passes into your large intestine (colon and rectum). Here, excess fluids are absorbed and any food residues that cannot be absorbed (mostly indigestible cellulose or fiber) are formed into feces (stools) and eliminated via the rectum and then the anus.

There is enormous variation between different people in "gut transit time" (that is, the length of time food takes to travel from the mouth to the anus), but the usual range is from one to three days.

Mouth and tongue disorders

Disorders of the mouth and tongue are common, and rarely serious. However, because you use your mouth for speaking, eating, swallowing, and for making facial expressions, these disorders can cause a great deal of discomfort and, in some cases, embarrassment.

Tongue conditions

Problems with your tongue may involve changes in its appearance and/or discomfort.

WHAT IS IT?

Your tongue may be affected by nutritional deficiencies, mouth ulcers, oral thrush (see below), and, rarely, cancer (see opposite). Other conditions that may cause your tongue to appear abnormal include:

Glossitis This is inflammation of the tongue due to injury (for example, scalding) or infection.

Geographic tongue This is a harmless condition in which irregular red, smooth patches appear on the tongue. It is not known what causes it.

Black hairy tongue In this condition dark, "hairy" areas appear on the tongue caused by bacterial growth on its surface.

WHAT NEXT?

Your doctor is likely to be able to diagnose your tongue problem by a simple visual examination.

MY TREATMENT OPTIONS

Treatment depends on the cause. Minor tongue conditions, such as glossitis and geographic tongue, usually get better without specific treatment. If your doctor suspects an infection, you may need to take antibiotics or antifungal medication, perhaps in the form of lozenges.

DO I HAVE THE SYMPTOMS?

Tongue disorders can appear as any of the following:
- Painless bald, smooth areas on the tongue
- Brown or black discoloration on the tongue
- White patches on the tongue
- Soreness.

See your doctor if you notice any of these symptoms.

Ask your doctor about any possible side effects of the medication.

HOW CAN I HELP MYSELF?

To keep your tongue healthy, pay attention to oral hygiene (see p68).

Oral thrush

Thrush (yeast) infection of the mouth usually occurs only if you're run down and the natural defenses of your body are disrupted.

WHAT IS IT?

This condition, in which you get white patches in your mouth, is more common if you have diabetes, are

---

DO I HAVE THE SYMPTOMS?

Oral thrush can be asymtomatic or cause these symptoms:
- White patches inside the mouth or on the tongue under which the area is red and sore.

See your doctor if you notice these symptoms.

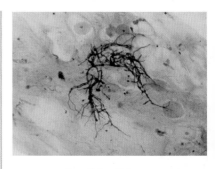

Candida albicans
Light micrograph of human saliva, showing the fungus that causes thrush.

malnourished, or have an immune deficiency, which can occur with age and with AIDS. You may also get this if you have poorly fitting dentures, have been taking antibiotics, have been treated with chemotherapy, or immunosuppressant drugs for autoimmune disorders.

WHAT NEXT?

Your doctor will confirm the diagnosis by doing a simple visual examination or by taking a sample of the plaque. If the cause of the thrush is not obvious, he or she will probably order tests to help identify the underlying cause of your infection.

MY TREATMENT OPTIONS

You will be prescribed an antifungal lozenges or paste.

HOW CAN I HELP MYSELF?

Use a soft toothbrush (change frequently) and avoid discomfort-causing acidic or spicy foods.

Leukoplakia and oral cancer

Both these conditions are characterized by abnormal-looking but painless areas in the mouth or on the tongue.

WHAT IS IT?

Leukoplakia is a condition in which painless white patches occur, often as a result of repeated damage to the mouth or tongue—for example, from a jagged tooth—

AM I AT RISK?

Both leukoplakia and oral cancer are more common in smokers and those who chew tobacco, and are more likely over the age of 40. Those who have an excessive intake of alcohol are also more susceptible.

but for which often no cause can be found.

Leukoplakia patches may clear up after the source of the irritation has been taken away. Very rarely, the patches may develop into oral cancer so you should be sure to see your dentist for a followup. Oral cancer, a rare condition that often first appears as a slowly growing sore or ulcer in the mouth that doesn't heal, may also develop without being preceded by leukoplakia.

WHAT NEXT?

Your doctor may arrange for a biopsy of the tissue to be taken from the affected area. The laboratory results from the sample will help your doctor make a firm diagnosis of the cause.

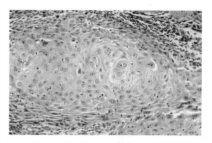

Oral cancer
Light micrograph of cancer cells (areas in pink) in the mouth of a patient.

MY TREATMENT OPTIONS

Leukoplakia patches often require no treatment, but your doctor may suggest that you have them regularly monitored. In some cases of leukoplakia, and often in the case of small oral cancers, the abnormal tissue may be removed surgically or by laser treatment. Follow-up treatment with X-rays may be advised in the case of oral cancer. Ask your doctor about any side effects of the treatment.

HOW CAN I HELP MYSELF?

To reduce your risk, don't smoke or chew tobacco, and keep your alcohol intake low. In addition, going for regular checkups at the dentist will help you to avoid leukoplakia caused by dental problems.

DO I HAVE THE SYMPTOMS?

The symptoms of these conditions are usually painless and may include the following:
- White patches in the mouth or on the tongue, which may have a hard surface, and that cannot easily be scraped away
- An isolated nodule inside the mouth that is perhaps slowly growing
- A persistent mouth ulcer that fails to heal

See your doctor if you notice any of these symptoms.

Gastroesophageal reflux disease

Heartburn caused by acid reflux is very common, especially when we have overindulged in food or have eaten too close to bedtime. Although not usually life threatening, frequent episodes of acid reflux can damage your esophagus.

WHAT IS IT?

Food travels from your mouth through the esophagus into your stomach via a valvelike muscle (the lower esophageal sphincter). The food starts to be broken down by the acid in your stomach, while the sphincter helps prevent food and acid flowing back into the esophagus. Unfortunately, the sphincter sometimes allows acid to flow back into the esophagus (acid reflux). Although your stomach is designed to withstand the acid, the lining of the esophagus is very sensitive to it, and when you have acid reflux, you'll be aware of heartburn—a burning sensation in your chest.

Heartburn affects many pregnant women. The increased pressure in the abdomen from the growing baby has a tendency to force the acidic stomach contents back into the esophagus.

Frequent and recurrent episodes of acid reflux (gastroesophageal reflux disease, or GERD) may damage the esophagus, causing inflammation and ulceration.

Although it causes discomfort, GERD rarely leads to any life-threatening complications. However, in Barrett's esophagus, the cells of the lower part of the esophagus change in response to repeated exposure to stomach acid. These cells are associated with an increased cancer risk, and if your doctor suspects this, he or she will monitor you by regular endoscopy. An endoscope is a small flexible tube that contains a tiny light and video camera and is used to examine various parts of the body. Here, it is passed down into the esophagus so that the doctor can inspect the lining of the esophagus. Persistent and untreated reflux can lead to scarring and narrowing of the esophagus, in which case the esophagus may need to be stretched using an endoscope.

AM I AT RISK?

Risk factors for acid reflux include:
- Being pregnant
- Being overweight or recent weight gain
- Eating a high-fat diet
- Consuming excessive amounts of alcohol or coffee
- Being a smoker
- Having a hiatal hernia.

WHAT NEXT?

You rarely need tests and exams to diagnose GERD and your doctor will be able to diagnose it from your description of your symptoms. If lifestyle changes and standard drug treatments do not help, or if you have additional symptoms, such as weight loss or vomiting blood, your

DO I HAVE THE SYMPTOMS?

Symptoms vary between people and between episodes. They are most noticeable after eating and may include:
- Heartburn or chest pain
- Acid taste in mouth
- Persistent sore throat
- Difficulty or pain during swallowing
- Persistent cough.

See your doctor if your symptoms are persistent, do not respond to self-help remedies (see opposite), or if discomfort from heartburn frequently interrupts your sleep.

HIATAL HERNIA

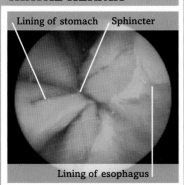

Lining of stomach   Sphincter

Lining of esophagus

Junction of the esophagus and stomach

A hiatal hernia occurs when the upper part of the stomach (dark pink) pushes upward through the lower esophageal sphincter into the esophagus (light pink). Having a large hiatal hernia makes it more likely that you will have GERD, but it does not cause the symptoms. If you need surgery for GERD (see right), your hernia will be repaired at the same time.

doctor will probably arrange for you to have a endoscopy. An endoscope is passed down your esophagus and into your stomach so that your doctor can inspect the stomach lining and also screen for Barrett's esophagus if indicated.

MY TREATMENT OPTIONS

There are three types of medication that are commonly prescribed in the treatment of GERD. Ask your doctor about any possible side effects when discussing your treatment options.

Antacids These quickly neutralize the acid from the stomach and prevent the esophagus from being damaged but have a short duration.

Histamine receptor blockers (H2 blockers) and proton pump inhibitors (PPIs) These reduce acid output and are the most effective acid reducers.

Promotility drugs These help the esophagus empty itself of any stomach contents.

Medication for GERD rarely has side effects. Although not licensed to be taken during pregnancy, most of these have not caused adverse effects to a developing baby. Nevertheless, always discuss any drug treatment with your doctor if you are pregnant.

Surgery Occasionally, surgery is necessary to tighten the lower esophageal sphincter.

HOW CAN I HELP MYSELF?

Lifestyle changes are the first course of action to improve your symptoms, particularly if they are mild and infrequent:

Watch your weight There is a close relationship between body weight and reflux symptoms and losing weight by diet and exercise (see pp52–7) may help. You should try to maintain your weight within a healthy range (see your body mass index, pp58–9).

Quit smoking (see p64) since smoking relaxes the sphincter between the stomach and the esophagus and encourages reflux.

Don't eat late at night Allow at least three hours between eating and going to bed, to allow your stomach to empty. It may help to have a light meal at night. Coffee, chocolate, and fatty foods may trigger symptoms, and should therefore be avoided by anyone with a tendency to acid reflux. Avoid tight-fitting clothing that increases pressure in the abdomen and promotes reflux.

Prop up your bed to raise the level of your head to help prevent nighttime acid reflux through the simple action of gravity.

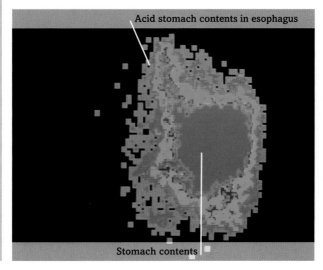

Acid stomach contents in esophagus

Stomach contents

Acid reflux on camera

Here, acid stomach contents can clearly be seen in the esophagus as a result of a hiatal hernia. The stomach contents are the red mass in the center; the area of reflux is the red "horn" in the upper left of the picture.

Indigestion and ulcers

Most of us have indigestion at some time and we can usually treat it with over-the-counter remedies. Having indigestion doesn't usually mean there is anything seriously wrong with you, but if you suffer from it frequently, you should ask your doctor to investigate it further.

WHAT IS IT?

Some people have indigestion because their stomach does not empty itself of its contents as fast as it should. Specific problems that may cause the symptoms of indigestion are gastroesophageal reflux disease (see pp290–1), ulcers in the upper intestine (peptic ulcers), or—in rare cases—cancer of the stomach or esophagus.

WHAT NEXT?

Your doctor may treat your indigestion without any further investigations. However, if you are over the age of 55 or have any of the symptoms in the right-hand column of the box below, you will usually need an endoscopy of your upper intestinal tract (see pp290–1)

before treatment to make sure nothing serious is causing your symptoms. Otherwise, your doctor may do a simple test to look for the bacteria *Helicobacter pylori*, which is the main cause of peptic ulcers. He or she may suggest lifestyle modification (see Am I at risk? right) and may prescribe acid-suppressing medication.

MY TREATMENT OPTIONS

Treatment depends on what seems to be the cause of the problem. Ask your doctor about any possible side effects.

A combination of antibiotics and acid blockers These are recommended if your bacteria test is positive; they kill the bacteria and heal any ulcers.

AM I AT RISK?

There are several lifestyle habits that often contribute to, or cause, indigestion. These include:

- Eating heavy meals, especially late in the evening (leave a four-hour interval between eating and going to bed)
- Irregular meal times
- Smoking
- Drinking excess alcohol
- Stress and anxiety
- Regular use of an analgesic such as aspirin or a nonsteroidal anti-inflammatory drug (often used for arthritis).

Acid blockers These treat peptic ulcers caused by aspirin and nonsteroidal anti-inflammatory drugs (NSAIDs). They also work when sensitivity to acid is the cause.
Promotility agents These help your stomach empty faster.
Lifestyle modification See Am I at risk? above.

HOW CAN I HELP MYSELF?

Check the risk factors identified in the panel (above) and if any of these apply to you, try to eliminate them from your lifestyle.

DO I HAVE THE SYMPTOMS?

If you have indigestion, you may feel the following:

- Pain or discomfort in the upper abdomen or chest often associated with eating
- Nausea
- Bloating
- Heartburn (see pp290–1)
- Belching

See your doctor if you have indigestion regularly and especially if episodes of indigestion are a recent development for you, are over 55 years of age, or have any of the following symptoms:

- Unintended weight loss
- Vomiting
- Difficulty in swallowing.

Esophageal disorders

If you have trouble swallowing, together with chest pain, it could be that the problem lies in the muscles of your esophagus. Although these often distressing disorders are not particularly common, they are more likely to occur in young and middle-aged women.

WHAT ARE THEY?

There are three main types of disorders that can prevent your food from passing normally from the esophagus into your stomach. They give you discomfort when you swallow.

Achalasia See the panel (right).

Diffuse esophageal spasm In this disorder, the muscles of the esophagus contract irregularly.

Hypertensive ("nutcracker") esophagus In this disorder, the contractions of the esophageal muscles are too strong.

WHAT HAPPENS IN ACHALASIA?

If you have achalasia, the muscles of your lower esophagus do not contract properly and the valve between the esophagus and the stomach (the lower esophageal sphincter) does not relax. This prevents food from passing through into your stomach.

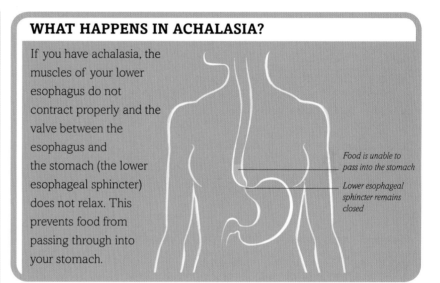

Food is unable to pass into the stomach

Lower esophageal sphincter remains closed

DO I HAVE THE SYMPTOMS?

If you have these disorders, you may notice the following:

● Difficulty swallowing, as though food, and sometimes liquid, is stuck behind your breastbone within seconds of swallowing

● Chest pain that feels as though it is coming from the heart area; this is more common in younger people.

See your doctor if you experience either symptom or you don't respond to therapy.

WHAT NEXT?

Most muscular disorders are diagnosed by barium swallow (you swallow a white chalky mixture, after which X-rays are taken) or by esophageal manometry (measuring the pressure in the esophagus using a pressure catheter passed through the nose or mouth and guided into the esophagus). Your doctor may recommend an endoscopy of your upper intestinal tract (see pp290–1). This test will also reveal if there is any narrowing of the esophagus or evidence of GERD (see pp290–1). It will also help the doctor exclude esophageal cancer as a cause of your symptoms.

MY TREATMENT OPTIONS

Treatment depends on the diagnosis.

Botulinum toxin injection to relax the muscle fibers.

Balloon dilation uses a small balloon at the end of an endoscope to stretch the muscle.

Myotomy disrupts muscle fibers by surgically cutting the muscle.

Medication to relax the muscles.

Ph Probe to test for and treat reflux.

HOW CAN I HELP MYSELF?

The following can often help:

Eat slowly and chew well.

Drink plenty when you eat.

Have a carbonated drink. This can help shift food that gets stuck.

Gallstones

It a common saying that the typical gallstone patient is female, fat, fertile, and forty, and there is some truth is this. It is a fact that women are twice as likely as men to develop gallstones, and the condition is more common in those who are overweight and middle-aged.

WHAT IS IT?

Gallstones are small, solid lumps—the most common type are made from cholesterol—that form in the bile (see pp286–7). They begin as tiny crystals, but then grow and may get as large as a few centimeters across. You may get one or several gallstones. Women are more often affected by this problem than men because the female hormones progesterone and estrogen tend to relax the gallbladder. This slows the flow of bile and makes it more likely that stones will form.

If a stone blocks one of the ducts that carry bile from your

DO I HAVE THE SYMPTOMS?

Those with gallstones may experience these common symptoms:
- Bouts of upper abdominal pain, often on the right
- Nausea and vomiting
- Yellowing of the skin or whites of the eyes
- Pale stools

See your doctor if you experience any of these symptoms.

AM I AT RISK?

The following are risk factors for developing gallstones:
- Being overweight and eating a high-fat diet: these two factors result in high levels of cholesterol being secreted in the bile, which increases the tendency of stones to form.
- Being on a very low-calorie diet: surprisingly, gallstones often develop during the first few weeks of a very low-calorie diet, perhaps because the gallbladder cannot contract and empty normally.
- Taking certain prescribed medications, including oral contraceptives, affect gallbladder functioning and may increase the risk of gallstones.
- Having a family tendency to develop gallstones.
- Being a woman: you're more likely to develop gallstones than a man with a similar lifestyle and genetic inheritance.

gallbladder to the intestines you may get symptoms, including mild to severe abdominal pain, nausea, and vomiting. These symptoms are known as biliary colic. You will feel the pain in your upper abdomen, more often on the right, and it may extend to your back. It may last between several minutes and several hours, and it can occur repeatedly. You may not feel any pain between "attacks." Only a small percentage of those with gallstones will develop symptoms.

Some sufferers from this condition also develop jaundice (yellowing of the skin and whites of the eyes), and

you may also notice that you pass pale feces. This is due to the lack of bile pigment in the gut. Gallstones can also cause inflammation of the gallbladder (cholecystitis) or pancreas (acute pancreatitis). If you have either of these complications, you are likely to have pain in your upper abdomen and you may also have a raised temperature. Each of these conditions needs urgent hospital assessment and treatment.

WHAT NEXT?

Gallstones don't always cause symptoms and they're often found while something else is being

WHERE DO GALLSTONES LODGE?

Gallstones form within the gallbladder and may remain there. However, they may also pass into the bile duct, where they cause problems if they become stuck. Small stones may simply pass into the intestine.

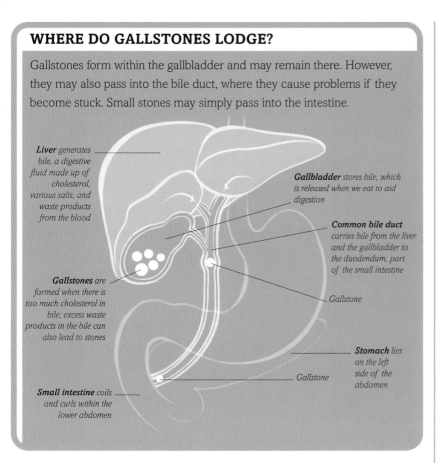

Liver generates bile, a digestive fluid made up of cholesterol, various salts, and waste products from the blood

Gallbladder stores bile, which is released when we eat to aid digestion

Common bile duct carries bile from the liver and the gallbladder to the duodendum, part of the small intestine

Gallstone

Gallstones are formed when there is too much cholesterol in bile; excess waste products in the bile can also lead to stones

Stomach lies on the left side of the abdomen

Gallstone

Small intestine coils and curls within the lower abdomen

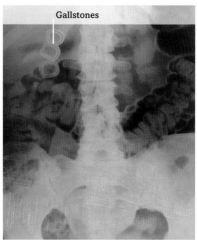

Gallstones

Gallstones

This colored X-ray of the abdomen shows three large gallstones (colored blue) in the gallbladder.

investigated. If you've been experiencing symptoms that may be caused by gallstones, your doctor will want to be sure of the cause before recommending treatment. An ultrasound examination of your gallbladder is usually the first test. You may also need blood tests and special X-rays or an endoscopy (see pp290–1), to see if gallstones have become lodged in your bile ducts.

MY TREATMENT OPTIONS

If you don't have any symptoms, you won't need treatment, otherwise your doctor will find the best treatment for you. Ask your doctor about any side effects when discussing treatment options.

More frequent meals If you don't have symptoms and the stones are small, your doctor may recommend you simply eat more frequent small meals. This will encourage the gallbladder to expel any stones that may have formed.

Surgery Your doctor will usually recommend removal of the gallbladder—which can usually be done by laparoscopic ("keyhole") surgery—only if there are signs of infection, cancer, or obstruction from gallstones. Most people who have had this treatment can leave

the hospital the next day and return to normal activities within two weeks. Removing the gallbladder can cause diarrhea due to bile draining into the digestive tract.

Dissolving the gallstones
Medication or mechanical methods to dissolve or fragment the gallstones while leaving the gallbladder in place are also occasionally used for the treatment of gallstones, but there is a risk that gallstones will form again.

HOW CAN I HELP MYSELF?

Most risk factors for gallstones are unavoidable, but you can reduce the chances of developing the problem by keeping to a healthy weight (see pp58–9) and sticking to a low-cholesterol diet (see p273).

"Because of our female hormones, women are twice as likely as men to develop gallstones."

Liver disorders

Your liver is your largest internal organ and plays an essential role in regulating many aspects of your digestion and the way your body uses the nutrients in your food. Liver problems—many of them caused by drinking too much alcohol—are becoming more common, and many more women are affected than they once were.

Hepatitis

The term hepatitis covers a group of conditions characterized by inflammation of the liver, which damages the liver cells.

WHAT IS IT?

Often caused by infection, hepatitis can be acute (starts suddenly and lasts less than six months) or chronic (long lasting). Common causes are:

- The hepatitis viruses A, B, C, D, and E
- Other viral diseases such as mononucleosis
- Overdose of drugs, such as acetaminophen
- Drinking excessive amounts of alcohol (see opposite)
- Cirrhosis (see p298).

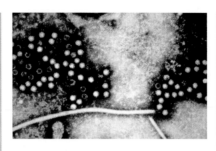

Hepatitis E virus
This virus, shown here as round particles (in purple), like Hepatitis A, is often spread via contaminated water.

The hepatitis A and E viruses only cause acute hepatitis, while the other hepatitis viruses can cause both acute and chronic hepatitis. If you have an episode of acute hepatitis, your liver will heal completely, whereas chronic hepatitis may eventually lead to permanent damage to the liver (see Cirrhosis, p298).

AM I AT RISK?

Hepatitis A is easily transmitted in contaminated water or food (often shellfish). If you travel to areas of high risk (Africa, Asia, South America), it is very important to be vaccinated against hepatitis A before you go.

Hepatitis B and C are transmitted through infected blood and blood products and, especially in the case of hepatitis B, through sexual intercourse. Intravenous drug users who share needles and people who have sex with an infected person are among those most at risk.

Hepatitis D only occurs in people who already have hepatitis B, and then usually only in drug addicts, while hepatitis E mainly occurs in Southeast Asia. It can be severe in pregnant women.

DO I HAVE THE SYMPTOMS?

Often the condition is symptomless. In the early stages of acute hepatitis, you may experience the following symptoms:

- Fatigue and aching muscles
- Jaundice (yellowish skin and whites of the eyes)
- Pale stools and dark urine
- Pain in the right of your upper abdomen.

Symptoms are similar in chronic hepatitis, but jaundice usually only develops in the late stages.

See your doctor if you have any of the symptoms described.

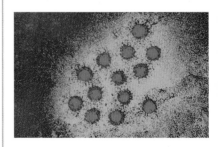

Hepatitis A virus
The hepatitis A virus (shown here as red dots) is a common cause of hepatitis infection for which you can be immunized.

WHAT NEXT?

Your doctor will diagnose hepatitis on the basis of your symptoms and the results of your blood tests. If you have chronic hepatitis, a liver biopsy is usually recommended to check for liver damage.

MY TREATMENT OPTIONS

Your doctor will work with you to find the best treatment.

Acute hepatitis There is no specific treatment.

Chronic hepatitis You may be prescribed antiviral drugs, and/or steroids or other drugs that suppress your immune system.

HOW CAN I HELP MYSELF?

For all forms of hepatitis, the best treatment is to rest, avoid alcohol, and eat well (see pp52–5).

Alcoholic liver disease

Alcohol-related liver disease is progressive liver damage caused by the excessive consumption of alcohol (see p299).

WHAT IS IT?

Alcohol affects the liver in the following ways:

Fatty changes in the liver This is the first stage of the disease and is reversible if you stop drinking. These changes do not cause symptoms and are often only revealed by blood tests that check your liver function (see also p298).

Alcoholic hepatitis If you continue to drink heavily, you can develop alcoholic hepatitis. In this condition your liver becomes enlarged and you get jaundiced. Alcoholic hepatitis can lead to the potentially life-threatening condition, cirrhosis (see p298). Women are more sensitive than men to the effects of alcohol (see p65 and p299) and some people have an inherited susceptibility to alcohol-related liver damage. However, in simple terms, the more you drink, the more likely you are to experience liver problems.

WHAT NEXT?

If you have a history of excessive alcohol consumption and abnormal results of blood tests for liver function, the diagnosis of alcoholic liver disease can usually be made from your symptoms Your doctor may also arrange for you to have an ultrasound examination of the liver and perhaps a liver biopsy, too.

DO I HAVE THE SYMPTOMS?

Symptoms of alcoholic liver disease may not appear for several years, but after less than 10 years of heavy drinking, you may experience:

- Nausea and occasional vomiting
- Discomfort in the upper right side of your abdomen
- Weight loss
- Fever
- Yellowing of the skin and the whites of the eyes
- Swollen abdomen.

See your doctor if you regularly consume alcohol and have noticed any of these symptoms.

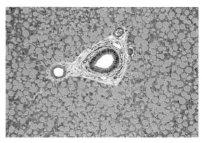

Liver changes in alcoholic hepatitis
This micrograph of a section through the liver shows how the normally regular cell structure of the liver is disrupted by fatty deposits (yellow areas).

MY TREATMENT OPTIONS

Once a diagnosis has been made, you may need to go into the hospital.

Medication This may be given to help you deal with alcohol withdrawal and prevent cravings.

HOW CAN I HELP MYSELF?

There are important lifestyle changes you can make:

Stop drinking alcohol This is key to halting the disease. Abstaining from alcohol gives your liver a chance to return to normal, otherwise you run the risk of developing cirrhosis (see p298). Consider joining a support group.

Eat a healthy diet A balanced healthy diet and vitamin supplements are also important (see pp52–5 for advice).

Fatty liver

This is yet another of those common conditions that you can have without realizing it. In fact, it's so common that, in developed countries, about one-fifth of the population has it.

WHAT IS IT?

Fatty liver occurs when there's an excessive buildup of fat in your liver cells. It's usually the result of too much fat being delivered to your liver, and your liver then being unable to process it normally. You're more likely to get it if you're obese or have diabetes, and a rare form can affect women during pregnancy.

DO I HAVE THE SYMPTOMS?

Usually there are no symptoms and the condition is usually detected during tests for other reasons or because your lifestyle leads your doctor to suspect that fatty liver is a possibility.

WHAT NEXT?

If blood tests reveal abnormal liver function and if a scan of your liver supports this, your doctor will suspect your liver is fatty. The only way definitely to prove the diagnosis of fatty liver is to perform a liver biopsy. However, this is not usually necessary if the blood tests reveal only a mild problem and the results of tests for other causes of liver disease are negative. Fatty liver caused by pregnancy corrects itself following the birth of the baby.

MY TREATMENT OPTIONS

There is much ongoing research into drug treatment for fatty liver, but the main treatment currently consists of measures you can take yourself (see How can I help myself?, below).

HOW CAN I HELP MYSELF?

Lose weight If you're overweight, it's vital to reduce your weight by lowering your calorie intake and increasing your physical activity (see pp56–7).

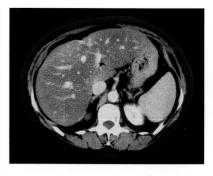

Fatty liver in cross section
This CT scan shows a cross section through the abdomen of a woman suffering from fatty liver. The liver is the large purple-colored organ. Fatty deposits show up as blue patches.

This will help improve the condition and may even reverse it in some cases.
Avoid alcohol to stop damaging the liver further (see p65).
Watch your diet A diet that's high in fiber and polyunsaturated fats but low in other types of fat (you should have less than 30 percent of your total calories as fat) will almost certainly help (see p173).
Watch your blood sugar Be sure to take measures to control your blood sugar levels if you have diabetes (see pp320–5).

Cirrhosis

This serious condition affecting the liver develops as a result of long-term damage.

WHAT IS IT?

The damaged liver cells are replaced by scar tissue and the remaining cells try to replace the dying ones, resulting in clusters

(nodules). The liver's abnormal structure then affects its blood flow, and the loss of healthy liver cells stops it from functioning normally.

Drinking excessive amounts of alcohol over many years is the most common cause of cirrhosis in the developed world, while long-standing hepatitis B or C infection is the most common cause worldwide. Hemochromatosis, a much more

rare cause, is an inherited disease. In this, your intestine absorbs too much iron from what you eat and you get deposits of iron in your liver, heart, pancreas, and pituitary gland. In the long term, the excess iron in your liver causes cirrhosis. Severe fatty liver (above) may also cause cirrhosis and there are other more rare causes, too. If you have cirrhosis, it can lead to liver cancer.

DO I HAVE THE SYMPTOMS?

You may experience very few symptoms until the late stages of the disease. The damaged liver is unable to function normally, leading to:

- Easy bruising
- Mild confusion
- Altered sleep patterns
- Jaundice (yellowing of the skin and whites of the eyes)
- Swollen abdomen
- Bleeding from the esophagus.

See your doctor if you have any of these symptoms

WHAT NEXT?

The only way to confirm that you have cirrhosis is by having a liver biopsy. However, blood tests and ultrasound or CT scans can often give your doctor all the information needed to make a diagnosis.

MY TREATMENT OPTIONS

The most important part of your treatment is to remove the underlying cause (see How can I help myself?, right). Other aspects of the treatment of cirrhosis include managing the symptoms and detecting complications early.

Diuretic pills Your liver helps the kidneys get rid of unwanted fluids, but cirrhosis impairs this function. Fluid can build up in the abdomen, and diuretic pills are often given to reduce excess fluids.

Checks on the esophagus
You may need an endoscopic

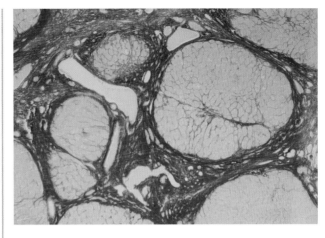

Cirrhotic liver tissue
This micrograph shows a section through liver tissue with alcohol-induced cirrhosis. The red areas are scar tissue. A cirrhotic liver has a knobby appearance.

examination (see pp290–1) of the lining of the esophagus and, if necessary, you'll be given medication to reduce the pressure in the blood vessels and to prevent bleeding from the esophagus.

Ultrasound Regular ultrasound scans are likely to be advised to check for any signs of liver cancer.

Vaccinations If you have cirrhosis, you'll be more susceptible to infection so your doctor may offer vaccinations against hepatitis A and B, pneumococcus, and influenza.

Liver transplant In advanced cases when liver function is dangerously reduced, a liver transplant may be offered.

HOW CAN I HELP MYSELF?

Whatever the cause of your cirrhosis, you must abstain from alcohol for the rest of your life.

HOW ALCOHOL AFFECTS THE LIVER

Once alcohol has been absorbed from the stomach and intestines (see p287), it goes straight to the liver via the bloodstream. Here it is broken down, in the same way as your other food and drink. If you consume more alcohol than your liver can process, the imbalance means that your liver cannot break down the protein, fats, and sugars in your food as it should.

The first and most common problem you get when you have had too much alcohol is that your liver is infiltrated by the excess fat that it cannot break down fast enough. This can develop in as few as eight days after the start of heavy drinking. It is reversible, but if you continue drinking, you will get more serious and irreversible liver damage.

Women are more susceptible than men to the effects of alcohol on the liver because they absorb alcohol more quickly, have a smaller volume of blood, have less alcohol dehydrogenase, and have a higher ratio of fat to lean tissue—and alcohol is relatively insoluble in lean tissue.

Gastroenteritis

If you've ever had a vacation intestinal bug with diarrhea and vomiting, then you've had gastroenteritis, which is most commonly caused by an infection. The condition, which affects women and men equally, usually subsides without requiring any specific treatment.

This common condition usually clears up without the need for medical treatment.

WHAT IS IT?

Gastroenteritis is inflammation of the lining of the stomach and intestines. It's usually caused by infection transmitted either from person to person or by eating contaminated food or drink. A variety of bacteria or viruses, among them staphylococcus, may be responsible. Most people in previously good health recover quickly, but the condition creates a potentially serious risk of

DO I HAVE THE SYMPTOMS?

The symptoms of gastroenteritis include:

- Diarrhea
- Vomiting
- Abdominal pain
- Fever.

See your doctor as a matter of urgency if you pass bloodstained diarrhea, are unable to keep fluids down, have not passed urine for over 6 hours, become drowsy, listless, or confused, or are in poor health.

PREVENTING GASTROENTERITIS

These measures help combat the spread of gastroenteritis from person to person or via contaminated food and water.

- Wash your hands thoroughly with soap and water before cooking and preparing food.
- Wash hands with soap and water after using the bathroom.

- Thaw frozen meat and poultry completely before cooking.
- Store cooked and raw foods in separate areas of the refrigerator.
- Cook meat and poultry thoroughly.

If you have gastroenteritis:

- Don't share towels or cutlery with other people.
- Disinfect the toilet after use.

dehydration for babies and those in poor health and pregnant women.

WHAT NEXT?

Your doctor is likely to diagnose gastroenteritis on hearing about your symptoms.

MY TREATMENT OPTIONS

You can usually manage the condition at home (see How can I help myself?, below). If you show serious signs of dehydration, you may need intravenous fluids.

HOW CAN I HELP MYSELF?

Follow the advice above to avoid spreading infection. Stay home from work until the symptoms have stopped completely. If your job involves handling food, ask your

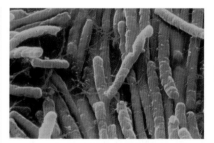

Clostridium difficile
These bacteria are sometimes the cause of gastroenteritis. There are normally small numbers of them in the human gut.

doctor's advice before returning to work. Pepto-Bismol has been shown to be helpful preventatively as well..

Drink plenty Try to drink 8–12 cups (2–3 liters) of fluids a day in frequent small amounts.

Use rehydration salts These help maintain the correct fluid and salt balance in the body (see p302).

Celiac disease

A condition that can only be controlled by diet, celiac disease often means that sufferers must make significant changes to their lifestyle. This uncommon disorder occurs in between 0.5 and 1 percent of the population. Women are, however, more often affected than men.

Celiac disease, or "gluten sensitivity," is the result of an abnormal reaction of the immune system that damages the lining of the small intestine.

WHAT IS IT?

In celiac disease, your immune system reacts against gluten—a protein contained in wheat, rye, and barley, and any foods that are made from these grains. This reaction damages the villi of your small intestine so that you can't absorb nutrients properly.

DO I HAVE THE SYMPTOMS?

The disease often reveals itself in infancy, but can also appear later in life. Symptoms may include:
- Mouth ulcers
- Loose, greasy-looking feces
- Iron-deficiency anemia
- Abdominal pain
- Bloating and flatulence
- Fatigue and weakness
- Persistent itchy rash on the knees, buttocks, elbows, and/or shoulders
- Weight loss.

See your doctor if you have any of these symptoms.

WHAT NEXT?

Your doctor will do a blood test to look for increased levels of a certain antibody (protein) as a first step. A biopsy of the lining of the small intestine is the only way to confirm the diagnosis. Your doctor will also take a blood sample to check for anemia (see p248). A DEXA scan (see p260) may be ordered to check for osteoporosis, which can occur because of reduced absorption of calcium and vitamin D. Your doctor may advise that your close relatives be tested for the disease.

MY TREATMENT OPTIONS

Steroids and immunosuppressives can help with severe cases of celiac disease. Your doctor may refer you to a dietician, though a change in diet may take three months to be effective. Endoscopy and blood tests should take place before dietary changes are made as well as after. Follow the advice given under How can I help myself?

HOW CAN I HELP MYSELF?

Self-management is the primary option for treating the symptoms.
Avoid gluten You must avoid this in your diet for the rest of your life, which will involve very major adjustments.

AM I AT RISK?

The disease seems to run in families, and many sufferers have at least one close relative with the condition. In the long term, you have a slightly increased risk of certain types of cancers if you have untreated celiac disease.

There are now plenty of gluten-free foods on the market, so you'll have a wide choice, but you'll need to watch what you eat carefully when you're eating out. Following a gluten-free diet is particularly important for the health of your baby if you're pregnant or are planning a pregnancy. There are a number of support groups that can offer information and advice.

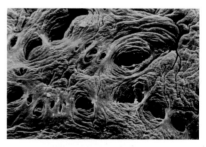

Celiac disease up close
Celiac disease leads to an unusually smooth wall of the small intestine caused by the loss of villi (see p287), as shown by this scanning electron micrograph (SEM).

Altered bowel habits

The majority of people move their bowels between three times a day and three times a week, but many have bowel movements more or less frequently than this and still have completely normal bowels. You only need to worry if there's a change in your normal habits.

Diarrhea

If you pass loose stools unusually frequently, either suddenly or over a long period of time, it's a sign that you may have an underlying problem that should be checked out.

WHAT IS IT?

Diarrhea is usually defined as passing loose or watery stools more than three times a day, or a large volume of stool. You might sometimes have it combined with stomach pains, nausea, or an urgent need to go to the bathroom. Acute diarrhea, which often starts suddenly, may be short-lived, lasting only a few days or up to three weeks. It's often due to an infection (see p300). If you have chronic diarrhea, it's persistent and often lasts longer than a few weeks. Many people with this condition are diagnosed with irritable bowel syndrome (IBS; see pp304–5), but there are many possible causes of diarrhea other than IBS. For example, it can be a side effect of some medications.

WHAT NEXT?

If you have chronic diarrhea, you should see your doctor so he or she can investigate the cause. This is especially important if you have a family history of inflammatory bowel disease (see pp310–11); colon cancer (see pp307–9); or celiac disease (see p301); if you're 45 or older, or if you've recently had abdominal surgery. Often you'll need nothing more than simple blood tests. Your doctor may want to test a stool sample for infection, particularly if you've been treated with antibiotics or have recently returned from abroad. Your doctor may also want you to have a colonoscopy to check your colon (see p308). You'll usually only need other tests if your blood tests are abnormal or your symptoms are particularly troublesome.

MY TREATMENT OPTIONS

The treatment of chronic diarrhea depends on the cause. If the problem

---

DO I HAVE THE SYMPTOMS?

Along with chronic diarrhea you may notice any of the following symptoms:
- Blood in the feces
- Weight loss
- The need to get up at night to move your bowels

See your doctor if you have any of these symptoms.

REHYDRATION SALTS

Diarrhea can deplete fluids and salts in your body, leading to dehydration. The signs of dehydration are passing small amounts of dark-colored urine, a dry mouth, thirst, and feeling weak. Rehydration salts help restore the natural balance. It's easy to make your own, and often cheaper than buying premade salts. You can buy the ingredients from any pharmacy and most supermarkets.

Ingredients
Glucose 20 g
Sodium chloride (table salt) 3½ g
Sodium bicarbonate
 (baking soda) 2½ g

Method
Add the powders to 3½ cups (1 liter) of tap water and stir. Drink small amounts regularly throughout the day. You will need to make a fresh solution each day.

is serious enough to bring to your doctor's attention, treatment options will be dicussed once a firm diagnosis is made.

HOW CAN I HELP MYSELF?

If you have acute diarrhea, follow the self-help measures advised for gastroenteritis (see p300), in particular, be sure to drink plenty of clear fluids such as water or dilute fruit juice. Be alert for any signs that you may be suffering from dehydration (see box, left). Some foods like raisins or dates can be particularly helpful, while calcium supplements can be binding.

Constipation

Not being able to pass a stool is one of the most common gastrointestinal complaints and, like diarrhea, is usually a symptom of something else. It's more common in women than in men, and is often a particular problem when you're pregnant.

WHAT IS IT?

Constipation is the infrequent passage of stools, or difficulty passing a stool because it's hard and dry. You may also feel bloated. The more constipated you are, the harder it is to pass a stool, which may put you at risk of hemorrhoids (see pp314–15) and a weakened pelvic floor (pp340–2).

It's usually caused by having a diet that doesn't contain enough fiber (roughage) and/or fluids.

Leading a sedentary lifestyle can be a contributory factor, too, and if you regularly resist the urge to defecate, you may lose your normal bowel reflexes. Constipation is much more of a problem for women than for men. Some women notice that their constipation is worse at particular times of the menstrual cycle and during pregnancy. This may be due to the effect of female hormones on the intestine.

WHAT NEXT?

Although there's rarely any serious underlying cause for constipation, if your bowel habits suddenly change, it's important to seek your doctor's advice, especially if you've noticed blood in your feces, severe abdominal pain, weight loss, or you're over 45 years old.

MY TREATMENT OPTIONS

Constipation often improves with a few simple lifestyle changes involving adding fiber to your diet and getting more exercise (see How can I help myself?, right).
Laxatives If your constipation is severe, your doctor may decide to prescribe a laxative. Ask about any possible side effects.
Specialized investigations If your constipation doesn't respond to these measures, you may need more tests to investigate in detail the way your bowel muscles are working and if the sphincter muscle in your anus relaxes as it should to allow normal passage of a motion.

DO I HAVE THE SYMPTOMS?

Constipation can be defined as any of the following:
● Passing fewer bowel movements than is normal for you
● Straining to pass a stool
● Passing feces that are hard and pelletlike
● A feeling of incomplete bowel emptying.
See your doctor as a matter of urgency if you also have blood in the feces or experience severe abdominal pain.

HOW CAN I HELP MYSELF?

Constipation can usually be alleviated by changes in your diet and lifestyle:
Eat plenty of fiber High-fiber foods include fruit, vegetables, legumes, and whole-grain cereals.
Drink plenty of water Liquids add fluid to the colon and bulk to the stools, making bowel movements softer to pass. Drink 5–7 cups (1.5–2 liters) of fluid per day. Avoid too many caffeine-containing drinks and alcohol, which can cause dehydration.
Exercise regularly Even gentle physical activity such as walking helps keep your digestive system active. Try to make time for exercise every day (see pp56–7).
Do not ignore the need to use the bathroom Always respond promptly to your body's natural signals. This helps your reflexes return to normal.

Irritable bowel syndrome

The pain and discomfort of this unpleasant condition can come and go and you may feel perfectly normal in between episodes. It can start at any age but mostly begins when you're a young adult. For reasons that aren't fully understood, irritable bowel syndrome (IBS) is more common in women.

IBS is a common condition of the intestines—it affects about 15 percent of people at some time in their lives. It comes under the umbrella term of "functional bowel disorders." In these disorders, although the intestine appears normal when examined by X-ray and endoscopy (see pp290–1), there is actually something wrong with its normal activity and sensitivity.

WHAT IS IT?

If you have IBS, you may have a variety of symptoms (see Do I have the symptoms?, below). These are the result of increased strength or frequency of the contractions of the muscles of your intestine, heightened sensitivity of the nerves of your intestine (intestinal hypersensitivity), or a change in the way in which your brain controls some of these functions. There is no single cause of IBS, but it's believed that stress or emotional upset may play a role. Some people get the symptoms after they've been having a particularly stressful time or have experienced a major life event.

Sometimes symptoms start after an intestinal infection, in which case it's called postinfectious IBS. About 10 to 20 percent of people develop IBS after they've had gastroenteritis (see p300), even though the bacteria or virus that caused the gastroenteritis is no longer present.

WHAT NEXT?

Your doctor will probably diagnose IBS based on your symptoms. He or she may have some simple blood tests done, for instance, to check for celiac disease (see p301) if you're mainly suffering from diarrhea.

You may need further investigations if your symptoms aren't typical of IBS, if you develop symptoms for the first time when you're over 45 years old, or if a close relative has a bowel problem, such as Crohn's disease (see pp310–11).

MY TREATMENT OPTIONS

There is no single treatment that is appropriate for everyone and you may have to try one or two before you find the one that helps you. The treatment will also depend on the particular type of symptoms you are having. If your symptoms aren't too troublesome, it's perfectly acceptable not to have anytreatment, but if you are prescribed medication, be sure to ask your doctor if there might be any side effects.

DO I HAVE THE SYMPTOMS?

IBS may cause one or more of the following symptoms, which may be present every day, or may come and go and be interspersed with periods of feeling completely well:

- Abdominal pain that may be mild or severe, often in the lower abdomen. The pain may be eased by passing gas or with passage of stool.
- Altered bowel habit, either loose, frequent stools, or hard, pelletlike stools. The stools may also vary, with alternating diarrhea and constipation, perhaps containing mucus. There may be urgency to defecate and a feeling of incomplete evacuation.
- Bloating of the abdomen
- Other symptoms may include feeling sick, belching, fatigue, and feeling full soon after eating.

See your doctor if you have any of the symptoms of IBS described.

Medication Many IBS sufferers manage their condition without the need for medication (see How can I help myself? right). Others benefit from one or more of the following drug treatments:

Antispasmodic drugs These can be useful for pain and are taken as needed. They may also be helpful if you take them about 30 minutes before you eat, if urgency to use the bathroom after mealtimes is a problem.

Antidiarrheal drugs If you suffer mainly from diarrhea, you may find an antidiarrhea medication, such as loperamide, is helpful. You can take this as needed.

Laxatives There are a variety of laxatives available if you suffer mainly from constipation; your doctor will recommend a product that is right for you.

Antidepressants These are used in low doses if you are suffering

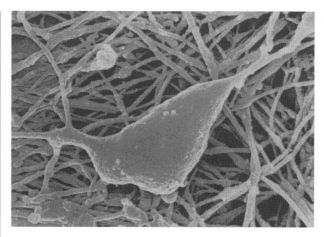

A nerve cell (neuron) in the intestine
In IBS, these nerve cells may be overly sensitive, causing irregular muscle contractions.

from intestinal hypersensitivity, since they slow down the movement of the bowel and may also alter the way the nerve impulses between the intestine and the brain are processed. They can be very effective if abdominal pain or diarrhea are your main symptoms.

HOW CAN I HELP MYSELF?
Many IBS sufferers manage their symptoms effectively without the need for medication.

Watch your diet There is no single food that has been shown to worsen or relieve symptoms, but a few people find that certain foods make them worse, so it may be worthwhile keeping a food diary for a few weeks to try to identify any culprits. Adjusting your diet is more likely to be helpful if your main symptom is diarrhea. Foods that seem to trigger symptoms are wheat and dairy, including milk, cheese, and yogurt. Soy products can be substituted for

dairy. A high-fiber diet may help if constipation is a particular problem, but this can make bloating and gas worse.

Keep hydrated Make sure that you drink enough fluids throughout the day but avoid caffeine-containing drinks since these may trigger the problem.

Make lifestyle changes Have regular mealtimes and avoid eating "meals on the go." Try relaxation techniques (see pp62–3) and regular exercise (see pp56–7) to help you to reduce and manage stress.

Try probiotics ("good bacteria") These are sold over the counter and may help to ease bloating and flatulence. You may need to try a number of different products before you find one that is right for you.

Try hypnotherapy This can help some types of IBS. You need to commit to it to complete the course.

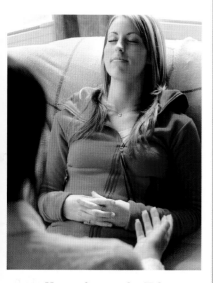

Hypnotherapy for IBS
Relaxation and visualization techniques can help you deal with your symptoms.

"Many IBS sufferers manage their symptoms effectively without medication."

Gastrointestinal cancer

Any part of the gastrointestinal tract may be affected by cancer. Some of these cancers are relatively common, others are quite rare. Fortunately, it is also the case that many of these cancers can be successfully treated if diagnosed early.

Cancers of the upper gastro-intestinal tract

Cancerous tumors may occur in almost any part of the digestive tract. Those affecting the esophagus, stomach, pancreas, bile ducts, liver, and small intestine are known collectively as upper gastrointestinal (GI) cancers.

DO I HAVE THE SYMPTOMS?

Symptoms vary according to the specific cancer, and are often mild and therefore overlooked.
The most common symptoms of upper GI cancers include:
- Upper abdominal pain
- Weight loss.
A symptom specific to esophageal cancer is increasing difficulty in swallowing over a short period of time.
Jaundice (yellowing of the skin and whites of the eyes) may occur in cases of cancer of the liver, bile ducts, and pancreas.
See your doctor if you notice any of the symptoms described.

WHAT ARE THEY?

Like other forms of cancer, these cancers occur when normal cell division and renewal are disrupted and abnormal cells multiply uncontrollably, forming a tumor that prevents the affected organ from functioning as it should. In some cases of liver cancer, the disease occurs as a result of the spread of abnormal cells from a tumor elsewhere in the body.

Luckily, most of these cancers are relatively rare. The exception is stomach cancer, which worldwide is the second most common cause of cancer death. However, the numbers affected by this cancer are diminishing, possibly due to changes in diet. In general, upper GI cancers tend to affect mainly people over the age of 50.

WHAT NEXT?

The initial tests your doctor suggests will depend on your symptoms, but usually include an endoscopy (see p290) of your upper gastrointestinal tract, or an ultrasound or CT scan of your abdomen. You may need a biopsy to confirm the diagnosis. If cancer is diagnosed, you will be referred to a specialized team of doctors.

AM I AT RISK?

You're more at risk from upper GI cancers if:
- You're over 50
- You smoke
- You're overweight
- You have a high alcohol intake.

Further tests may be needed to find out how far the cancer has developed and whether the tumor is confined to its original site or has spread beyond it to affect other organs.

MY TREATMENT OPTIONS

Your treatment will depend on the stage of the disease and your general health. In the case of medication, ask your doctor about any possible side effects.
Surgery Tumors that are confined to the original site can usually be removed by surgery. If you have a primary liver tumor, in a few selected cases, you may be given a liver transplant.
Chemotherapy and/or radiation therapy are often given before or after the surgery to improve your overall outcome. Tumors that have spread beyond

the original site cannot be removed surgically and are usually treated with chemotherapy.

Other treatments may be used to improve your symptoms. For instance, depending on the part of the body affected, stents (see pp170–1) may be inserted in your esophagus during an endoscopy to help with swallowing, or into in the bile ducts to relieve jaundice.

HOW CAN I HELP MYSELF?

A few simple lifestyle changes may reduce your risk of developing this type of cancer:

Stop smoking. GI cancers are more common in smokers.

Maintain a healthy weight within the recommended range for your height (see pp58–9). Many forms of GI cancer are more prevalent in those who are seriously overweight.

Reduce your alcohol intake to within recommended limits (14 units a week for a woman).

Colorectal cancer and polyps

Cancer of the large intestine is one of the most common of the gastrointestinal cancers. The good news is that a recently introduced screening program is detecting and treating the disease at an early stage when treatment is most likely to be successful.

WHAT IS IT?

The colon is the section of the gastrointestinal tract that connects the small intestine to the final section of the large intestine— the rectum.

Cancer in any part of the body develops when the process of cell division, repair, renewal, and development of new cells becomes uncontrolled for some reason. In some cases these abnormal cells form a tumor (a growth or lump).

In the early stages of colorectal cancer, the tumor is confined to the colon or rectum, while more advanced cancers are likely to spread into the lymph nodes, or at an even later stage into the liver and/or lungs. In some people, cancer may start within an intestinal polyp (see p309).

Colon cancer is equally common in men and women, but is more common among older people. In fact, it is extremely uncommon in anyone under the age of 40, unless there is a family history of the disease at a young age.

Rectal cancer is slightly more common in men, and in a small percentage of sufferers, there is a genetic tendency to develop this form of cancer. Brothers, sisters, and children of people with colorectal cancer are thought to be more likely to get the disease in later life. They may be advised to

> ### DO I HAVE THE SYMPTOMS?
>
> Colorectal cancer is likely to cause one or more of the following common symptoms:
> - Bleeding from the rectum
> - Abdominal pain
> - A change in bowel habit.
>
> **See your doctor** if you develop any of these symptoms.

> ### AM I AT RISK?
>
> Although the exact cause, or causes, of colorectal cancer is not yet understood, there are certain lifestyle factors that are thought to contribute to this condition. These include:
> - A high-fat, low-fiber diet
> - Smoking
> - Not getting enough exercise
> - Obesity.
>
> In addition, you are at increased risk of developing colorectal cancer if you have intestinal polyps or if a close family member has had the disease.

go for regular screening (perhaps including a colonoscopy) to detect polyps or an early cancer— particularly if they had a relative who developed cancer before the age of 45.

WHAT NEXT?

After assessing your symptoms in the context of your age and your medical and family history, your doctor will decide whether you need further investigations.

WHAT HAPPENS DURING A COLONOSCOPY

Colonoscopy is the most commonly used technique for examining the colon and rectum to detect early colorectal cancer and polyps, for taking biopsies (tiny tissue specimens), and for removing polyps if they are present. The day before you have the colonoscopy, you will be given strong laxatives to empty your colon so the lining can be clearly seen. On the day of the procedure, you will normally be given a mild intravenous sedative. Once you are sedated, a small flexible tube (colonoscope) with a light source and a camera is passed via the anus into the rectum and colon, and then to the junction of the colon and the small intestine. The specialist can see on a monitor what is going on in your colon and rectum and can remove any polyps. If these are attached to blood vessels, the blood vessels will be cauterized to prevent bleeding. The whole procedure usually only takes about 30 minutes.

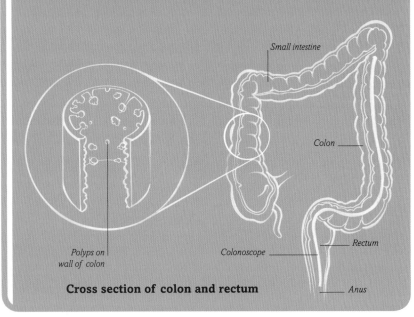

Small intestine

Colon

Polyps on wall of colon

Colonoscope

Rectum

Anus

Cross section of colon and rectum

COLOSTOMY

The type of stoma known as colostomy is when an opening is made in the large intestine and abdominal wall so that feces can be collected in a colostomy bag outside the abdomen before they enter the anal canal. A colostomy is usually a temporary surgical procedure to enable the colon to heal, or other corrective surgery to be undertaken, but in some cases it can be permanent.

colon will need to be flushed out the day before using strong laxatives so that the lining of the colon can be clearly visualized. Of these three methods, colonoscopy is the most common technique.

If you have colorectal cancer and no symptoms, it may be picked up when you are having other tests, for example if you have a family history of the disease and are being routinely screened.

MY TREATMENT OPTIONS

If cancer is diagnosed, you'll be advised to have further tests. You may need to have a CT scan of your chest and abdomen to check if the cancer has spread and to identify the stage it has reached. If you have rectal cancer, you will usually also need an MRI or ultrasound scan. Your treatment will depend on the stage of the disease. When discussing your options, ask your doctor about any possible side effects.

The symptoms of colorectal cancer (see Do I have the symptoms? p307) are not specific to the condition, but may be caused by many less serious diseases, such as ulcerative colitis and Crohn's disease (see pp310–11).

Further investigations will involve taking a look at what is going on in the colon. This can be done by one of the following three methods: colonoscopy (see box, above), barium enema (when a white, chalky, barium-containing mixture is placed in the colon, which is then X-rayed) or by a special CT scan called a CT colonography or virtual colonoscopy.

Whichever method is used, the

Colon or rectal surgery Part of your treatment will usually be surgery to remove the tumor from your colon or rectum. Sometimes you will also need a stoma—an opening in your abdomen for feces to leave your body, bypassing the colon—either temporarily or permanently. If you need this procedure, your surgeon and a specialized stoma nurse will discuss it with you in advance.

Medication and radiation therapy Sometimes chemotherapy (treatment with cancer fighting drugs) or radiation is advised before or after surgery to improve your overall outcome.

HOW CAN I HELP MYSELF?

There are several lifestyle changes you can make that may help improve your health and reduce your risk of developing colorectal cancer:

Eat a healthy, balanced diet that includes plenty of fiber (roughage) (see pp52–5).

Maintain a healthy weight within the normal range for your height (see pp58–9).

Get regular exercise For more information, see pp56–7.

Avoid or quit smoking For more information, see p64.

Limit your alcohol intake For more information, see p65.

See your doctor if you have a family history of colon cancer. He or she will advise you if you need to be screened.

Take part in the recommended bowel cancer screening program.

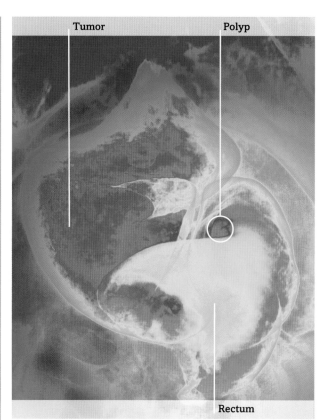

Tumor   Polyp

Rectum

Colon cancer and polyp
This X-ray shows a tumor at the junction of the rectum (lower right) and the colon (center left). The patient also has a polyp—the dark circle in the bright part of the colon just to the right of the tumor.

INTESTINAL POLYPS

In many cases, colorectal cancer develops from polyps—growths in the lining of the colon and rectum. Most polyps are not malignant, but some have the potential to develop into a cancer if they aren't removed. Polyps can range in size from ¹⁄₁₆–2 inches (a millimeter to several centimeters), and you may have just one or several hundred. You are more likely to develop polyps as you get older. You often don't have any symptoms from them, and they are then detected only when your colon is examined for other symptoms, such as diarrhea, or during

screening for colorectal cancer.

Some people have bleeding from the rectum, which may be caused by polyps. The time between a polyp first developing and later turning into cancer can take months or years. Once a polyp is completely removed from the colon, the risk of cancer in that polyp is also removed, and it won't grow back.

If you have had polyps removed, you will usually be asked to return for a further colonoscopy (see opposite) several months or years later (depending on the type and size of the polyp) to check that no more polyps have developed.

Inflammatory bowel disease

Inflammatory bowel disease (IBD) is an umbrella term that includes two separate conditions: Crohn's disease and ulcerative colitis. Often affecting young adults, both disorders can cause distressing symptoms. Once diagnosed, these conditions can be successfully treated in most cases.

Often similar in terms of the symptoms they cause, ulcerative colitis and Crohn's disease have different causes and treatment.

WHAT IS IT?

Both of these conditions cause inflammation and ulceration in the intestine. One person in every 400 has IBD, and women are as likely to be affected as men. It's most likely to be first noticed between the ages of 10 and 40, but symptoms of the condition can appear at any age.

WHAT NEXT?

IBD can often be confirmed by a colonoscopy (see p308). During this procedure, the doctor will usually take biopsies of your colon to decide which type of inflammation you have. If your doctor suspects that your small intestine is affected, you may be given a barium X-ray, during which you drink a thick, white solution of barium that reveals the outline of your small intestine on an X-ray. Alternatively, you may have video capsule endoscopy; in this, you swallow a capsule-like camera that produces pictures of your small intestine. These are captured on a data recorder that you wear as a belt for 24 hours. You excrete the capsule with your stools. Sometimes ultrasound, CT, or MRI scans are advised.

DO I HAVE THE SYMPTOMS?

The symptoms of ulcerative colitis are:
- Diarrhea with or without blood
- Fatigue and lethargy.

Symptoms of Crohn's disease usually include:
- Diarrhea with or without blood
- Weight loss
- Abdominal pain.

Both can also cause inflammation in the eyes, joints, and skin, fevers, and mouth ulcerations.

See your doctor if you have one or more of these symptoms.

ULCERATIVE COLITIS OR CROHN'S DISEASE?

Ulcerative colitis affects only the colon (large intestine). Inflammation always begins in the lower colon (rectum) and spreads around the colon in a continuous pattern. Crohn's disease can affect any part of the intestine, but most commonly affects the end of the small intestine and the colon. Inflammation is patchy. Crohn's disease also causes narrowing of the bowel, which can cause abdominal pain.

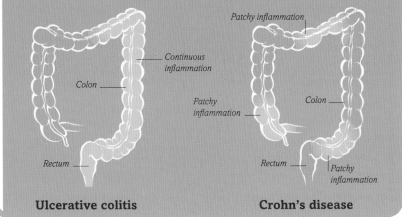

Ulcerative colitis — Continuous inflammation, Colon, Rectum

Crohn's disease — Patchy inflammation, Colon, Rectum, Patchy inflammation

Ulcerative colitis　　　　**Crohn's disease**

MY TREATMENT OPTIONS

If you have ulcerative colitis, your doctor may advise one or more of the following treatments.

Medication Your doctor may try one or more of the following drug treatments, depending on your condition and symptoms. Ask about any possible side effects.

- 5-ASA (5-aminosalicylate) medicines such as mesalazine and sulfasalazine are often used to treat and prevent flare-ups.

- Steroids can be given to treat more serious flare-ups, and then tapered off when symptoms subside. If you have a very severe flare-up, they may be given intravenously in the hospital. If inflammation is confined to the lower part of your colon, these drugs can be administered as suppositories or enemas.

- Immune-system suppressants are used if you are unable to taper off steroids. They prolong symptom-free periods if you continue to have frequent attacks despite 5-ASA treatment.

IBD AND PREGNANCY

Most women with IBD do not have reduced fertility or any difference in the progress of their pregnancy. Although most IBD drugs are safe, you should consult your doctor if you are planning a pregnancy, or if your partner has IBD, because a few of the drugs are best avoided in the months before conception and during pregnancy.

AM I AT RISK?

The exact cause of IBD is uncertain, but a combination of three factors is thought to be responsible: having a family predisposition (genetic factors), having an abnormal immune response in the intestine, and environmental triggers.

- Family predisposition means that there's a greater chance of developing the disease if your brother, sister, either of your parents, or your child is affected. The inherited risk is greater with Crohn's disease than with ulcerative colitis, and overall you're 10 times more likely to develop IBD if you have one close relative with the condition; your risk is greater if two or more relatives are affected.

- An abnormal immune response occurs as a result of oversensitivity of your immune system, Normally activated as a response to invading bacteria in your intestine, the activated immune cells release special proteins that not only kill the virus or bacteria but also give you some of the symptoms of infection, mainly fever and fatigue. In IBD your oversensitive immune system attacks the beneficial bacteria that normally live in the intestine, causing inflammation and ulceration of your intestine.

- Environmental factors play a part. Smoking, for example, has a role in Crohn's disease; smokers have a higher risk of developing Crohn's, have more frequent attacks, and respond less well to treatment. Stress may also trigger the IBD and also increases the chances of a relapse in those who have had the condition before.

Surgery The colon may need to be removed if drugs don't offer enough relief (see Colostomy, p308).

Surgery may be curative in ulcerative colitis but should be avoided in Crohn's disease—unless there are strictures causing obstruction—because the disease can recur at the surgery site. Medication options are similar to those for ulcerative colitis. In addition, a new range of drugs has recently been introduced, which deactivate the immune response. Methotrexate—used in the treatment of autoimmune disease—is sometimes prescribed.

HOW CAN I HELP MYSELF?

You can increase the effectiveness of IBD treatment with lifestyle changes:
Stop smoking. This is particularly important if you have Crohn's disease. For help quitting, see p64.
Eat a healthy, well-balanced diet with plenty of nutrients and vitamins (see pp52–5). During flare-ups eat a bland diet, avoiding fresh fruit, vegetables, and dairy products. In Crohn's disease a simple liquid diet may be recommended for a time.
Avoid aspirin and NSAIDS.
Learn to manage stress, perhaps by going to relaxation classes or by practicing yoga.

Diverticular disease

Diverticular disease is one of those complaints that you are more likely to experience as you get older. As with many other conditions affecting the bowel, you can reduce your chances of developing the disease in later life by making sure that you eat a healthy, high-fiber diet.

This condition is mainly a problem in industrialized societies, where diets that are high in processed food are more common. It occurs in over half of people in their 80s in the West, but is rare in most of Asia and Africa.

WHAT IS IT?

In diverticular disease, small pouches, known as diverticula (singular diverticulum), develop in the wall of your colon. The exact

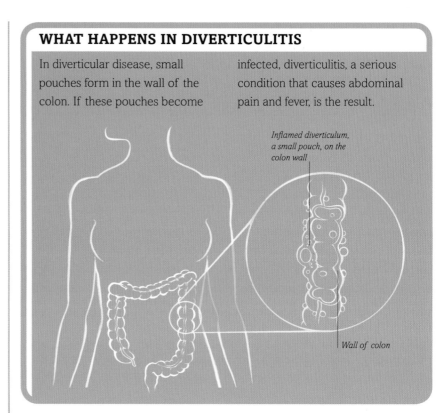

WHAT HAPPENS IN DIVERTICULITIS

In diverticular disease, small pouches form in the wall of the colon. If these pouches become infected, diverticulitis, a serious condition that causes abdominal pain and fever, is the result.

Inflamed diverticulum, a small pouch, on the colon wall

Wall of colon

DO I HAVE THE SYMPTOMS?

It is common for diverticula to cause no obvious symptoms. Some sufferers, however, have the following:
- Crampy abdominal pain
- Altered bowel habits such as diarrhea or constipation
- Bleeding from the rectum.

If the diverticula become inflamed (diverticulitis), you may experience:
- Intense pain on the left side of the lower abdomen
- Fever.

See your doctor if you have any of these symptoms.

cause is not known, but it's thought that a low-fiber diet and the constipation likely to result create increased pressure in the colon. This increased pressure may force the inner lining (mucosa) through the outer muscle layer, leading to formation of diverticula.

Diverticula can exist in the bowel with painless rectal bleeding or without any symptoms. This is known as diverticulosis. Treatment

for bleeding includes a high-fiber diet, endoscopic therapy, angiography (injection of dye into the vessels), or surgery. Occasionally, diverticula can become inflamed—a condition known as diverticulitis. This can lead to intense abdominal pain and fever. Rarely, an inflamed diverticulum can burst, which can lead to an abscess, peritonitis (inflammation of the lining of the abdominal cavity), or the formation of an abnormal connection (fistula) with the bladder or another section of intestine.

WHAT NEXT?

If your doctor suspects you've got diverticular disease, you will probably be advised to have some tests, such as a barium enema (see p308) or colonoscopy (see p308). In some cases a CT scan maybe recommended.

MY TREATMENT OPTIONS

If your diverticular disease isn't causing symptoms or if the symptoms are mild, you are unlikely to be offered medical treatment. Instead, you'll probably be advised to adopt a high-fiber diet (see How can I help myself? below right). The following may be recommended in certain situations. Ask your doctor about possible side effects of any medication prescribed:

Antispasmodics if you have cramping pains in the abdomen.

Laxatives if you are suffering from severe constipation.

Antibiotics are often used to treat diverticulitis. In mild cases, you can take these by mouth, but for more severe diverticulitis, you may be admitted to the hospital so that

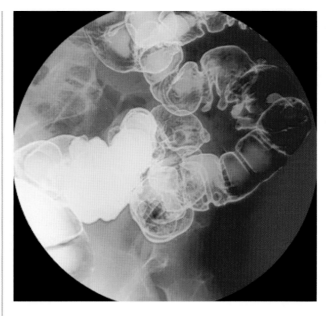

Colon affected by diverticular disease
This colored X-ray shows several diverticula (in blue) protruding from the wall of the colon in a person with diverticular disease.

antibiotics and fluid can be given via an intravenous drip.

Surgery may occasionally be necessary to drain an abscess or repair a fistula. If you have diverticula that are bleeding, you may need to stay in the hospital for observation and in severe cases, you may need a blood transfusion.

If part of your bowel is especially badly affected by the disease, you may be advised to have that part removed surgically. After the surgery, the healthy sections of the intestine will be joined together.

HOW CAN I HELP MYSELF?

There are plenty of nonmedical measures you can take, mainly to reduce any tendency to constipation. These can help minimize your risk of getting

diverticular disease and—if you have it already—can reduce the severity of your symptoms:

Eat a high-fiber diet that contains plenty of fruit, legumes, and vegetables. Choose whole-grain products, such as whole-wheat bread and pasta. (See pp52–5 for further advice on a healthy diet.

Drink plenty of fluid, up to 5–7 cups (1.5–2 liters) a day to help keep your bowel movements soft.

Get regular exercise (see pp56–7) to maintain regular bowel action.

For pain relief take acetaminophen, if necessary, and avoid nonsteroidal anti-inflammatory drugs (for example, ibuprofen and indomethacin). These medications have been linked to an increased risk of developing complications of diverticular disease.

AM I AT RISK?

The likelihood of developing diverticular disease is increased if:
- You're over 50
- You've suffered from constipation for long periods.

"In the industrialized West, diverticular disease affects over half of those in their 80s."

Hemorrhoids and anorectal conditions

Hemorrhoids (piles) and other minor problems of the anal region are extremely common conditions, but people are often too embarrassed to talk about them to anyone. The problems are rarely serious, but the symptoms can be irritating and can take a long time to clear up.

Hemorrhoids

Hemorrhoids (also called piles) are enlarged veins, similar to varicose veins, around the anus. Although they are a common problem for both sexes, they are a particular problem for women during pregnancy.

WHAT ARE THEY?
Hemorrhoids form when the blood in the veins around the anus slows down or stops flowing. This is often caused by constipation and straining when you use the bathroom.

When you are pregnant, you are particularly susceptible to hemorrhoids because of the increased pressure on the pelvic veins caused by enlargement of the uterus. Pregnancy also brings an increase in the amount of blood circulating through your body and hormonal effects on the walls of the veins make them weaker. In addition, your hormones have a relaxing effect on the muscles of the intestine and slow down the movement of food residue through the gastrointestinal tract, which can lead to constipation.

Although hemorrhoids are usually only a minor complaint, they can become very painful if a blood clot (thrombosis) forms within the vein.

WHAT NEXT?
You will be examined with a proctoscope (a hollow tube with a light source), passed into the anus, or with an endoscope. Hemorrhoids that protrude from the anus can be seen without a proctoscope.

> **DO I HAVE THE SYMPTOMS?**
> Symptoms range from temporary and mild, to persistent and painful (some people do not have any symptoms):
> - Rectal bleeding—usually seen as a small amount of blood in the toilet bowl or on toilet paper after wiping
> - Anal itching
> - Pain
> - Awareness of a lump in the anus.
> **See your doctor** if you experience persistent bleeding or pain.

> **THE SITE OF HEMORRHOIDS**
> Hemorroids form in the anus—either just inside or around the oustide of the opening.

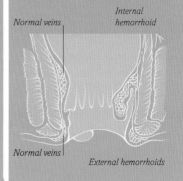

Normal veins

Internal hemorrhoid

Normal veins

External hemorrhoids

MY TREATMENT OPTIONS
Mild cases require no treatment.
Creams You can buy over-the-counter creams to reduce discomfort.

In more severe cases, you may be advised to have hemorrhoids removed by one of these methods:
Band ligation A rubber band is placed around the base of the hemorrhoid, cutting off the blood supply to the swollen vein.
Infrared light or laser in which the hemorrhoids are destroyed by the burning action of the rays.

Injection of a sclerosant solution into the hemorrhoid, which makes the vein wither away. **Surgery** to remove hemorrhoids is reserved for those whose symptoms persist in spite of treatment, or when a hemorrhoid has become clotted with blood. **Over-the-counter suppositories** treat internal hemorrhoids.

HOW CAN I HELP MYSELF?

Follow your doctor's advice and most importantly, avoid constipation and straining (see p303) when you use the toilet.

Anal fissure

Like many other bowel conditions, anal fissure is associated with constipation and a low-fiber diet.

WHAT IS IT?

An anal fissure is a tear in the lining of the anal canal. Most are caused by local trauma, such as passing hard stools. The sphincter muscle may then go into spasm and pull the edges of the fissure apart, preventing healing.

WHAT NEXT?

Your doctor will make a diagnosis based on an external examination. Most fissures are not serious.

DO I HAVE THE SYMPTOMS?

Typical symptoms include:
● Tearing pain on opening the bowels
● Rectal bleeding
● Itching around the anus.
See your doctor if you experience any of these symptoms.

MY TREATMENT OPTIONS

Simple treatment is effective in most cases. Ask your doctor about any possible side effects.
Laxatives These soften the stools and prevent constipation.

Local treatment The two most commonly used preparations are nitroglycerin and diltiazem cream used topically. These help relax the sphincter muscle and prevent spasm. Some specialists recommend an injection of botulinum toxin (Botox) into the sphincter, which has a similar relaxing effect on the sphincter.
Surgery Only in rare cases is surgery needed.

HOW CAN I HELP MYSELF?

The most important measures you can take are those to help you avoid constipation and straining on the toilet, as described for hemorrhoids (see above).

Pruritus ani

A minor condition affecting the anal area, pruritus ani can usually be relieved by simple measures.

WHAT IS IT?

Pruritus ani is itching and irritation around the anus. It may be due to fissures and hemorrhoids (see above and opposite), to skin problems, such as eczema, in the anal area, or infection with pinworms. Often no definite cause can be identified.

WHAT NEXT?

Your doctor will make a diagnosis based on your symptoms, and will perhaps do a physical examination.

MY TREATMENT OPTIONS

Having eliminated any treatable cause, your doctor will probably advise self-help measures (below) and may recommend that you use a steroid-containing cream.

HOW CAN I HELP MYSELF?

The following self-help measures are usually effective:

Avoid irritants Remove all possible irritants, such as soap, from the skin around the anus.
Keep clean Rinse the anal area thoroughly after you have opened your bowels. Use non-irritant water-based cream instead of soap when you wash yourself.
Keep dry Dry the skin gently without rubbing after bathing and going to the bathroom.
Avoid scratching.
Stay cool Wear loose-fitting underwear made of a natural fiber such as cotton.

Endocrinology and metabolism

Beatriz Rodriguez Olson MD FACP
Clinical Assistant Professor
Yale University School of Medicine

Your hormones and metabolism

Much of the way in which your body functions depends on your hormones. These are chemical messengers that initiate and regulate many of your bodily functions, including your fertility, growth, and energy needs. They are produced in glands situated throughout the body, known collectively as the endocrine system, and are released into the bloodstream, where they are carried to the various cells and tissues on which they have a specific influence.

There are a number of hormones that are produced in very different amounts in women and men. Sex-specific hormones are discussed in Chapter 5 (see pp86–141), but this chapter deals with hormones and any problems related to their production, which are common to both men and women. However, some of these disorders can have a different incidence in women, or they may affect women in a different way from men.

Your body produces several hormones that control the way the body burns fuel for energy, lays down fat, and influences the rate at which many chemical processes occur. The umbrella term used to describe this complex collection of functions is metabolism—and many of the disorders in this chapter affect metabolic processes.

CAUSES OF HORMONAL PROBLEMS

Many hormone problems are related to autoimmune disease, in which the body's own immune system, which normally fights off infection, turns against one or more of its own organs (see pp259, 266–71). Hormonal

---

GLANDS AND HORMONES

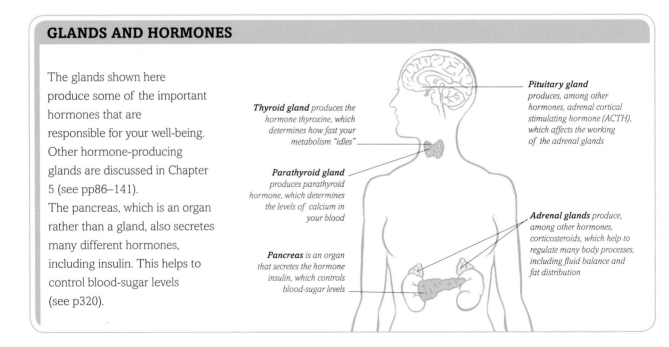

The glands shown here produce some of the important hormones that are responsible for your well-being. Other hormone-producing glands are discussed in Chapter 5 (see pp86–141).
The pancreas, which is an organ rather than a gland, also secretes many different hormones, including insulin. This helps to control blood-sugar levels (see p320).

Thyroid gland produces the hormone thyroxine, which determines how fast your metabolism "idles"

Parathyroid gland produces parathyroid hormone, which determines the levels of calcium in your blood

Pancreas is an organ that secretes the hormone insulin, which controls blood-sugar levels

Pituitary gland produces, among other hormones, adrenal cortical stimulating hormone (ACTH), which affects the working of the adrenal glands

Adrenal glands produce, among other hormones, corticosteroids, which help to regulate many body processes, including fluid balance and fat distribution

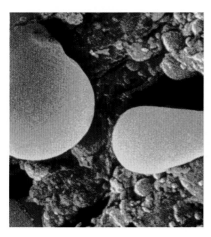

Thyroid gland
The tissue of the thyroid gland secretes thyroglobulin (colored orange), from which the hormones thyroxine (T3) and triiodothyronine (T4) are released. These hormones control your body's metabolism.

I'M EXHAUSTED!

Complaints of being "tired all the time" are one of the most common problems that doctors come across, and women present with it far more often than men.

Tiredness is an extremely vague diagnosis, and it's often not clear what's causing it. However, in women, the most common causes include thyroid problems (see pp326–9) and anemia (see pp248–9).

Other hormone problems that cause tiredness are diabetes (see pp320–5) and Addison's disease (see p331). Although simple exhaustion, inadequate or impaired sleep, stress, or depression can often be an underlying cause in our multitasking, fast-moving world—making it a requirement to take time out for yourself and relax—consult your doctor if you are consistently tired and lack energy.

disorders that have an autoimmune cause include underactive and overactive thyroid glands (see pp326–8) and Type 1 diabetes (see pp320–1). With the notable exception of Type 1 diabetes, women are much more prone than men to most of these disorders, although we don't yet know why this is so. These disorders are often linked and may run in families, so if you or other members of your family suffer from a hormonal or autoimmune problem, your risks of developing other, similar problems are increased.

HORMONES AND FERTILITY

Given how crucial your female hormones are in determining whether and when you ovulate, it's hardly surprising that the other hormones your body produces can have an impact on your fertility. Even a slightly over- or underactive thyroid gland can reduce your chances of conceiving. So if you have a known thyroid problem, you will be referred to an endocrinologist or reproductive specialist more quickly than usual if you're having trouble getting pregnant. Likewise, if you have diabetes, you're likely to be referred if you've been trying to get pregnant unsuccessfully for a year. If you have such a condition, it's crucial to talk to your doctor in advance about your plans to become pregnant.

PREVENTING HORMONAL DISORDERS

Type 2 diabetes is the most preventable of the hormone disorders that are discussed in this chapter. It is almost exclusively a problem among people who carry excess weight, so it can usually be avoided by paying attention to particular aspects of your lifestyle—for example, making sure that you exercise regularly, ensuring that your weight is within the recommended limits for your height, and being sure that you have healthy eating habits (for more advice on a healthy lifestyle, see Chapter 3, pp50–69).

While most hormone disorders are not preventable, adequate nutrition with sufficient vitamin D and iodine intake may decrease the risk. You can be aware of the symptoms, especially if you're at particular risk of a specific disorder. It's always worth explaining your symptoms to your doctor if you think you might have a hormone problem. He or she may be able to rule it out with a blood test, or explain to you why you don't need to worry. Smoking may increase your risk of developing some hormone problems, and it can greatly increase your risk of developing the complications that are often associated with hormonal diseases.

> "Women are more prone than men to hormonal disorders, although we don't know yet why this is so."

Diabetes

"Sugar" diabetes, or diabetes mellitus, is one of the best-known hormone disorders. There are two main forms of the condition, and although both have serious risks, the good news is that these risks can be greatly reduced if you stick carefully to your treatment plan and make lifestyle changes.

The key feature of diabetes mellitus is excess glucose in the blood. When we eat, food is broken down in the gut into sugars. The main sugar is glucose. This passes from the gut into the bloodstream. The pancreas responds to increased levels of glucose in the blood (blood sugar) by releasing the hormone insulin, which helps the body absorb the glucose and turn it into energy. In the two main types of diabetes mellitus—type 1 and type 2—either the pancreas produces insufficient amounts of insulin or body cells are resistant to insulin's effect.

THE LONG-TERM RISKS OF DIABETES

Diabetes that remains undiagnosed or uncontrolled will directly cause:

- Eye retinal damage causing loss of vision
- Kidney damage, diminishing toxin clearance
- Nerve damage, causing loss of sensation or increased pain and slow digestion:
- Diabetes can also promote high blood pressure and elevation of cholesterol and triglycerides, which can harm blood vessels and increase the risk of:

- Heart attack
- Reduced circulation in limbs, ulcers, poor healing, and limb loss
- Stroke
- Kidney failure and need for dialysis
- High-risk pregnancy

Diabetics must have these regular checks to avoid complications:

- Blood pressure checks
- Blood sugar level checks
- Cholesterol level checks
- Annual retina examination
- Kidney function tests
- Foot examination.

Type 1 diabetes

This form of diabetes mellitus used to be known as "insulin-dependent diabetes," because everyone who gets it needs to take insulin every day. It usually first develops in childhood, adolescence, or young adulthood.

WHAT IS IT?

Type 1 diabetes develops when the insulin-producing cells in your pancreas stop producing insulin. It's an "autoimmune" condition (see pp259, 266) with several possible causes; it's probably a combination of genetic susceptibility and triggers in the environment. In this form of diabetes, the insulin-producing cells of the pancreas are totally destroyed. Once insulin production stops, you are likely to develop the symptoms described in the panel (opposite). You may also develop a condition called ketoacidosis. This is caused by the release of toxic chemicals, which occurs when—

because of the lack of insulin—your body is forced to burn fat for energy rather than the sugars in your blood. Ketoacidosis causes nausea and vomiting, abdominal pain, and confusion, and often leads to your breath smelling of acetone (like nail-polish remover). This condition requires urgent medical help.

WHAT NEXT?

If your symptoms suggest type 1 diabetes, your doctor is likely to arrange for tests to determine the

DO I HAVE THE SYMPTOMS?

In Type 1 diabetes, symptoms tend to come on over days rather than weeks or months. These symptoms include:

- Intense thirst
- Passing water very frequently
- Tiredness and lack of energy
- Blurry vision
- Rapid weight loss
- Poor concentration and sometimes collapse.

See your doctor if you have any of the above symptoms.

levels of sugar in your blood and urine to confirm the diagnosis. Blood tests may also indicate how much insulin is being produced by your pancreas.

MY TREATMENT OPTIONS

If you have type 1 diabetes, you'll certainly need insulin injections.
Medication There are both short- and long-acting forms of insulin. You'll be taught how and how often to self-administer insulin using either a syringe, a pen, or an insulin pump.This enables you and your doctor to see if the treatment is controlling your blood sugar effectively. You may need extra medication to treat any complications, such as high blood pressure or raised cholesterol (My treatment options, p323).
Surgery In rare cases, a pancreas transplant may be offered, but it carries a high risk of rejection.

HOW CAN I HELP MYSELF?

You must regulate your food intake to minimize blood-sugar level fluctuations. Much of the advice on diet for type 2 diabetics (see pp324–5) will also help you.
Monitor your blood sugar When you're on insulin treatment, you must check your blood sugar, usually daily. Use a digital meter to prick your finger painlessly to release a drop of blood that you smear onto a test strip. Inserted into the meter, this shows your current blood-sugar level. The results will tell you if you need to adjust your insulin dose. Be sure to learn to recognize symptoms of excessively low blood sugar (hypoglycemia). This can occur if your food intake, insulin levels, and energy output get out of balance. Always have readily absorbed sugar available (such as glucose tablets or sweet drinks) in case this happens.

AM I AT RISK?

The risk factors for type 1 diabetes, include:

- A family history of type 1 diabetes: you are at greater risk of developing it if your father suffered from it than if your mother did.
- Your sex: males and females are diagnosed at about the same rate under the age of 15. Over the age of 15, men are about 50 percent more likely to be diagnosed with type 1 diabetes than women.

INSULIN SELF-TREATMENT

These days, there are lots of convenient and almost painless ways of injecting yourself with insulin, using a syringe, pen, or insulin pump. The highlighted areas below show the best places for safely injecting insulin. You will need to change the site every few days.

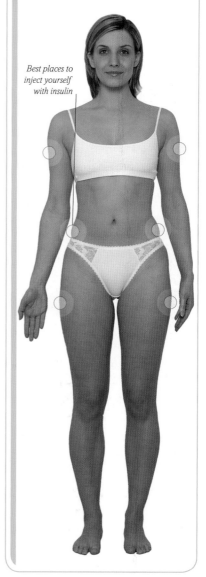

Best places to inject yourself with insulin

Type 2 diabetes

Type 2 diabetes accounts for 90–95 percent of adult-onset diabetes. The vast majority of those affected are overweight. Type 2 diabetes in younger people in the US has also significantly increased.

Type 2 diabetes is preventable through lifestyle changes that promote weight loss.

WHAT IS IT?

Type 2 diabetes occurs when your body gradually stops responding normally to insulin—a condition known as insulin resistance—so your pancreas needs to release higher and higher "doses" to keep your blood sugar at a normal level. Eventually, the insulin-producing cells in your pancreas are unable to keep up with your body's need for insulin. When you have a combination of insulin resistance and decreasing production of insulin, your body's blood-sugar levels can no longer be controlled and you develop the symptoms of type 2 diabetes.

WHAT CAUSES IT?

Four out of five people diagnosed with type 2 diabetes are overweight or obese. Obesity is traditionally measured using the BMI, or body mass index, which is a ratio of your weight to height (see pp58–9). This doesn't mean that everyone who is obese will develop diabetes, but they are at much greater risk. As a woman, if your BMI is over 35, you're 90 times more likely to develop diabetes than someone with a BMI of only 22.

These days, we've also learned that it's not just how much you weigh, but where that weight sits that matters. Your abdominal circumference could be the key to your risk of developing diabetes. Those who tend to lay down fat in the abdominal area are at a far greater risk of developing type 2 diabetes (as well as a number of other disorders) than those who tend to put on weight on their hips, bottoms, and thighs.

Women with central obesity (a waist measurement of over 35 inches) are also are more likely to develop elevated triglycerides.

DO I HAVE THE SYMPTOMS?

The symptoms of Type 2 diabetes are easily overlooked. They tend to come on gradually and can include:
- Needing to pass urine often (including needing to get up at night)
- Constant thirst
- Recurrent yeast infections, boils, or minor skin infections
- Feeling generally tired and run down.

See your doctor if you have any of the above symptoms.

AM I AT RISK?

The risk factors for type 2 diabetes include:
- A family history of developing type 2 diabetes
- Having "gestational diabetes" in pregnancy (see p324)
- Being overweight or obese (especially if you put on weight mainly in your abdominal area)
- Your ethnic background (Native Americans, Hispanic, African-American, Pacific Islanders)
- Taking certain medications (chronic steroids, some psychiatric/antipsychotic medications, as well as some blood pressure medications)
- Having PCOS (see p95).

Smoking is a risk factor for type 2 diabetes that seems to affect women more than men. Women who smoke heavily are up to 75 percent more likely to develop diabetes than those who've never smoked; in men, that figure is just under 50 percent. And if you do have diabetes, smoking amplifies the associated risks.

WHAT NEXT?

Diagnosing diabetes at an early stage is crucial if you want to avoid the serious complications it causes;

"Smoking is a risk factor for Type 2 diabetes that seems to affect women more than men."

as long as diabetes is undiagnosed, your body is living with damagingly high levels of blood sugar, and probably raised cholesterol and blood pressure as well. The early symptoms of type 2 diabetes are often very mild and non-specific; sadly, this means that all too many people ignore the early symptoms, or put them down to stress.

MY TREATMENT OPTIONS

Your doctor will advise on lifestyle changes (see p324). In addition to such changes, a number of drugs can help regulate blood-sugar levels:

Antidiabetic medications

The drug metformin increases the sensitivity of tissues in the body to insulin. Drugs from a family of medicines called sulfonylureas may be prescribed as an alternative, or together with metformin. These stimulate the pancreas to produce increased levels of insulin. Other drugs that may be prescribed include glitazone, insulin sensitizers, and the gliptins, the postprandial glucose regulators. Your doctor will explain the possible side effects of each of these options and work with you to find a drug-treatment regime that is best suited to your circumstances and condition.

Other forms of medication

Further drug treatment is aimed at treating possible complications.

- If you have raised blood pressure, the level for treatment is anything over 140/90 for diabetes. Your doctor will want your blood pressure kept to a level of 130/80 or below. If you have high blood pressure, two groups of related drugs called the ACE inhibitors (see p170) and the ARBs, or sartans, can also help to protect your kidneys from damage.
- If you have raised cholesterol levels, you are likely to be prescribed statins (see p170), though you may need to stop taking them before you consider getting pregnant (see p324). A healthy lifestyle can delay or even prevent the need for this medication. If you're over 40, you'll probably be prescribed a statin as a matter of course.
- To help you lose weight, your doctor may consider prescribing you a drug that helps you to control your weight.

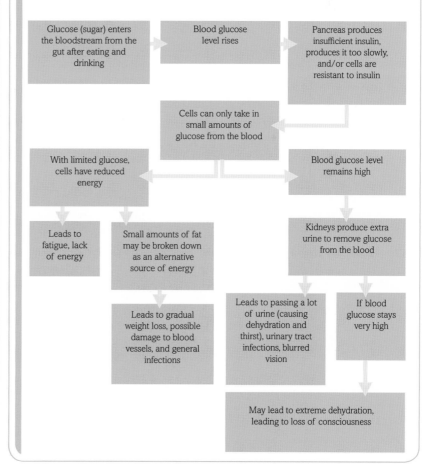

TYPE 2 DIABETES: HOW YOUR BODY USES GLUCOSE

In type 2 diabetes, your pancreas doesn't produce sufficient insulin, produces it too slowly, or your body cells are resistant to it. As the diagram below illustrates, this in turn affects the body's ability to use blood glucose (sugar) properly, resulting in a range of health problems.

Glucose (sugar) enters the bloodstream from the gut after eating and drinking

Blood glucose level rises

Pancreas produces insufficient insulin, produces it too slowly, and/or cells are resistant to insulin

Cells can only take in small amounts of glucose from the blood

With limited glucose, cells have reduced energy

Blood glucose level remains high

Leads to fatigue, lack of energy

Small amounts of fat may be broken down as an alternative source of energy

Kidneys produce extra urine to remove glucose from the blood

Leads to gradual weight loss, possible damage to blood vessels, and general infections

Leads to passing a lot of urine (causing dehydration and thirst), urinary tract infections, blurred vision

If blood glucose stays very high

May lead to extreme dehydration, leading to loss of consciousness

> "Reduce your weight to a healthy level through regular exercise and diet."

HOW CAN I HELP MYSELF?

Being diagnosed with diabetes is always a shock, but it's important to keep things in perspective. If lifestyle change goals are met, people with type 2 diabetes have the potential to come off of medication. There's a lot you can do to help yourself, alongside taking any medication your doctor may prescribe for you.

Lose weight One of the most important things you can do is to reduce your weight to a healthy level through regular exercise (see pp56–7) and a healthy diet (pp52–5). This will help you to avoid the complications of diabetes.

Control your blood sugar Keeping blood-sugar levels stable helps the effectiveness of any medication you are taking and reduces the risk of complications. Tips for regulating your blood sugar include:

- Eat regularly—don't go more than four hours between meals.
- Choose foods that release their energy slowly (see opposite).
- Avoid high sugar or long shelf-life processed foods containing either high fructose corn syrup or partly hydrogenated fats.
- Be aware that your female hormones, which vary with your menstrual cycle, can affect your blood-sugar control. You may be more prone to both low blood sugar and raised blood sugar around the time of your period.

Lower your cholesterol level

The risks of high cholesterol levels are discussed in Chapter 7. These risks are much higher for women than for men. That makes reducing your levels of cholesterol even more crucial than it is for a man. Diet and exercise can make a big difference (see pp52–7). Your abdominal fat (see p322) has a huge impact on your cholesterol levels. Reducing your weight by just 10 percent can reduce your abdominal fat by a massive 30 percent. Your doctor may also recommend that you take medicine to reduce your cholesterol (see p323).

Control your blood pressure

After raised cholesterol, raised blood pressure (see p161) is one of the most important risk factors for heart disease, and particularly for stroke. This is especially true if you have diabetes, so it's crucial to get your blood pressure checked at least twice a year. You may need to take a blood-pressure lowering drug (see p170).

DIABETES AND PREGNANCY

Pregnancy can cause gestational diabetes. It affects one in 25 women. In most cases, dietary changes with or without insulin will be needed until the birth. However, a history of gestational diabetes increases your risk of developing type 2 diabetes in the future, so you'll probably need a blood test for diabetes once a year for the rest of your life.

If you're already taking drugs for type 2 diabetes, you may need to change medication before getting pregnant. Insulin, though, is perfectly safe during pregnancy, and is likely to be recommended as a substitute.

METABOLIC SYNDROME

Also known as insulin resistance syndrome, metabolic syndrome is a cluster of risk factors that significantly increase your risk of both diabetes and heart disease. The problem centers around excess fat that is laid down in the abdominal area. This fat affects the way your body metabolizes fat and sugar. It predisposes you to the following conditions:

- Insulin resistance and diabetes
- Higher levels of "bad" cholesterol, lower levels of "good" cholesterol
- Raised blood pressure
- Polycystic ovary syndrome. Metabolic syndrome itself doesn't usually cause symptoms, but because of the health risks, it's important to know if you are at risk. If you think you have abdominal obesity (see pp58–9), seek medical advice.

Slow energy-release foods

If you have either type of diabetes, controlling your blood glucose (blood sugar) will be much easier if your diet consists mainly of foods that release their energy slowly. These are sometimes called "low GI" foods. Some examples of these foods are shown below.

Beans

Pulses are the ideal low GI food. They supply a steady release of energy, with protein and plenty of fiber, and are low in fat.

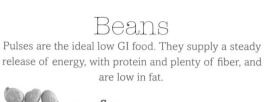

Soy beans

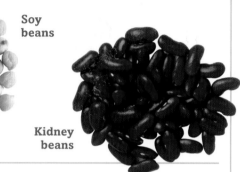

Kidney beans

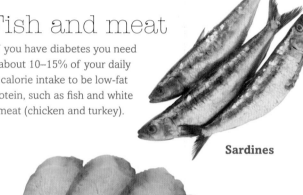

Mackerel

Fish and meat

If you have diabetes you need about 10–15% of your daily calorie intake to be low-fat protein, such as fish and white meat (chicken and turkey).

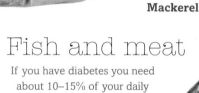

Sardines

Vegetables

Vitamin-rich vegetables are broken down slowly into glucose by the body, so they supply higher levels of energy for longer. Fresh fruit (not juices) works in a similar way.

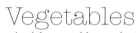

Broccoli

Chicken

Bread and cereals

White bread and many wheat- or corn-based cereals are high GI: they raise your blood sugar quickly, making it harder to control your overall sugar levels. Whole-grain bread and cereals based on whole grains, like oats, are much better.

Rolled oats

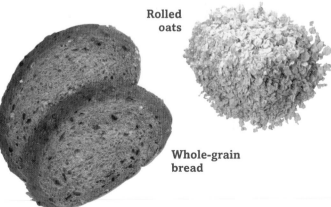

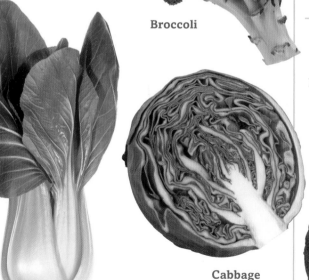

Bok choy

Cabbage

Whole-grain bread

Disorders of the thyroid gland

The hormone thyroxine is produced by the thyroid gland, which is located at the front of your neck. This hormone plays a major part in determining how fast your metabolism (the body's chemical processes) "runs." Problems can occur if the body produces either too much or too little of this hormone.

The thyroid gland is one of the main glands in the endocrine system, which helps to regulate the body's energy levels. With up to ten times as many women as men affected by thyroid problems, the thyroid is a gland that every woman should be aware of.

Many of the cells and tissues in our bodies need sufficient amounts of thyroxine if they are to work correctly. If your thyroid gland produces too little thyroxine, many of your body's natural functions slow down; if it produces too much, many aspects of your metabolism speed up. Normally, your body's production of thyroxine is controlled by a feedback mechanism of interacting hormones (see left). Some types of thyroid imbalances are caused by disruption to this process resulting from problems with the pituitary gland.

Disorders of the thyroid gland usually come on slowly, and it is possible to overlook the symptoms for months or even years. However, once your doctor suspects you have a problem with the proper functioning of your thyroid, the initial diagnosis is usually easily made by a blood test. Sometimes further tests may be needed in order to determine the underlying cause of the problem. Once over- or underactivity of the thyroid gland is confirmed, the condition is usually easily treated with drugs, which often produce a rapid improvement in symptoms. Sometimes, however, treatment needs to continue indefinitely.

THYROXINE PRODUCTION

The hypothalamus, situated at the base of the brain just above the pituitary gland, secretes the thyrotropin-releasing hormone (TRH), which triggers the pituitary gland into producing a thyroid-stimulating hormone (TSH). This in turn tells the thyroid gland to start secreting thyroxine into the bloodstream. When levels are high enough, the hypothalamus and pituitary glands reduce their output of TRH and TSH until the thyroxine levels drop again. The hypothalamus, pituitary, and thyroid glands work together to ensure the right levels of thyroxine are produced.

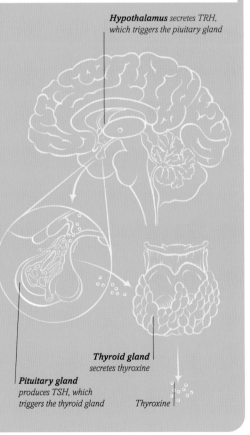

Hypothalamus secretes TRH, which triggers the piuitary gland

Thyroid gland secretes thyroxine

Pituitary gland produces TSH, which triggers the thyroid gland

Thyroxine

Underactive thyroid

This highly treatable condition is ten times more common in women than in men, and particularly affects people over 50.

WHAT IS IT?

When you have an underactive thyroid (hypothyroidism), it does not produce enough of the hormone thyroxine. This causes a slowing down of many processes in the body, leading to many of the symptoms in the panel (right).

Worldwide, the most common cause of hypothyroidism is a lack of iodine (one of the components of thyroxine) in the diet. In most of the Western world, however, the main cause is inflammation of the thyroid, often caused by an autoimmune response (see pp259, 266). It can raise your blood cholesterol and therefore your risk of heart disease.

HYPOTHYROIDISM IN PREGNANCY

It's common for women to develop hypothyroidism in pregnancy—it affects up to 1 in 40 pregnant women. If it's not treated, it can increase the risk of complications in pregnancy, including premature labor, raised blood pressure, anemia, stillbirth, and serious bleeding after the birth.

This is one of the few types of hypothyroidism that can get better by itself. However, it can recur later in life, so if you've had hypothyroidism in pregnancy, you should have your thyroid checked once a year for the rest of your life.

If you are already taking thyroxine, the dose will likely need to be increased during pregnancy.

WHAT NEXT?

You will have blood tests to check TSH levels in your body.

MY TREATMENT OPTIONS

Once you're diagnosed with hypothyroidism, you'll be treated with thyroxine pills. Be sure to discuss any side effects with your doctor. You'll probably be started on a low dose to see how your body responds. The dose may be increased later.

In most cases, you'll be given a blood test every few weeks to check the blood levels of thyroxine. Once your levels are stable, you'll probably only need a blood test every year or so, but in most cases, you'll need treatment for life.

HOW CAN I HELP MYSELF?

Follow your doctor's advice on your medication program, and make sure you have a healthy lifestyle (see Chapter 3, pp48–69).

DO I HAVE THE SYMPTOMS?

The most common symptoms of hypothyroidism include:
- Tiredness and sleeping longer
- Weight gain without overeating
- Susceptibility to the cold
- Constipation
- Dry skin and coarse hair
- Depression
- Mental slowness
- Fluid retention.

Less common symptoms of the condition include:
- Irregular or heavy periods
- Problems getting pregnant
- Hoarse voice
- Forgetfulness
- Enlargement of the thyroid gland (see Goiter, p329).

See your doctor if you have two or more of these symptoms.

AM I AT RISK?

Aside from being a woman, risk factors for hypothyroidism include:
- Being over 50 years old
- Pregnancy
- A history of hypothyroidism
- A history of an overactive thyroid gland (see pp328–9) due to an autoimmune cause
- Having another autoimmune disease (see pp259, 266–71)
- Having certain inherited conditions, such as Down syndrome or Turner's syndrome
- Taking certain medications such as amiodarone (to treat heart rhythm disorders), lithium (to treat bipolar disorder), or sunitinib or interferon alfa (to treat cancer).

Overactive thyroid

Hyperthyroidism, or an overactive thyroid gland, is also known as thyrotoxicosis. It affects about ten times more women than men. This manageable condition is most likely to develop between the ages of 20 and 40.

WHAT IS IT?

One in 50 women has hyperthyroidism. In up to four out of five of those women affected, the malfunction of the thyroid has an autoimmune cause, in which the body's antibodies cause excessive production of thyroxine. Graves' disease (see opposite) is a common cause of overactivity of the thyroid.

The course of hyperthryoidism is highly variable. In many of those affected, the condition settles by itself within one and half to two years. If this happens to you, you'll still need to make sure you get your thyroid function checked regularly, since the condition can recur. However, for others, treatment needs to continue for many years.

WHAT NEXT?

Hyperthyroidism is diagnosed with blood tests to check your body's levels of thyroxine (which are high in hyperthyroidism) and TSH (which are low). Sometimes, hyperthyroidism can be associated with transient thyroid inflammation as a result of a virus or bacterial infection or in association with the postpartum period. In addition, some benign thyroid nodules can produce too much thyroxine.

MY TREATMENT OPTIONS

You'll need to see an endocrinologist or thyroidologist to discuss

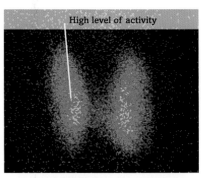

High level of activity

Scan of a normal thyroid gland
This scintogram shows hormone-producing activity in a healthy thyroid gland. The bright green areas are the most active, the blue areas are the least active.

ways to address the cause of hormone overproduction:
● Observation
● Medication
● Surgery
● Radioactive iodine.
Each of these treatments is appropriate in different circumstances, and each has its pros and cons. Your doctor will work with you to choose the best treatment for your circumstances; be sure to discuss any side effects.
Medication The most common antithyroid medications used in the US to treat hyperthyroidism due to Graves' disease or autoimmune thyrotoxicosis are carbimazole and propylthiouracil (PTU), the latter in particular during pregnancy.

While you're waiting for the carbimazole to take effect, you may need to take other drugs, such as beta blockers, to help control your symptoms. You'll also need to seek urgent medical advice if you develop any other symptoms of infection, such as a fever or sore throat. This is because very

> "One in fifty women develops overactivity of the thyroid gland."

DO I HAVE THE SYMPTOMS?

Symptoms of hyperthyroidism may include some or all of the following:
● Irritability and anxiety
● Weight loss, despite increased appetite
● Poor sleep
● Palpitations
● Diarrhea
● Shortness of breath
● Light or absent periods
● Tremor (especially of the hands)
● Dislike of heat, and excess sweating
● Itching
● Thinning of the hair or patchy hair loss
● Enlarged thyroid gland (called a goiter), causing a visible swelling in the throat
● Bulging eyes.

See your doctor if you have two or more of the above symptoms.

GRAVES' DISEASE

This is an autoimmune disease that accounts for at least two thirds of cases of hyperthyroidism. The condition occurs when your body starts producing antibodies that stimulate your pituitary gland to produce TSH, even when your body's levels of thyroxine are normal or high. About half of those who have Graves' disease develop prominent, bulging eyes, dryness and soreness of the eyes, and/or double vision. Smoking and treatment with radioactive iodine increase the risk of Graves' eye disease. Unfortunately, lowering your thyroid levels doesn't reverse the eye changes. Some people notice the onset of eye symptoms even after starting treatment for the disease.

For most people affected, using artificial tears, wearing sunglasses, and using eye protectors when asleep control the symptoms adequately. However, if you have severe eye changes, you'll need to have regular checks. Sometimes fatty tissue builds up behind the eyeballs, and this may need to be removed by surgery. Alternatively, your specialist may recommend X-ray therapy or steroids.

occasionally (in less than 1 in 200 people taking it), carbimazole and PTU can adversely affect the white blood cells in your blood, which help to combat infection.

After about 12–18 months, your doctor will probably recommend tailing off your dose of carbimazole or PTU to see if your condition has settled on its own. However, you may need to take further courses of the drug in the future if the condition flares up again. If the condition doesn't fix itself naturally, your doctor may suggest another recommended treatment option.

Surgery Some kinds of hyperthyroidism cause a large swelling of your thyroid, called a goiter (see below). In these cases, surgery, which has a 98 percent success rate, is an option. There is a small risk of complications, such as bleeding, and problems with low calcium and vocal cord dysfunction. It's also common to develop hypothyroidism after surgery, but this can be treated in the same way as other causes of hypothyroidism.

Radioactive iodine In this form of treatment, you simply swallow a liquid or capsule of radioactive iodine. The radioactive iodine concentrates in your thyroid gland, reducing its ability to make thyroxine. One treatment is usually sufficient to improve your symptoms. In the long term, between half and three quarters of those treated with radioactive iodine develop hypothyroidism, but this is easily treated with supplements of thyroxine.

HOW CAN I HELP MYSELF?
There is no specific self-help advice for those who have an overactive thyroid gland. Be sure to follow the treatment program prescribed by your doctor and be vigilant for any complications.

GOITER

A goiter in the throat can range in size from a small lump to a large swelling. It may indicate an under- or overactive thyroid.

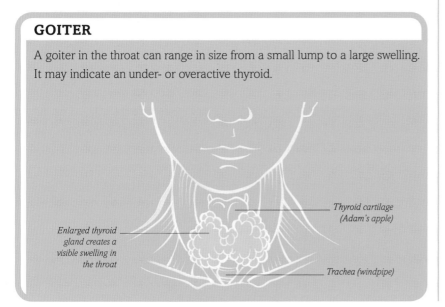

Thyroid cartilage (Adam's apple)

Enlarged thyroid gland creates a visible swelling in the throat

Trachea (windpipe)

Disorders of other glands

The parathyroid, pituitary, and adrenal glands may be less well known than some other hormone-producing glands, such as the thyroid gland, but the hormones they produce are nevertheless vital. Over- or underproduction of any of these hormones can occur, but fortunately such conditions are rare.

Parathyroid gland disorders

Located in the neck behind the thyroid gland, the parathyroid glands produce parathyroid hormone. Sometimes too much hormone is produced (hyperparathyroidism), or too little (hypoparathyroidism).

WHAT IS IT?

Parathyroid hormone determines the calcium levels in your body. Over-production can lead to excess calcium in the blood, which can cause the formation of calcium-rich "stones" in the kidneys (see pp346–7) and fragile bones.

WHAT NEXT?

You may need a blood test to check the levels of parathyroid hormone.

MY TREATMENT OPTIONS

Parathyroid overactivity is treated with surgery to remove excess glandular tissue, while underactivity of the gland is usually treated with dietary supplements of calcium and vitamin D.

HOW CAN I HELP MYSELF?

Take 1000 IU of vitamin D_2 or D_3 daily to avoid overworking the gland.

DO I HAVE THE SYMPTOMS?

An overactive parathyroid gland may cause:
- Abdominal pain, nausea, and constipation
- Loss of appetite and weight
- Tiredness and depression.

An underactive parathyroid gland may cause:
- Muscle spasm
- Numbness or tingling.

See your doctor if you experience any of the above symptoms.

Pituitary gland disorders

DO I HAVE THE SYMPTOMS?

If you have a problem with your pituitary gland, it can cause a wide variety of different symptoms, including:
- Headaches
- Disturbances in vision
- Irregular periods.

See your doctor if you experience any of the above symptoms.

The tiny pituitary gland is deep inside the brain. It is often called the master gland because its hormones govern many different body processes. Many of these hormones regulate the levels of other hormones in the body. For example, it produces adrenal cortical stimulating hormone (ACTH), which acts on the adrenal glands (see opposite). The pituitary gland also produces several hormones involved in the reproductive processes.

WHAT IS IT?

Pituitary gland disorders are rare, but growths can occur within the gland. Although usually benign, these growths can produce hormone oversecretion. They can also grow, causing undersecretion of one or many pituitary hormones, headache, visual changes, and/or a change in thirst.

A common effect of this tumor is that too much prolactin—the milk-producing hormone—is made. The result is that women who aren't pregnant stop menstruating and produce breast milk.

WHAT NEXT?

If your doctor suspects a pituitary gland problem from an account of your symptoms, the diagnosis can be confirmed by blood tests and possibly MRI or CT scans. In some cases you may be asked to undergo tests on your field of vision, if a tumor is thought to be creating pressure on the part of the brain that governs vision.

MY TREATMENT OPTIONS

Tumors of the pituitary gland are commonly treated with surgery and radiation (X-rays). Many pituitary tumors can be treated with medication.

HOW CAN I HELP MYSELF?

There are no adjustments to lifestyle that can prevent or treat pituitary problems.

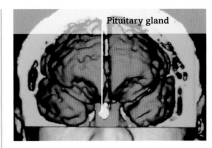

Pituitary gland
The location of the pituitary gland in the brain, as shown on a colored 3-D CT scan. The gland is about the size of a pea.

Adrenal gland disorders

The adrenal glands produce corticosteroids (or steroids), which help maintain muscle and fat structure and fluid balance. They also influence blood pressure, blood-sugar, and bone density.

WHAT IS IT?

Adrenal gland disorders include:
Cushing's disease This results from excess production of corticosteroid hormones by the pituitary gland. It may also be caused by a tumor or adenoma in the adrenal gland, or Cushing's disease.
Addison's disease Usually the result of an autoimmune problem (see pp259, 266), it causes adrenal underactivity.

WHAT NEXT?

Adrenal hormone levels can be checked with blood, urine, or saliva tests. More tests may be needed.

DO I HAVE THE SYMPTOMS?

Cushing's disease may cause symptoms that include:
- Weight gain around the abdomen
- Reddening and rounding of the face
- Increased hairiness of the face and body.

Addison's disease may cause:
- Tiredness
- Weight loss
- Irregular periods
- Skin darkening.

See your doctor if you have any of the above symptoms.

MY TREATMENT OPTIONS

Treatment for Cushing's may involve surgery on the pituitary or adrenal glands. Hydrocortisone or prednisone with fluodrocortisone are used to replace missing steroids in Addison's disease.

HOW CAN I HELP MYSELF?

Follow the treatment program prescribed by your doctor.

STEROIDS—THE RISKS FOR WOMEN

Steroid drugs are given by mouth to treat a wide variety of medical problems. But high levels of steroids in your body, especially over more than a few months, can bring a variety of unwanted effects and make you prone to:
- High blood pressure
- Raised blood sugar (see Diabetes, pp322–5)
- Wasting of the muscles of the arms and legs
- Easy bruising

- Thinning of the skin and stretch marks
- Laying down of fat around the stomach
- Filling out of the cheeks, resulting in a "moon faced" appearance
- Frequent infections of all kinds. In addition, prolonged steroid treatment makes you more prone to osteoporosis (see pp260–2). If you have to take steroid tablets in the long term, talk to your doctor about measures to prevent osteoporosis.

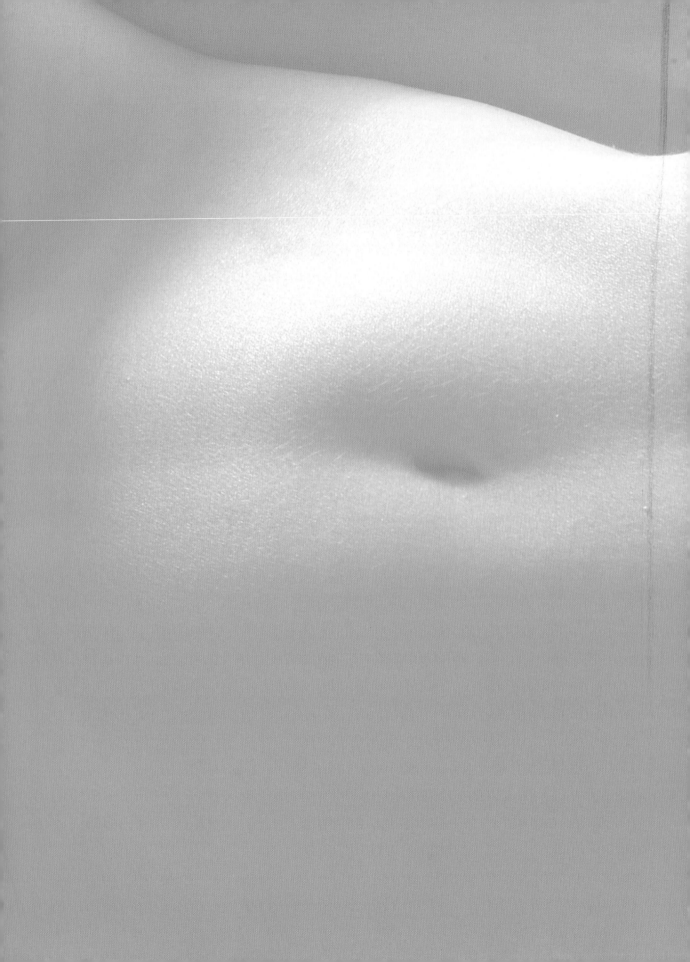

Bladder and urinary tract

Lindsey A. Kerr MD
Director, Center for Continence Care and Sexual Medicine
Louisville, KY

Bladder & urinary tract

Your urinary tract consists of a pair of kidneys, a pair of ureters, a bladder, and a urethra. Its main function is to get rid of the waste products that accumulate in your body, regulate water levels, and make sure your bodily fluids are kept in balance. The key organs are the kidneys, which carry out the process of filtering out wastes and excess water from the blood to produce urine. The urine then flows down the ureters to the bladder and is passed out of the body through the urethra.

THE FEMALE URINARY SYSTEM

Your kidneys are situated on either side of the spine, at the back of the abdomen just below the diaphragm. Each adult kidney is a reddish brown bean-shaped organ about 4 in (12 cm) long and 2¾ in (7 cm) wide. Each kidney is connected to a ureter, a muscular tube about 10 in (25 cm) long that carries urine to the bladder. Essentially a muscular bag, the bladder stores urine until it is passed out of the body through the urethra, a tube about 1½ in (4 cm) long.

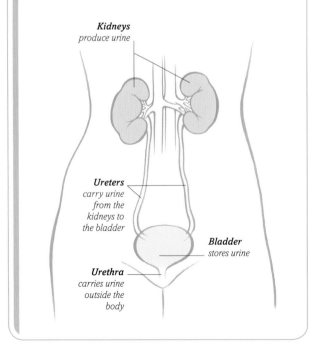

Kidneys
produce urine

Ureters
carry urine from the kidneys to the bladder

Bladder
stores urine

Urethra
carries urine outside the body

THE URINARY TRACT

Your kidneys are designed to filter your blood but they do so selectively, removing waste products and excess water but retaining useful substances, such as glucose (blood sugar). The liver has a similar waste removal function, but it removes different waste products. The filtered waste products and water are what make up your urine. Together, the kidneys produce approximately 1 fl oz (30 ml) of urine every hour, and this amount increases the more you drink. By regulating the amount of water lost from the body in the urine, your kidneys keep your body fluids balanced so you don't get dehydrated or overhydrated. Your kidneys also play an important role in the production of red blood cells and in making vitamin D. If your kidneys stop working, you will become overloaded with fluid, anemic, and be very ill due to the build up of waste products in your body. You may also develop other problems, such as high blood pressure and osteoporosis (thinning of the bones).

The ureters are muscular tubes that transport the urine from your kidneys into your bladder. They run alongside the bones of your spine and then turn inward at the level of your pelvis to pass obliquely into your bladder. The tunnel formed by the oblique passage of the ureters acts as a one-way valve. This stops urine from flowing back up into the kidneys when your bladder contracts to empty out the urine.

The bladder is a muscular bag that is lined with specialized waterproofed cells. It is designed to store urine and to let it out when required. Usually we pass about

14–18 fl oz (450–500 ml) each time, although this varies according to how big you are—small people have smaller bladders! It's normal to pass urine about every four hours during the day, but this becomes more frequent the more you drink and even more frequent if you drink diuretic fluids (fluids that increase urine flow), such as coffee, tea, and alcoholic drinks. Before you are 50 years old, it isn't normal to have to get up to go to the bathroom during the night, but as you get older it becomes increasingly common. In fact, it is considered normal to get up in the night once in your 50s, twice in your 60s, and up to three times in your 70s.

DIFFERENCES BETWEEN WOMEN AND MEN

Up to the bladder, the urinary tracts of men and women are similar. It is the structure beyond that point—the urethra, which carries urine from the bladder to outside the body—that differs. In women, the urethra is about 1½ in (4 cm) long and is surrounded by a muscle called the urethral sphincter. It passes in the front wall of the vagina and exits in the midline between the clitoris and vagina.

In men, the urethra is longer—about 10 in (25 cm) long—and S-shaped. It has a sphincter (ring of muscle) both where it joins the bladder and below the prostate gland, and passes through the penis. In both men and women ejaculate (the fluid produced during orgasm by men in the prostate or by the contraction of glands near the urethra in women) and urine leave the body via the urethra.

DISORDERS OF THE URINARY TRACT

The most common urological disorders that affect women are urinary tract infections (also called bladder infections, UTIs, or cystitis), kidney infections (pyelonephritis), urinary incontinence, and bladder pain syndrome (interstitial cystitis). Other conditions include urinary tract cancers, especially those of the bladder and kidneys, inflammation, and stones in the urinary tract.

> "Your kidneys not only remove waste products and excess water from the body, but also help in the production of red blood cells."

KIDNEY CROSS SECTION

The kidney has an outer cortex that filters blood to produce urine, which passes into the medulla, then the pelvis, and then out through the ureter.

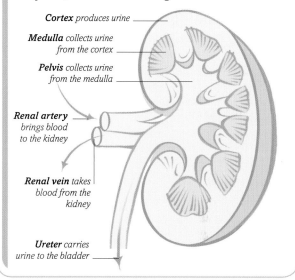

Cortex produces urine
Medulla collects urine from the cortex
Pelvis collects urine from the medulla
Renal artery brings blood to the kidney
Renal vein takes blood from the kidney
Ureter carries urine to the bladder

FEMALE AND MALE URETHRAS

The female urethra runs from the bladder to leave the body between the vaginal opening and the clitoris. The male urethra runs from the bladder, through the prostate gland, and exits via the penis.

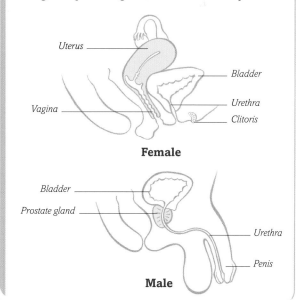

Uterus
Vagina
Bladder
Urethra
Clitoris
Female

Bladder
Prostate gland
Urethra
Penis
Male

Urinary tract infection

About half of all women get a urinary tract infection (UTI) at least once in their lives, and some women suffer repeated infections. However, it is usually easily treated with a short course of antibiotics. You will only need further investigation and treatment if you keep getting infections.

DO I HAVE THE SYMPTOMS?

The most common symptoms of a UTI are a sudden onset of:

- Burning pain when you pass urine
- Needing to urinate very frequently
- Passing only small amounts of urine
- Difficulty in delaying urination
- Blood in urine
- Pain or discomfort just above your pubic bone

See your doctor if your UTI doesn't clear up using self-help measures (see What Next?, right). Seek medical advice immediately if there is blood in your urine.

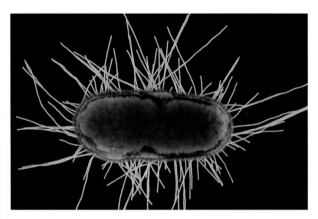

E. coli bacterium
This usually harmless inhabitant of the intestine is the cause of most urinary tract infections.

WHAT IS IT?

The term "UTI" is usually used to refer to cystitis (a bacterial infection of the bladder), but it may be used to talk about an infection anywhere in your urinary tract, from your kidneys to your urethra. Urine is normally sterile so the presence of any bacteria in it is abnormal. A UTI is diagnosed when the urine contains a significant number of bacteria. The bacteria—usually the ones living in your intestine, such as *Escherichia coli* (usually known simply as E. coli)—may enter your urinary tract through your urethra. This may happen during sex.

WHAT NEXT?

When you first develop symptoms, you should increase the amount you drink—try drinking 1 pint (600 ml) of water immediately, then 10 fl oz (300 ml) every 30 minutes. This will increase your production of urine and the number of times you urinate. Taking cranberry extract pills, eating blueberries, or drinking full-strength cranberry or blueberry juice is also helpful. You should also avoid having sex until the infection has cleared up if it is uncomfortable.

You should see your doctor as soon as your symptoms develop. He or she will prescribe antibiotics based on symptoms, and if necessary, test your urine for infection.

If there's a delay before you can see the doctor, then you can try over-the-counter urine alkalizers, such as potassium citrate and sodium citrate, and painkillers such

"To help prevent a UTI, you should increase your daily fluid intake to approximately 2.5–3.5 pints."

as ibuprofen or to help relieve symptoms. A word of caution, though. If you're pregnant, breast-feeding, or are taking any other medications, ask your doctor or pharmacist before trying these over-the-counter remedies.

If your UTI doesn't respond to treatment or it recurs more than three times in six months, your doctor will refer you to an urologist for further investigation.

MY TREATMENT OPTIONS

If symptoms persist or have not subsided with self-help measures (see right), your doctor will probably prescribe medication.
Medication Your doctor will prescribe a short (3–5 day) course of antibiotics. A corresponding course of probiotics (acidophilus) may help prevent developing a secondary yeast infection as a result of using antibiotics. Ask your

doctor about any side effects and make sure you tell him or her if you are pregnant or breast-feeding.
Further treatment If your UTI recurs, your doctor may give you a six-week course of vaginal estrogen cream or suppositories plus more antibiotics.

For some women who have recurrent UTIs, the doctor may recommend dilation (stretching) of the urethra to help with emptying the bladder, a monthly course of antibiotics along with a short course to treat your partner, or a course of six weekly instillations of sodium hyaluronate (Cystistat) into your bladder to improve the protective layers of the

lining of the bladder (see also p344).

HOW CAN I HELP MYSELF?

There are lots of measures you can take to help prevent a UTI.
Drink more Increase your fluid intake to about 2.5–3.5 pints (1.5–2 liters) per day.
Sex Before having sex, drink a glass of water and gently wash the perineal area to get rid of any bacteria. Make sure you urinate within about an hour of sex, to flush out any remaining bacteria.
Drink cranberry juice A large glass of cranberry juice per day may reduce the number of UTIs you have if you get them often.

AM I AT RISK?

All women are at risk of UTI because their urethras are located in moist environments, which are more susceptible to bacteria, and may incur trauma during intercourse. You may also be at risk if:

- You are sexually active
- You are pregnant
- You are postmenopausal
- You have problems with urinary incontinence (see pp339–41)

DEALING WITH AN ACUTE ATTACK OF UTI

If you are suffering from an acute attack of UTI, even if it's during the night, then:

- Immediately drink 1 pint (600 ml) of water, then drink 10 fl oz (300 ml) every 30 minutes
- If you're in pain, fill two hot water bottles, wrap them in towels, and put one on your lower back and one between your thighs
- Mix 1 teaspoon of bicarbonate of soda with some water and drink it; repeat every three hours. If you have high blood pressure, you should talk to your doctor before you take bicarbonate of soda. Alternatively, if you've had UTI attacks in the past, keep a supply of urine alkalizers from

your pharmacist at home and take one as soon as an episode starts

- Take one or two analgesics to help with the pain. If you are pregnant, you should talk to your doctor before taking analgesics
- Try to relax with activities that take your mind off the symptoms.

You may find that the symptoms start to subside after three hours of this routine, but call your doctor if the episode continues for longer than a day, if you're pregnant, or if you notice blood in your urine. Call your doctor as soon as possible if these self-help measures do not ease your discomfort.

Pyelonephritis

Painful urination, together with intense pain in your lower back, could mean you have the kidney disorder known as pyelonephritis (PN). This serious condition is usually easily treated and can clear up in a few days. But prompt attention is needed, since untreated PN can lead to kidney damage and may be fatal.

WHAT IS IT?

PN, which is an inflammation of one or both of kidneys, is usually caused by a bacterial infection. The disorder often follows a urinary tract infection (see pp336–7). More rarely, pyelonephritis may occur if there is a blockage in the urinary tract, such as a kidney stone (see p346–7). Occasionally, PN can become a long-term disorder, especially if it is associated with abnormalities of the bladder. Recurring inflammation (chronic PN) although unusual, may be the result of an underlying anatomic defect.

WHAT NEXT?

If you have the symptoms of PN, consult your doctor the same day. He or she will test your urine for an infection and start treatment (see below). If PN persists, your doctor will refer you to an urologist. This specialist may do blood tests, an ultrasound scan of your kidneys, and a CT scan if your symptoms are acute.

MY TREATMENT OPTIONS

PN needs immediate treatment to prevent kidney damage and the systemic movement of symptoms.
Medication A 7–14 day course of antibiotics is usually effective in treating the infection. Ask your doctor about possible side effects.
Hospital If you are very unwell, you may be admitted to the hospital for emergency treatment with intravenous antibiotics.

HOW CAN I HELP MYSELF?

If you develop the symptoms of PN, you should start drinking plenty of water. For long-term protection, you need to drink at least 2½–3½ pints (1.5–2 liters) a day—more in hot weather or if you are particularly active.
Drink cranberry juice In people who suffer from recurrent PN, drinking a large glass (over 12 fl oz/ 350 ml) of cranberry juice per day may reduce the frequency of infections.

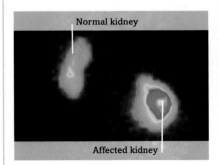

Pyelonephritis
This scan shows the inflamed area (red) in a kidney affected by PN. Recurrent and/or prolonged PN may cause serious damage.

Urinary incontinence

The loss of bladder control—urinary incontinence (UI)—and overactive bladder are extremely common in women, yet many are too embarrassed to talk about it. Left untreated, UI can seriously affect your quality of life. There's no need to suffer in silence. There are many effective treatments available.

DO I HAVE THE SYMPTOMS?

The most common symptoms of urinary incontinence are:
- Involuntary leakage of urine following a cough, sneeze, or during strenuous exercise
- Frequent, sudden urges to urinate
- Difficulty in delaying urination
- Complete inability to control urination once the flow of urine has started.

See your doctor as soon as possible if you think that you may have UI.

WHAT IS IT?

Urinary incontinence (UI) is the involuntary loss of urine from the bladder. This very common problem affects between 25 and 45 percent of women of all ages.

There are different types of UI, which occur for a variety of reasons. These include:
- Urge incontinence—the sudden urge to pass urine, often followed by uncontrollable emptying of the bladder. In most cases, urge incontinence occurs without any identifiable underlying cause.
- Stress incontinence—leakage of small amounts of urine when you cough, sneeze, or exercise.

This is the most common type of UI. It is caused by weak pelvic floor muscles failing to hold the bladder in the correct position. Stress incontinence may follow pregnancy or pelvic surgery, or occur in older women who have lost muscle tone.
- Mixed incontinence—this disorder is a combination of urge and stress incontinence
- Overflow incontinence—when blockage effectively prevents normal urination, so urine continually overflows.
- Overactive bladder—urgency with or without urge leakage.

SOME COMMON TYPES OF UI

Urge incontinence, failure to "make it" to the bathroom in time, is caused by uncontrollable contractions of the bladder muscles. This is usually because the bladder has become overactive. Stress incontinence, the involuntary leakage of urine when you cough, sneeze, or exercise, is the result of weakened pelvic floor muscles. Loss of support causes the neck of the bladder and urethra to drop down, which makes it impossible for the muscles that control urine flow to close properly.

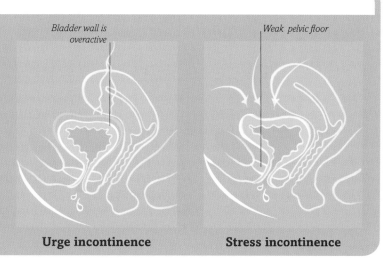

Bladder wall is overactive

Weak pelvic floor

Urge incontinence

Stress incontinence

"There are a number of excellent treatments available that can either greatly improve or even cure urinary incontinence."

WHAT NEXT?

If you develop UI you should talk to your primary care doctor. Don't let embarrassment prevent you from getting the help you need. Your doctor will assess the type and severity of your incontinence, check for any associated symptoms that may need further investigation, and test for hematuria (blood in the urine) and bacturia (bacterial infection). You may be referred to a continence specialist, who will do a pelvic and abdominal exam, and do an internal examination to assess the strength of your pelvic floor muscles. He or she may perform tests to measure the flow rate of your urine and to check whether you are completely emptying your bladder. You may also have an ultrasound scan of your bladder, and a sample of your urine may be tested for evidence of bleeding and infection.

MY TREATMENT OPTIONS

Treatment depends on what type of UI you have. Your doctor will be able to advise you on the relative effectiveness and possible side effects, if any, of each treatment. Some options may involve minimally invasive surgery. To treat stress UI:

Kegel exercises While Kegel exercises (see right) may be taught during treatment for stress UI, it is unlikely that these will provide sufficient improvement.

Injections Collagen is injected into the bladder neck to bulk up the tissues and improve closure of the outlet.

Suburethral sling A special piece of tension-free vaginal tape is placed around your urethra. Insertion of the tape involves a relatively straightforward surgery that may be performed under local anesthetic.

Pubovaginal sling In this rare surgery, tissue from another part of the body, such as the abdomen, is wrapped around the neck of the bladder to form a supporting sling.

Colposuspension This surgery involves lifting up the vagina and attaching it behind your pubic bone. The top of the vagina stretches across the bladder opening to reposition the bladder and urethra.

PELVIC FLOOR MUSCLES

The pelvic floor muscles act as a supportive sling that holds the bladder, vagina, uterus, and rectum in place. Loss of muscle tone, often due to overstretching during childbirth but also because of aging, can cause the pelvic floor to become slack. If this happens, the pelvic organs sag, and problems such as incontinence occur. Exercises can help to restore the strength of the pelvic floor muscles (see opposite).

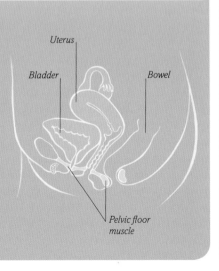

Uterus

Bladder

Bowel

Pelvic floor muscle

KEGEL EXERCISES

Also sometimes called pelvic floor exercises, Kegel exercises help strengthen the muscles and tighten the ligaments at the base of the abdomen. Kegel exercises are best done preventively during pregnancy and in the postpartum period. The exercises can be done standing, sitting, or lying down and don't need any special equipment, although some women find that using a vaginal cone (a small weight shaped like a tampon that is placed in the vagina) is helpful. The exercises should be done every day, and it may take several months before you notice any benefit. To perform Kegel exercises, you should do the following:

Identify the muscles Tighten the muscles around your vagina and anus and lift upward and inward. Alternatively, try to stop the flow of urine when you are on the toilet. To check that you're using the right muscles, put two fingers in your vagina when trying to tighten the muscles; you should feel a gentle squeeze.

Contract the muscles Having found the right muscles, you need to do both fast and slow contractions. Ideally, you should do a set of slow contractions plus a set of fast contractions six times every day. Some women find that using biofeedback while doing the exercises helps them make sure the correct muscles are being used. The exercises should not be done while urinating since this may lead to abnormal urinary retention.

To do slow contractions, slowly tighten the pelvic floor muscles to a count of 10, hold them contracted for 10 seconds, then relax and rest for 10 seconds. Do this sequence 10 times to complete one set.

To do fast contractions, tighten your pelvic floor muscles quickly, hold them contracted for one second, then relax and rest for one second. Do this sequence 10 times to complete one set.

Alternatives to Kegel exercises Some people have found that electrical stimulation helps to improve bladder control. A probe is inserted into your vagina to the muscles around the bladder and a weak electric current is passed through the probe. This causes a tingling sensation but is not painful. It may take daily sessions of up to an hour each for several months to produce noticeable results.

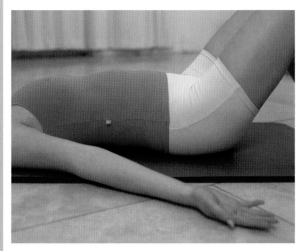

Pelvic tilts
Step 1 This simple exercise is another way to strengthen your pelvic floor muscles, while also toning your lower abdominal muscles. Lie on your back, and take a big breath in.

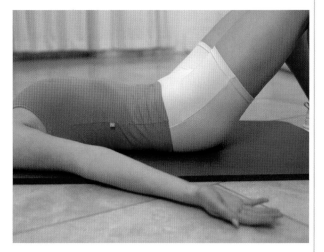

Step 2 Breathe out, squeeze your pelvic floor muscles and draw your lower abdominal muscles toward your spine—think "navel to spine"—as you curl your buttocks slightly off the floor. Keep your buttocks relaxed. Repeat 5–10 times.

Artificial urinary sphincter

Used only as a last resort, this method employs an inflatable cuff that wraps around the neck of the bladder to keep it closed. This is connected to a pressure regulating balloon placed in the abdominal cavity and a tiny pump implanted in the labia majora. Pressing the pump with a finger releases the cuff to let urine flow out.

To treat urge UI:

Bladder training The initial treatment is often bladder training (see below) with some lifestyle changes.

Medication Your doctor may give you antimuscarinic pills, which help reduce involuntary contractions in the bladder muscles. If these don't work or you can't tolerate the side effects, you'll be referred to a specialist for further treatment.

Botulinum toxin (Botox) injections Injected into the lining of your bladder, these drugs block muscle contractions.

Sacral neuromodulation An implant is inserted near your bladder. This sends out mild electrical impulses that stimulate the nerves to the bladder and give you better bladder control.

Clam cystoplasty A patch of tissue taken from the intestine is inserted into the bladder to lessen the impact of muscle contractions.

HOW CAN I HELP MYSELF?

If you have a mild form of UI, there are a number of self-help measures that you can take to improve your condition:

> "Practicing Kegel exercises regularly, stopping smoking, and eating a healthy diet may help to prevent urinary incontinence."

Adjust your lifestyle Eat plenty of fiber-rich foods, such as bran, whole-wheat bread, whole-grain cereals, fruit, leafy vegetables, beans, and lentils, and keep active to prevent constipation (see also pp52–7, 303). Straining the bowels puts stress on the pelvic muscles.

Drink more To stop your urine from becoming too concentrated and irritating the bladder, try to drink about 2½–3½ pints (1.5–2 liters) of fluid a day.

Cut down on caffeine and carbonated drinks Reduce or eliminate these types of drinks since they tend to overstimulate both the bladder and the kidneys.

Stop smoking This irritates the bladder lining and makes UI worse.

BLADDER TRAINING

If you suffer from urge incontinence, you may be able to improve your bladder control with a method known as bladder training. This technique needs perseverance—you will not see results overnight—but many women find it very effective.

Set times Bladder training involves visiting the bathroom only at fixed intervals. The idea is to train yourself to delay emptying your bladder for gradually extended periods.

Starting with an empty bladder, decide on an interval during which you will resist the urge to urinate. At first, try to "hold on" for five minutes before going to the bathroom. When you can manage this, gradually extend the interval—to 10 minutes, 15 minutes and so on—until you can delay urinating for two to three hours. As your bladder is re-educated, the urge to urinate will occur less often. It may take several weeks, or even months, to achieve your goal.

Distraction techniques You can try various ploys to keep your mind off wanting to "go" during intervals between bathroom visits. Some women use relaxation techniques, such as deep breathing, to control their urges. You could also take the opportunity to do some Kegel exercises to help things along.

Getting help Your doctor or incontinence nurse will help you work out a personal bladder training schedule. They will probably suggest that you monitor your progress by keeping a diary of both successes and leakages.

Painful bladder syndrome

This long-term bladder problem causes pain in the lower part of the abdomen and a frequent urge to urinate. Since these symptoms are shared by various other urinary tract disorders, such as cystitis, painful bladder syndrome is difficult to diagnose. Treatment is aimed at relief of discomfort, rather than cure.

DO I HAVE THE SYMPTOMS?

The symptoms of bladder pain syndrome vary from person to person, but the most common are a sudden or gradual onset of:

- Pain on passing urine
- Increased frequency of urination
- Pain, sometimes severe, in the lower abdominal area, just above the pubic bone
- Blood in the urine
- Pain or discomfort felt in the urethra or vagina
- Pain during sexual intercourse

See your doctor as soon as possible if you experience any of the above symptoms.

WHAT IS IT?

Painful bladder syndrome (PBS) generally refers to a collection of symptoms affecting the pelvic area. The disorder is also known as abacterial cystitis, interstitial cystitis, chronic pelvic pain syndrome, and painful bladder syndrome. Its symptoms are similar to those of some UTIs (see p336), but bacteria aren't involved.

Little is known about the causes of PBS. It could be a mucosal defect, or a disease of the nervous system, immune system, or integement.

WHAT NEXT?

If you develop symptoms of PBS, you should see your doctor for a pelvic exam. Your doctor will also send a urine sample to the laboratory for testing to exclude infection and cancer, and to look for cells in the urine, such as white blood cells, that indicate inflammation. If your samples don't grow any bacteria, you will be sent to an urologist for further examination. He or she will examine your abdomen and pelvis, and perform an internal vaginal examination to ensure that there aren't any other possible causes for your symptoms.

The urologist will also send a urine sample to look for cancer cells, and a blood sample to check that you are not diabetic and have normal kidney function. You will also have a cystoscopy, and if needed, an X-ray, an ultrasound scan of your urinary tract, and an ultrasound scan of your bladder after you have urinated to ensure you have no other urinary problems. You will be asked to keep a diary to see how often you urinate and how much you pass.

MY TREATMENT OPTIONS

There are many treatments available—each with a varied success rate. Your doctor will work with you to find the best treatment for you personally. Ask your doctor about any side effects if you are prescribed medication.

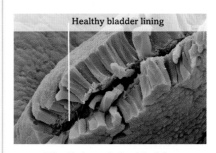

The lining of the bladder
A section of the lining of a healthy bladder. The cells are very tightly packed to prevent damage from urine.

"Stress may aggravate your symptoms, so try to make sure you have plenty of relaxation time in your life."

> "A number of treatments are often used at the same time to tackle successfully the different symptoms associated with bladder pain."

Tests The initial treatment done under a local anesthetic is to look into your bladder via your urethra with a cytoscope—a type of viewing instrument. The doctor may gently stretch your bladder by filling it with sterile liquid to see how much fluid it will hold, to see whether there are any signs of discomfort, and to look for evidence of inflammation when your bladder is emptied after the gentle stretch. The doctor may also take a biopsy of your bladder to rule out cancer and to look for inflammatory cells, and may also gently stretch your urethra. If you have urethral discomfort, the doctor may inject a local anesthetic and steroid around your bladder. This procedure is performed for diagnosis and treatment, and provides 6–12 months' relief of symptoms in about 50 percent of women. You'll be reviewed about six weeks afterward to see how you are—and additional treatment will be started as required.

Medication If you still have symptoms, antihistamine medication may be started for a minimum of six weeks to reduce the inflammation in your bladder. If this fails, or simultaneously, you may also be given a nerve-blocking painkiller along with an anti-inflammatory painkiller. If frequent urination is a particular problem, antimuscarinic pills are added. You may also be given antibiotics to try to eliminate bacteria that may be present and contributing to the PBS.

Pain specialist You may be referred to a pain specialist. He or she will help to manage the pain with strong nerve-blocking painkillers, local and spinal nerve-block injections, and superficial neuromodulation (TENS). This uses electrical stimulation to confuse nerves into not sending pain signals. The specialist may also involve a psychologist, who can offer you techniques to help you cope with PBS.

Bladder instillations If you don't respond to oral medication, your bladder may be filled with a solution containing the drug RIMSO. This is done via a catheter. The catheter is then removed and the drug stays in the bladder for 20 minutes and is then passed out as though you were passing urine. If this fails, instillations of sodium hyaluronate (Cystistat) may be tried.

Acupuncture If the bladder instillations fail or if they aren't acceptable, then a course of acupuncture (see below) may help.

Injections Botulinum toxin injections into your bladder lining may help control severe urgency and frequency. This procedure needs you to be able to insert a catheter into your own bladder in order to empty it if needed.

Electrical stimulation If these treatments fail sacral neuro-modulation (see p342) can be used to relieve frequency.

Surgery In rare cases, if all these treatments fail, and the pain is very severe, then surgery might be suggested. The possibilities are clam cystoplasty (see p342),

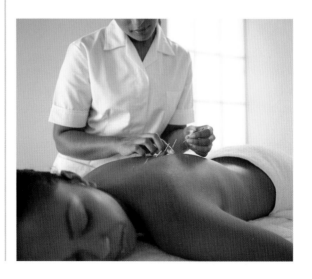

diversion of the urine into a special bag (stoma, or urostomy, bag) that is worn outside the body on the abdomen, or the surgical removal of the bladder with or without the urethra. Reconstruction of a new bladder from bowel tissue may be suggested.

HOW CAN I HELP MYSELF?
The following may help:
Keep a diary (see below.)

Avoid stress Stress exacerbates the problem, so it's wise to try to de-stress your life (see pp62–3).
Try acupuncture This may be help both the symptoms and to aid relaxation and de-stressing.

Foods that may trigger bladder pain

Many women who suffer from bladder pain syndrome agree that certain foods and drinks can irritate a sensitive bladder. Some of the most common triggers are detailed below. Keep a diet and symptom diary over a few weeks to try to identify dietary factors that may be triggering your symptoms. Avoiding these foods may help ease your symptoms.

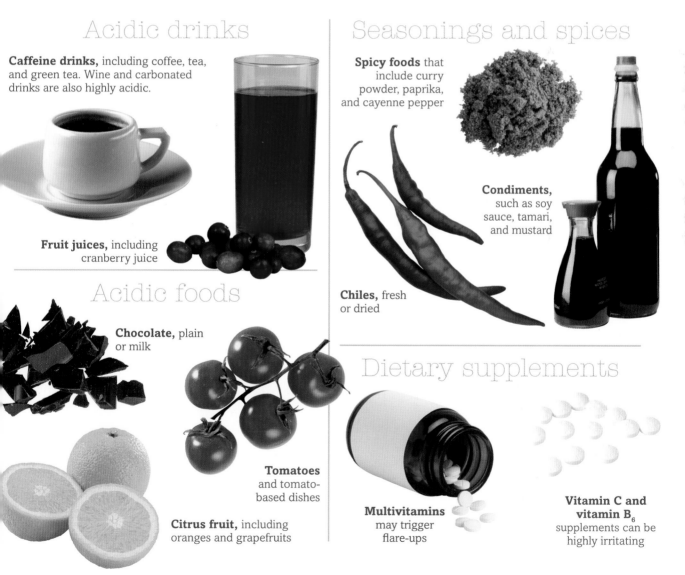

Acidic drinks

Caffeine drinks, including coffee, tea, and green tea. Wine and carbonated drinks are also highly acidic.

Fruit juices, including cranberry juice

Acidic foods

Chocolate, plain or milk

Tomatoes and tomato-based dishes

Citrus fruit, including oranges and grapefruits

Seasonings and spices

Spicy foods that include curry powder, paprika, and cayenne pepper

Condiments, such as soy sauce, tamari, and mustard

Chiles, fresh or dried

Dietary supplements

Multivitamins may trigger flare-ups

Vitamin C and vitamin B$_6$ supplements can be highly irritating

Urinary tract stones

The most noticeable symptom of a stone in the urinary tract, commonly known as a kidney stone, is excruciating pain in the back. Many women have said that the pain of passing a stone is worse than childbirth!

WHAT IS IT?

Urinary tract stones are small, solid masses—some are as small as a grain of sand, others are much larger—that form in one or both of your kidneys. They are caused by substances in your urine turning into crystals.

The stones may either stay in your kidney and in the top end of the ureter or they can travel down into your bladder. Most stones are small, less than ¼ in (5 mm) across. Stones smaller than 2mm usually pass out of your body in the urine without causing problems. However, if a stone is large, it is more likely to get stuck and cause symptoms (see Do I have the symptoms?).

WHAT NEXT?

If you develop the symptoms of a urinary tract stone you should first take a simple over-the-counter nonsteroidal analgesic, such as ibuprofen, and then consult your doctor immediately.

Your doctor will test your urine for blood and to check for infection. If he or she suspects a stone, you will be referred to an urologist—as a matter of urgency if simple anagesics are not controlling your pain and/or if you have a high temperature.

The urologist will also perform tests, including a blood test to check kidney function, and urine tests to look for any blood in the urine and to check for the possibility of a UTI (see p336). A specialized X-ray will also be done to look for stones in your kidneys, ureters, and bladder; this X-ray may be a CT scan, KUB (a type of abdominal X-ray), or an intravenous urogram (IVU). An IVU involves a series of X-rays taken before and after you have had an injection of a special dye. If you pass any stones, the urologist will also examine these to identify the precise type of stone.

DO I HAVE THE SYMPTOMS?

The symptoms of a urinary tract stone are a sudden onset of:
- Severe colicky pain on one side of your back, often radiating to the front of the abdomen toward the groin
- Nausea and vomiting
- Blood in urine
- Increased frequency of passing urine.

See your doctor immediately if you have any of these symptoms.

SITES OF URINARY TRACT STONES

The most common sites of stones are the major and minor calyces (the urine-collecting areas) and the renal pelvis, which channels urine to the bladder.

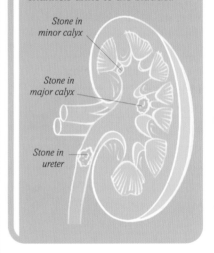

Stone in minor calyx

Stone in major calyx

Stone in ureter

"Stones can be as small as a grain of sand and pass out of your body naturally."

MY TREATMENT OPTIONS

There are a number of treatment options available depending on the size and type of your kidney stone. If the stone is small, you may require only pain relief; you will also be advised to drink plenty of fluids to help flush out the stone. Larger stones or stones that have become stuck may need lithotripsy or ureteroscopy (minimally invasive surgery) to break up the stones so that they can be passed out naturally or be easily removed. Drainage of the kidney may be needed.

Pain relief This first treatment you will be offered is medical expulsive therapy to get stones to pass on their own. Doctors also advise using narcotic analgesics to relieve pain.

Lithotripsy Also known as external shock wave lithotripsy (ESWL), this is the most common method of treating larger stones or those that are stuck in the urinary tract, although it is not suitable in all cases. Lithotripsy is a minimally invasive procedure in which focused sound waves are used to break up the stones into small fragments that can be passed out naturally when you urinate. Painkillers are usually given before the procedure, as it may cause some discomfort. For a few days after the procedure you may have blood in your urine and there may be tenderness over the treated area.

Ureteroscopy If a stone is stuck in your ureter, a small viewing tube (called a ureteroscope) is inserted into your ureter via your bladder and urethra, and a laser is used to break up the stone so that it can be passed out naturally.

Surgery If a stone is stuck in your kidney, a viewing tube (called a nephroscope) is inserted into your kidney and upper ureter through an incision in your back. The stone is pulled out or broken up via the nephroscope. Most urinary tract stones that require surgical treatment can be treated using minimally invasive techniques. Only rarely is it necessary to remove stones by open surgery.

Drainage Very rarely, a stone-related blockage can cause a serious kidney infection that may be life-threatening and requires emergency drainage of the kidney. Drainage may be carried out under local anesthesia and involves inserting a drainage tube through your skin into your kidney. Alternatively it may be done via the bladder, in which case general anaesthia is used.

HOW CAN I HELP MYSELF?

You can help prevent stones by eating a healthy diet (see pp52–5) and avoiding becoming dehydrated. It is generally advised that you should drink 2.5–3.5 pints (about 1.5–2 liters) a day if you've never had a stone, or 3.5–5 pints (about 2–3 liters) a day if you have had stones before.

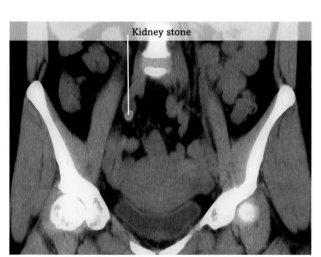

A kidney stone
This MRI scan clearly shows the presence of a kidney stone (red) in the woman's right ureter. (the tube that channels urine from the kidney to the bladder).

> ### AM I AT RISK?
>
> You may be at risk of urinary tract stones if you have:
> - Dehydration
> - A diet that is high in protein and low in fiber
> - A sedentary lifestyle
> - High calcium levels in your blood, which may be associated with parathyroid gland problems
> - Other metabolic abnormalities, such as hyperuricemia (associated with gout) and an inherited condition called cystinuria
> - An untreated long-term urinary tract infection.

Urinary tract cancer

Although serious, there's a good chance that urinary tract cancer can be treated successfully, particularly if it's detected early. The crucial thing is to see your doctor as soon as possible if you notice any symptoms. There may be nothing to worry about, but you should get a medical checkup to make sure.

WHAT IS IT?

Urinary tract cancer refers to cancer of your bladder, kidney, and ureters. Bladder cancer usually starts in the lining of the bladder, and it ranges from small warts to large tumors. There are several types of kidney cancer but the most common is renal cell cancer, which affects the cells that make up the main body of the kidney. Cancer of the ureter affects the tube that carries urine from the kidney to the bladder. In all types, there are often no symptoms in the early stages. If you do have any symptoms (see Do I have the symptoms?), you should make an immediate appointment to see your doctor.

Of the three types of urinary tract cancer, bladder cancer is the most common in women and ureter cancer the least common. The causes of urinary tract cancer aren't known, but it's thought that smoking and exposure to certain chemicals may increase the risk of developing it. The risk also increases with age.

WHAT NEXT?

Your doctor will ask about your symptoms and examine your abdomen and pelvis. He or she will do an internal examination to make sure your symptoms aren't due to a gynecological problem, and will do a dipstick test on a urine sample to check for blood. If these tests indicate cancer may be a possibility, you'll be referred to a urologist. The urologist will send a urine sample to the laboratory to see if there are any cancer cells, and a blood sample to check your kidney function. The urologist may look into your bladder using a flexible viewing instrument (called a cystoscope) that is passed through your urethra into the bladder. This is done under a local anesthetic. If abnormalities are found, you'll be given a general anesthetic and a rigid cystoscope will be used to take a tissue sample from your bladder and to remove any small tumors. You'll also have an X-ray taken of your kidneys, ureters, and bladder (called a KUB) and an intravenous urogram (IVU; see p346) of your urinary tract. You may also have a CT scan of your

DO I HAVE THE SYMPTOMS?

You may not have any symptoms with urinary tract cancer. However, the most common symptoms are:

- Blood in your urine
- Needing to urinate frequently
- Pain when you urinate
- Difficulty in delaying urinating
- A constant feeling of needing to urinate.

If you also have either or both of the following symptoms, this may be an indication of kidney cancer:

- Pain in your side that won't go away
- A lump in your abdomen.

See your doctor as soon as possible if you experience any of these symptoms.

AM I AT RISK?

You may be at increased risk of contracting cancer of the urinary tract if:

- You smoke
- You are obese
- You have a poor diet
- You have been exposed to any cancer-causing materials, such as asbestos.

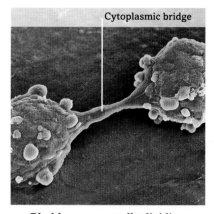

Cytoplasmic bridge

Bladder cancer cells dividing
This color-enhanced scanning electron micrograph (SEM) shows the final stage of a bladder cancer cell dividing. The two cells that are produced are attached by a cytoplasmic bridge (thin thread).

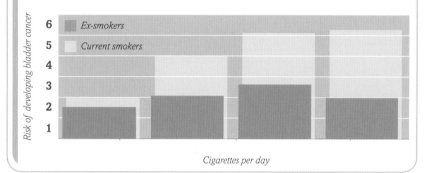

THE RISK OF BLADDER CANCER FROM SMOKING

The biggest risk of developing bladder cancer comes from smoking. The more cigarettes you smoke and the more deeply you inhale, the greater the risk of developing bladder cancer. However, as the graph shows (on a scale of 1 to 6), the risk reduces if you stop smoking.

Risk of developing bladder cancer

6 — Ex-smokers
5 — Current smokers
4
3
2
1

Cigarettes per day

urinary tract, and an X-ray of your lungs to see if cancer has spread.

MY TREATMENT OPTIONS
Treatment will depend on the type of urinary tract cancer, but there are a number of treatment options:
Surgery If you have bladder cancer and it's in the early stages, the tumor can usually be removed with minimally invasive surgery using a cytoscope. However, if the cancer is more advanced, you'll need more invasive surgery to remove the bladder. If you have kidney or ureter cancer and the tumor hasn't spread, you'll usually have surgery to remove the tumor. You may also have all or part of your kidney removed. However, if you have only a small tumor in your ureter, it may be possible to remove only the affected part and rejoin the ureter.
Laser therapy If you have a tumor on the surface of your ureter and it's in the early stages, it may be possible to remove it by laser therapy.
Radiation therapy In rare cases, if surgery isn't an option or the cancer has spread, radiation therapy may be recommended.
After surgery Depending on the type and severity of your cancer, other treatments may be given after surgery, including chemotherapy, radiation therapy, and immunotherapy (treatment to stimulate your immune system to destroy cancer cells).
Follow-up After treatment you'll have regular checkups to monitor your recovery.

HOW CAN I HELP MYSELF?
You can reduce the chance of developing urinary tract cancer by stopping smoking if you smoke (see p64), and by eating healthily (see pp52–5) and getting regular exercise (see pp56–7) to maintain a healthy weight.

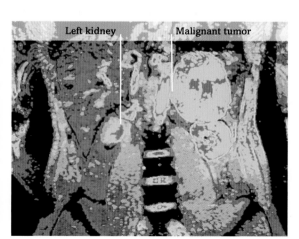

Left kidney   Malignant tumor

Cancer of the kidney
This color-enhanced MRI (magnetic resonance imaging) scan of the abdomen shows a large malignant tumor on the right kidney. The pelvic area is at the bottom and parts of the arms are upper left and right. The the central black areas are the lower part of the spinal column.

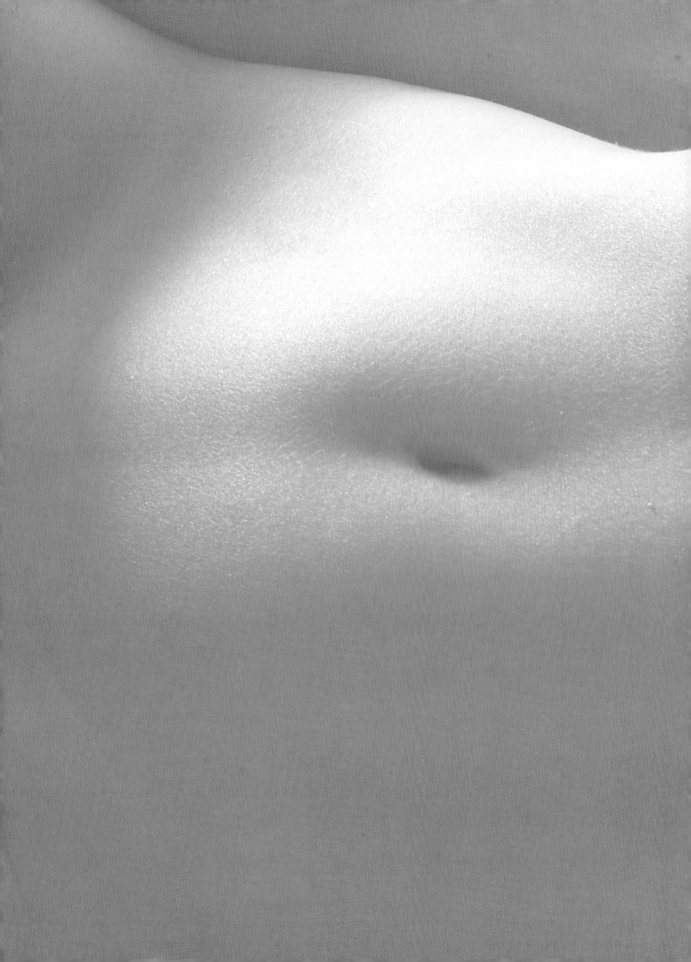

Skin and hair

Debra Jaliman MD
Assistant Professor, Department of Dermatology
Mount Sinai School of Medicine

Your skin and hair

Think of your skin and hair as an external reflection of your health and lifestyle. If you are full of zest for life and are taking care of yourself, eating well, being active, and making sure you have some "me time," it is likely that your skin will be radiant and your hair will be lustrous. Neglect yourself or indulge in bad habits, such as smoking or crash dieting, and your skin will pay the price with accelerated aging and premature wrinkles, and your hair may start falling out in clumps. It is never too late to start a good skin and hair care regimen (see pp66–7).

WHAT IS SKIN MADE OF?

The skin is the largest organ in the body, covering, on average, 2½ sq ft (2 sq m). This physical barrier—even at just ¼ in (6 mm) thick—protects our bodies from the outside environment. The base ingredient for skin is the fibrous protein keratin, which is made by the keratinocyte skin cells in the epidermis (the uppermost skin layer).

The skin's dermis lies beneath the epidermis and houses the cells that make elastin and collagen to give skin its plumpness and elasticity. This layer also contains blood vessels, nerve endings, hair follicles, and the other elements that are needed in order to maintain healthy skin.

Skin cells, along with hairs, follow a cycle: growth, no-growth, and then shedding. Disruptions or upsets to the cycle can worsen conditions such as psoriasis (see p356) or alopecia (hair loss, see p368).

HOW SKIN CHANGES AS WE AGE

The major cause of aging is ultraviolet light from the sun. You probably know that UV light produces extra pigmentation, which results in a sun tan or burn; less well known is that it can also result in age spots,

WHAT LIES BENEATH THE SURFACE?

In this cross-sectional view through the skin, you can see the elements contained within the two basic layers of the epidermis and the dermis.

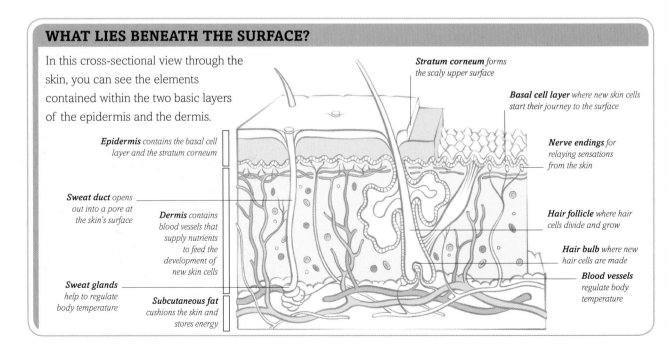

Epidermis contains the basal cell layer and the stratum corneum

Sweat duct opens out into a pore at the skin's surface

Dermis contains blood vessels that supply nutrients to feed the development of new skin cells

Sweat glands help to regulate body temperature

Subcutaneous fat cushions the skin and stores energy

Stratum corneum forms the scaly upper surface

Basal cell layer where new skin cells start their journey to the surface

Nerve endings for relaying sensations from the skin

Hair follicle where hair cells divide and grow

Hair bulb where new hair cells are made

Blood vessels regulate body temperature

broken blood vessels, and wrinkles, as well as drying out the skin generally. Super-hydrated skin appears to be firm and youthful, so if you want to appear younger, make sure you use an effective moisturizer and reapply it frequently.

HOW ARE WOMEN DIFFERENT?
Some small anatomical differences explain why women's skin is different from men's.

Women's skin tends to secrete a little less oil from the sebaceous glands than men's, due to the effects of estrogen. Having less oily skin has its benefits: you're less likely to have acne and other blemishes. However, drier skin is more prone to wrinkles.

Overall, women have thinner skin than men and so are more susceptible to the damaging effects of the sun's ultraviolet rays. The thickness of skin starts to decline after menopause. Collagen content is lower to start with and collagen degradation occurs to a greater extent in women's skin, meaning that women often look older than men of the same age.

WHAT IS HAIR MADE OF?
As with skin, the base ingredient for hair is the protein keratin. Each strand of hair consists of three concentric layers:
- The cuticle—this thin, colorless outer layer protects the inner layers
- The cortex—this thick layer contains melanin, which gives hair its color. Eumelanin produces brown or black hair; pheomelanin produces red hair. Blonde hair results from low amounts of melanin
- The medulla—this innermost layer reflects light, giving hair its various tones of color.

HOW HAIR CHANGES AS WE AGE
The most obvious sign of getting older is graying hair. Over time hair follicles stop making melanin and white or gray hairs start to appear. Much of how you age is genetically determined, so think about how your parents aged in terms of their hair. What's more, your hair becomes thinner and may even become quite sparse in places (female-pattern baldness, see p371).

SKIN THROUGH THE AGES
Genetics, hormonal changes, and the sun all play a part in how your skin changes through the decades. So what can you expect from your skin as you get older? Read on to find out.

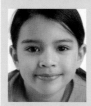

Under 11
This nearly perfect skin has a smooth overall texture with small pores. Hydration is good, the activity of the sebaceous glands is low, and healing capability is excellent.

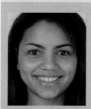

11–25
Sebaceous gland activity is high, helping cause bouts of acne that can affect the texture and color of the skin. Later, the first fine lines start to appear and pore size increases.

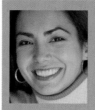

25–45
A noticeable drop in skin hydration causes more fine lines to appear, and even the first wrinkles. There are early signs of the skin sagging around the eye area as it loses some of its elasticity.

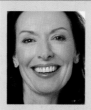

45–55
The skin is drier and the epidermis thins. The texture of the skin becomes rougher and pores enlarge as the skin loses elasticity. Age spots appear and the skin sags near the eyes and cheeks.

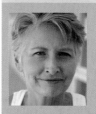

55–65
Wrinkles and fine lines are abundant. Skin color is uneven and sagging worsens. Oil production is low and the skin's ability to repair itself after injury is diminished.

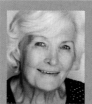

Over 65
The skin is more transparent and fragile as collagen diminishes. Numerous wrinkles are now apparent and sagging is pronounced. Skin growths and pigment spots are more noticeable.

Dermatitis

Substances in perfumes, cosmetics, detergents, jewelry, and clothes can irritate your skin or even, if you are abnormally sensitive, prompt an allergic reaction. In many cases, once the offending substance has been identified, avoiding it and using some simple treatments will be enough to solve the problem.

WHAT IS IT?

Dermatitis, literally meaning "inflamed skin," is a common skin condition. It's very likely that you'll know of someone with dermatitis: 1 in 10 people have it at any one time and 40 percent of the population will experience it during their lifetime. It's also known as eczema and the terms can be used interchangeably. While it's not dangerous, it can cause a lot of discomfort.

There are two types of dermatitis: irritant dermatitis and allergic dermatitis.

WHAT NEXT?

Your doctor will want to have a good look at the affected skin. More often than not, he or she will be able to identify dermatitis based on the pattern of redness and the appearance of the rash.

Next, your doctor will probably ask some questions about your skin-care regimen as well prompting you to remember anything new that you've used or worn in the past weeks or months since you've noticed the change in your skin—laundry detergent, costume jewelry, perfume, and hand soap, for example.

If nothing obvious springs to mind, your doctor may then arrange a test to find the allergen (the substance that is causing your

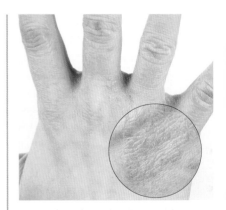

Checking for dermatitis
Early signs of dermatitis often occur between the fingers, encroaching down the tops of the hands.

allergic reaction). He or she may either perform a patch test in the office or refer you to a dermatologist for an allergy test. This very simple test is safe and effective. A series of chemicals on small disks is taped to your back and left in place for 48 hours. After this time, your doctor examines the skin on your back, looking for any area that has turned red, which would indicate that your skin is sensitive and you're allergic to that particular chemical.

DO I HAVE THE SYMPTOMS?

If your dermatitis is the result of contact with an irritant, you may have:

- Dry, red patches of skin (commonly between the fingers, in elbow creases, behind the knees, and on the neck)
- Scaling or blistering skin
- Itchy skin.

If your dermatitis is an allergic reaction, it may sometimes occur up to two or three days after you have been in contact with the substance. You may have:

- Red, swollen patches of skin
- Scaling or blistering skin
- Itchy skin
- Swollen eyes (if the dermatitis is very severe, your eyes may be swollen shut).

"It's possible you may have developed an allergy to a product you have used without problem for a long time."

In many cases, your doctor will be able to give you a list of products that the offending chemical is in so that you can avoid it in the future. Common allergens include:

- Poison ivy
- Nickel, often found in costume jewelry
- Fragrance, used in perfume, skin-care products, soap, air fresheners, and many other household products
- Certain foods: chocolate, eggs, milk, and peanuts
- Latex, present in disposable gloves and condoms
- Pet dander—the skin that sheds from pets and their fur
- Dust mites.

MY TREATMENT OPTIONS

It's a good idea but not enough just to avoid the irritant or allergen causing your dermatitis. There are

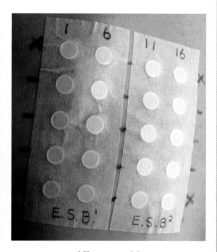

Allergy grid
To test for allergies, a grid consisting of disks with chemicals applied to them will be taped to your back for 48 hours. Reddening of your skin will identify your chemical sensitivities.

ATOPIC DERMATITIS

Atopic dermatitis, also known as eczematous dermatitis, is a condition in which there is an inherited tendency toward sensitive skin. Such sensitivity usually occurs early in life and is often associated with hay fever and asthma (see pp238–9). Atopic dermatitis can be exacerbated by excessive bathing with hot water and detergent soaps, and irritating fabrics such as wool. It's best treated by keeping skin hydrated (use a humidifier or put saucers of water on the radiators), showering with warm rather than hot water, and using emollient foams and creams, and a steroid cream.

---

some effective treatments, with minimal side effects.

Steroid creams The reaction occurring in your skin needs to be treated with a steroid cream, such as hydrocortisone.

Antihistamines Your doctor may also prescribe some antihistamine pills to counter any itchiness

Anti-inflammatories You may also be given prednisolone pills to further reduce inflammation and help relieve discomfort.

Antimicrobials If the affected area becomes infected, your doctor will also give you some antimicrobial medication. This may be oral antibiotics, antibiotic cream or ointment to apply to the skin, or antifungals for a fungal infection.

HOW CAN I HELP MYSELF?

There are several ways in which you can take steps to ease your dermatitis at home.

Check your beauty products
Does your bathroom cabinet look like a miniature version of the beauty section in a department store? If so, perhaps now is a good time to assess your products, identify which of your many lotions and potions may be responsible for causing your dermatitis, and get rid of them. In addition, the most practical thing to do is steer clear of the cause of your dermatitis.

Choose fragrance-free products
Fragrance is the most common cause of allergic reactions in the skin. Women are more likely to have allergic reactions from products because they use more than men. Read the manufacturers' labels on your cosmetics and household products carefully. Be aware that even products that can legally claim to be unscented may contain "masking fragrances."

Keep your skin moist Use emollients (moisturizers) to reduce water loss from your skin. These provide a thin film of ointment or cream to keep the water in and any infection and irritants out. Emollients aren't drugs and aren't absorbed by the skin, so there's no need to worry that you might be using them too much.

Psoriasis

Cold, windy weather, or even indoor heating, can result in dry, red skin. But if your skin starts scaling, cracking, or itching, psoriasis rather than environmental issues may be the cause.

WHAT IS IT?

Psoriasis is an autoimmune disease (see pp259, 266-71) in which a type of white blood cell called a T-lymphocyte, or T-cell, attacks healthy skin cells. The overactive T-cells prompt other immune responses that lead to more healthy skin cells and more T-cells being made, in a vicious circle that ultimately results in scaly, shiny patches of dead skin (see box below). While psoriasis can occur on any part of the body, the elbows, knees, and scalp are the usual sites.

People who suffer with psoriasis often have flare-ups. It appears to have a genetic component, but this is not yet well understood. However, there are well-known triggers of psoriasis to be aware of (see box opposite).

WHAT NEXT?

Your doctor will usually be able to diagnose the most common type of psoriasis (chronic plaque psoriasis) based on a physical examination of some affected skin. Rarely, he or she may want to take a small skin sample to send off for laboratory testing to confirm psoriasis. If your doctor suspects you have psoriatic arthritis, he or she will take a sample of blood to rule out other conditions.

(see pp259, 266-71)

(see box opposite)

DO I HAVE THE SYMPTOMS?

Psoriasis symptoms can vary but generally include:
- Pinkish red patches of skin covered with silvery scales
- Dry, cracked skin that may bleed
- Itchy, burning, or sore skin.

If, in addition to skin changes, you notice thickened, pitted, or ridged nails and swollen and painful joints, you may well have psoriatic arthritis. One person in 20 with psoriasis develops this inflammatory condition.

See your doctor if you have any of the above symptoms.

MY TREATMENT OPTIONS

Your doctor will work with you to find the treatment with the greatest benefits and fewest side effects. Treatments aim to interrupt the cycle that causes overproduction of skin cells. The traditional approach is to start with the mildest—creams you apply to the affected skin and phototherapy (UV light therapy)—and progress to stronger ones as necessary.

Creams, ointments, and solutions If you have mild to moderate psoriasis, your skin can be improved with creams and ointments alone. Some can also be combined with phototherapy.
- Steroid creams slow cell turnover by suppressing the immune system, reducing inflammation and itching.

CELL TURNOVER IN PSORIASIS

Cells in the the epidermis change gradually as they move toward the surface where they are shed continually in a process that normally takes three to four weeks. In skin affected by psoriasis, the rate of cell turnover speeds up so that the process takes only three to four days. Dead skin can't slough off quickly enough and builds up in thick, scaly patches on the skin.

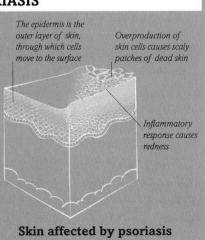

The epidermis is the outer layer of skin, through which cells move to the surface

Overproduction of skin cells causes scaly patches of dead skin

Inflammatory response causes redness

Skin affected by psoriasis

- Vitamin D analogues are synthetic forms of vitamin D, such as calcipotriene (Dovonex). They reduce inflammation and help stop cells from reproducing.
- Vitamin A analogues normalize DNA activity in the skin cells. Tazarotene (Tazorac) has been developed specifically for psoriasis. Tell your doctor if you plan to become pregnant while taking tazarotene.
- Anthralin ointment can smooth skin by removing scales, but stains everything it touches.
- Calcineurin inhibitors (tacrolimus and pimecrolimus) disrupt T-cells and are effective in the treatment of psoriasis.
- Coal tar is an old, but effective treatment for psoriasis. How it works is unknown, but it's messy, malodorous, and stains clothing.

Phototherapy This treatment uses natural sunlight or artificial ultraviolet (UV) light, either alone or in combination with medication.

- Sunlight, on even a brief daily basis, can destroy the super-active T-cells, reducing scaling and inflammation.
- UVB phototherapy, or broadband UVB therapy, uses controlled doses of UVB radiation. It can be used to treat single patches, widespread psoriasis, and psoriasis that resists creams or ointments.
- Narrowband UVB therapy is given two to three times a week until the skin improves, then weekly. However, it increases your risk of skin cancer.

- PUVA photochemotherapy involves using psoralen, either topically or orally, before exposure to UVA light and is a more aggressive treatment. Again, it increases your risk of skin cancer.
- Excimer laser is a beam of UVB light aimed at psoriatic skin to control scaling and inflammation.

Medication If you have severe psoriasis or it's resistant to other treatments, your doctor may prescribe drugs in pill form or as injections. Unfortunately, many come with serious side effects.

- Retinoids may reduce skin cell production, but because they can cause severe birth defects, you should avoid getting pregnant for six months after receiving this therapy.
- Immunosuppressants, such as methotrexate and ciclosporin, decrease skin cell production, suppress inflammation, and reduce the release of histamine (a chemical involved in allergy).
- Cytotoxic drugs, such as hydroxycarbamide, destroy cells and can be used in conjunction with phototherapy. Do not take them if you are pregnant or plan to become pregnant.
- Immunomodulators, such as alefacept and infliximab, block interactions between immune cells and are given as an intravenous infusion or injection.
- Azathioprine, a potent anti-inflammatory drug, may be used to treat severe psoriasis when other treatments fail.

HOW CAN I HELP MYSELF?
A few simple measures can improve your skin's appearance.

Bathe daily in warm, not hot, water and add oiled oatmeal, bath oil, Epsom salts, or Dead Sea salts. Blot your skin before applying a heavy, ointment-based moisturizer or oil while your skin is still moist.

Relieve redness and scaling by applying an ointment-based moisturizer and wrapping with plastic wrap overnight. Rinse off the next morning.

Expose your skin to small amounts of sunlight, but wear a sunscreen of at least SPF 15.

Cortisone cream (0.5% or 1%) bought over the counter will help when symptoms flare up.

Avoid alcohol during treatment since it can interfere with the effectiveness of some medications.

> **TRIGGERS FOR PSORIASIS**
>
> Episodes of psoriasis are typically triggered by:
> - Infections, such as strep throat or thrush (yeast)
> - Injury to the skin, such as a cut, insect bite, or severe sunburn
> - Stress
> - Cold weather
> - Smoking
> - Heavy alcohol consumption (four to six drinks a day)
> - Some medications, including lithium, beta-blockers, and antimalarial drugs.

Skin cancer

In these days of easy-to-use tanning lotions and sprays, there really is no excuse to bake in the sun and risk sunburn, which is actually a type of skin damage. Not only is it painful, but repeated sunburn can increase your risk of skin cancer—basal cell carcinoma, squamous cell carcinoma, and melanoma.

AM I AT RISK?

Risk factors for non-melanoma skin cancer include:

- Year-round sun exposure
- Childhood sunburns
- Fair skin, especially with blonde or red hair and freckles
- A large number of moles
- A suppressed immune system (e.g. due to HIV/AIDS or medication)
- Scars (burns, vaccinations) or leg ulcers are at risk of becoming cancerous
- Radiation therapy

Risk factors for melanoma include:

- Fair skin, especially with blonde or red hair and freckles
- A history of blistering sunburn
- Use of tanning beds
- Excessive sun exposure
- More than 50 moles
- A family and/or personal history of melanoma
- A suppressed immune system (e.g. due to HIV/AIDS or medication)
- Exposure to environmental chemicals such as creosote
- Genetic diseases associated with sun sensitivity.

UV LIGHT AND YOUR SKIN

Skin cancer is mainly caused by overexposure to ultraviolet (UV) light from the sun and other sources. There are three types of UV light—UVA, UVB, and UVC. The earth's ozone layer screens out UVC but UVA and UVB rays penetrate the atmosphere and can damage your skin. UVA penetrates deep within the skin to damage DNA in skin cells, making them more susceptible to cancer, especially melanomas (see p360). UVB rays cause sunburn and also increase the risk of skin cancer, particularly basal cell and squamous cell carcinomas.

Weather forecasts often include a sun or UV index so you can take the action needed for the different categories (see below):

Minimal You can safely stay outside with no protection.

Low to moderate Limit exposure between 10 am and 4 pm. Wear protective clothing, including a hat and UVA/UVB sunglasses; a regular T-shirt has an SPF of 6, but you can buy T-shirts with an SPF of 30. Use sunscreen of at least SPF 15.

High to very high Avoid the sun as much as possible between 10 am and 4 pm and cover up as above.

MY TREATMENT OPTIONS

Most skin cancers can be treated successfully by:

Excisional surgery The cancerous tissue is removed, together with a margin of healthy skin around it.

Freezing Small, early skin cancers can be destroyed with liquid nitrogen.

Laser therapy A laser beam vaporizes the cancerous cells.

Mohs surgery This is used for cancers in certain locations, such as near the nose, upper lip, and eye, as well as for recurring or difficult-to-treat cancers and for basal or squamous cell cancers.

Curettage Once the growth is removed your doctor can scrape away layers of cancer cells using a curet (circular blade).

Radiation therapy If surgery isn't possible, radiation can be used to destroy basal or squamous cell cancers.

Chemotherapy A specific combination of drugs is used to kill the cancer cells; these can be given as a cream or lotion in some cases.

Basal cell carcinoma

Basal cell carcinoma is the most common type of skin cancer, but fortunately it's also one of the most easily treated and least likely to spread around the body (metastasize).

WHAT IS IT?

As its name implies, this cancer arises from the basal cells within the skin's epidermis.

Basal cell carcinoma (BCC) is most common on areas that are exposed to the sun, such as your face, neck, hands, and ears. It can sometimes look like other skin conditions such as eczema or psoriasis, so you should always have any skin complaints checked out to be on the safe side.

WHAT NEXT?

Your doctor may be able to make a diagnosis during the consultation, but it's likely that a biopsy will be necessary if he or she suspects BCC. A small sample of the affected skin may be taken or the whole area cut out (known as an excision biopsy).

MY TREATMENT OPTIONS

Basal cell carcinomas may be treated by freezing, chemotherapy, excisional surgery, or curettage. If they're in a difficult location, your doctor may recommend a Mohs procedure (see opposite). About 94–99 percent of people with BCC are successfully treated, and this cancer is rarely life-threatening.

DO I HAVE THE SYMPTOMS?

A basal cell carcinoma may appear as:
- A scab that bleeds from time to time but doesn't heal properly
- A flat, scaly red mark
- A shiny bump
- A growth with elevated rolled edges, like a crater.

See your doctor if you notice any of the above.

HOW CAN I HELP MYSELF?

Check your skin regularly for any changes such as marks that are growing. Protect yourself from the sun (see opposite).

Squamous cell carcinoma

This less common skin cancer is a tumor of the squamous cells that lie just below the surface of the epidermis.

WHAT IS IT?

Squamous cell carcinoma (SCC) is more likely to spread to other parts of your body than basal cell carcinoma, but is easily treated if it's detected early. They can occur anywhere on the body but, like basal cell carcinomas, are most common in areas that get the most sun exposure: the face, neck, ears, and hands. They can also appear on scars or ulcerated skin, as well as chronic wounds.

WHAT NEXT?

If you've noticed any unusual changes in the texture of your skin, visit your doctor. An immediate diagnosis may be possible but you will probably need to have a small sample of the affected skin taken (a biopsy) or the whole area cut out (an excision biopsy) for examination under a microscope. When your doctor gets the results, he or she will be able to advise you on further treatment.

MY TREATMENT OPTIONS

These cancers are usually treated surgically. In some cases, if they're in a difficult location, your doctor may recommend a Mohs procedure (see opposite).

HOW CAN I HELP MYSELF?

Check your skin regularly for any changes such as a blemish that won't heal. Protect yourself from the sun (see opposite).

DO I HAVE THE SYMPTOMS?

A squamous cell carcinoma typically appears as:
- A raised, rough, scaly lump that may sometimes bleed and doesn't heal properly.

See your doctor if you have such a lump.

Melanoma

Melanoma is the most serious form of skin cancer. Unless treated early, it can metastasize and is potentially fatal. Even after treatment, it can recur.

WHAT IS IT?

Malignant melanomas often develop in or near a mole, but they can appear anywhere on the skin. The cancerous cells then spread to the surrounding skin and possibly to the lymph nodes and other areas of the body.

WHAT NEXT?

If you've noticed any changes in a mole, consult your doctor as soon as possible. Unless he or she can rule out melanoma, you'll be sent to have the mole removed and examined under a microscope.

MY TREATMENT OPTIONS

In general, your treatment options are as outlined on p358. If a melanoma is caught early while its effects are superficial, it can still be removed surgically as an outpatient. If the cancer goes deeper, then it must be removed in the hospital. In such cases, lymph nodes are investigated also to check for any spread of cancer cells; if affected these may need to be removed as well. You may also have an ultrasound or CT scan to check for any further spread of cancer cells.

HOW CAN I HELP MYSELF?

Every hour one person in the US dies of a malignant melanoma, because it wasn't discovered early enough and had spread to the lymph nodes and then to the rest of the body. That shocking statistic should be enough reason to make sure you check your skin every few months (get your partner or a friend to check your back and hard to see areas) and immediately report anything untoward to your doctor.

Most importantly, always protect yourself in the sun (see p358).

DO I HAVE THE SYMPTOMS?

Symptoms may include:
- A mole that changes color, size, or shape, or the appearance of what looks like a new mole.
- If it is untreated, a melanoma may become lumpy and ooze or bleed.

See your doctor if you have any of the above symptoms.

WATCH OUT FOR WARNING SIGNS

Doctors have a simple way of remembering what to look for in a mole that could be undergoing cancerous changes—and it's as easy as ABCDE.

A is for asymmetry; if a mole grows on one side more than the other, it warrants investigation since they are normally symmetrical.

B is for border; if the outer edge becomes irregular and not round, get your doctor to check it out.

C is for color; if the color of a mole becomes uneven or darker (even black), show it to your doctor.

D is for diameter; if a mole grows larger than ¼ in (6 mm) it needs medical examination.

E is for elevation; if a mole that was flat becomes raised or uneven on its surface, see your doctor.

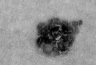

Asymmetry
A mole grows more on one side.

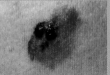

Border
The outer edge of a mole is irregular.

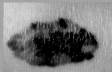

Color
The color varies from one shade to another.

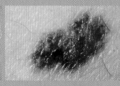

Diameter
The mole grows larger than ¼ in (6 mm).

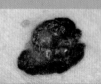

Elevation
A mole that was flat becomes raised.

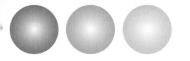

Pigmentation problems

Skin color is determined by your genes and the amount of pigment—melanin—your skin makes and stores. Normally, your skin has even coloring, so when patches of skin become much lighter or darker than usual, there may be a problem with pigment production.

Vitiligo

This patchy, often symmetrical, white discoloration commonly affects the face and hands.

WHAT IS IT?
Vitiligo occurs when the pigment-producing cells malfunction. The cause is not known but there is a genetic component; the immune system may also be involved.

WHAT NEXT?
Your doctor will make a diagnosis based on your medical and family history, and an examination.

MY TREATMENT OPTIONS
There is no cure, but there are some medical options you can try. **Steroid creams** can help return color to your skin if started early. **Repigmentation** Controlled exposure to sunlight or narrowband UVB (see p357) may cause pigment to return. **Depigmentation** This involves fading the rest of your skin to match the white areas.

(see p357)

DO I HAVE THE SYMPTOMS?
The symptoms may include:
- Usually symmetrical white areas on the face, hands, armpits, groin, feet, elbows, and knees.
- Whitening of your hair.

See your doctor if you have any of the above symptoms.

HOW CAN I HELP MYSELF?
You can use camouflage makeup.

Melasma

This patchy brown discoloration that mainly affects women appears on various areas of the face.

WHAT IS IT?
Melasma is due to melanocytes producing too much melanin. It's most likely to develop when you're pregnant and it usually appears on your cheeks, forehead, chin, and upper lip. It often develops gradually and may fade once the baby's born. It may also sometimes occur with the contraceptive pill or as a reaction to cosmetics.

WHAT NEXT?
Your doctor will make a diagnosis based on examining your skin.

MY TREATMENT OPTIONS
Consider stopping the pill and any causative cosmetics. If melasma doesn't fade after pregnancy, you may benefit from treatment. **Topical medication** Azelaic acid or retinoids are usually the first option. **Bleaching** Hydroquinone may be used, but its effects are permanent. **Light chemical peels** These remove the outer skin layers. **Non-ablative laser treatment** This blends back skin color.

HOW CAN I HELP MYSELF?
Sun exposure worsens melasma, so sunscreen with good UVA and UVB protection is vital (note that UVA can penetrate glass). It may help to avoid using cosmetics or anything else that may irritate your skin.

DO I HAVE THE SYMPTOMS?
The symptoms may include:
- Dark irregular patches on your face.

See your doctor if you have the above symptoms.

Acne and rosacea

Many teenagers suffer from acne vulgaris, the most common form of acne, which is triggered by hormonal changes at puberty; it usually clears up as people reach their 20s, although it can come and go during adult life, too. Rosacea is a skin condition that usually affects people in middle age.

Acne vulgaris

WHAT IS IT?

Skin with acne vulgaris is very oily with blackheads, whiteheads, cysts, and pimples. Women have both estrogen and testosterone, a male hormone that circulates in our bloodstream and that is partly responsible for acne. It seems that testosterone stimulates the sebaceous (oil) glands in the skin, which results in excess production of waxy, oily sebum.

As if oily skin were not enough, skin with acne cannot exfoliate dead skin cells properly. This is known as faulty keratinization. Every day our skin makes new cells and we need to shed old or dead ones, otherwise they clog up the pores on our skin. Clogged pores appear as stubborn whiteheads and blackheads.

There is a bacterium called *Propionobacterium acnes* that lives and multiplies in the sebum on the skin, causing inflammation and redness. With the helping hand of colonies of this bacterium, your skin then develops not only the blackheads and whiteheads, but also pimples and pustules. Large acne cysts develop if there is a lot of inflammation. If you squeeze any of these pimples, you risk scarring your skin.

WHAT NEXT?

Your doctor will examine your skin carefully since the treatment depends on the combination of acne features predominant on your skin.

MY TREATMENT OPTIONS

There is an array of treatments available for acne vulgaris. Your doctor will work with you to find one that produces the best results with the least side effects.

Gels, creams, and washes Many products called topicals are available to apply to your skin. There are two main types:
- Benzoyl peroxide works best

> ### DO I HAVE THE SYMPTOMS?
>
> Acne vulgaris concentrates in areas with lots of sebaceous glands and appears as:
> - Excessive oiliness of the face
> - Tiny blackheads
> - Small whiteheads
> - Red pimples
> - Painful large red lumps
> - Tender lumps beneath the skin without any heads (cysts)
> - Pus pimples.
>
> **See your doctor** if a symptom causes you problems.

> ### SAFETY OF RETINOID DRUGS
>
> Retinoid drugs, which are derived from vitamin A, can potentially cause serious side effects. They should not be used during pregnancy because they may cause birth defects in the unborn baby. Any woman who is of childbearing age and is prescribed a retinoid must be monitored with blood tests to ensure that she is not pregnant and must use appropriate contraception. Retinoids may also cause dryness of the skin and may increase the skin's sensitivity to sunlight so a sunscreen should be used at the same time as the retinoid medication. Isotretinoin may also raise cholesterol levels. Women with a history of depression should tell their doctor if he or she is considering prescribing isotretinoin.

HOW PIMPLES APPEAR

Your skin contains hairs that grow up through the epidermis from the dermis. A sebaceous gland around each hair produces sebum (oil) that waterproofs and lubricates the skin. When the gland is blocked, excess oil is trapped, the epidermis becomes inflamed, and a pimple results.

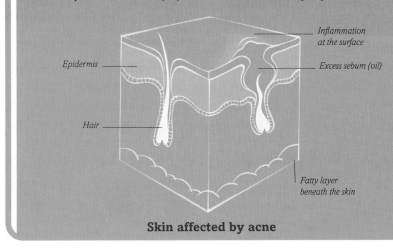

Epidermis

Hair

Inflammation at the surface

Excess sebum (oil)

Fatty layer beneath the skin

Skin affected by acne

with an antibiotic, such as clindamycin or erythromycin
- Retinoids, such as retinoic acid and adapalene gel, help unclog the pores by promoting the sloughing off of dead skin cells. If you have dry and sensitive skin, your doctor will probably start you on a cream and a low dosage to be used every other night. Retinoids should be applied only at night because they interact with sunlight. A non-pore-clogging sunscreen of SPF 30 should be used every day.

Light chemical peels To help remove dead skin cells and improve exfoliation, your doctor may refer you to a dermatologist for a light chemical peel (using 30 percent glycolic or salicylic acid, 4–6 percent). During such medical facials, the whiteheads and blackheads are removed and any cysts can be injected with hydrocortisone to decrease inflammation and help prevent scarring.

Oral contraceptives To counter the effects of testosterone, you can take oral contraceptive pills, which are very effective in the treatment of acne. The current trend is for doctors to prescribe those that have a low estrogen dose (20–30 mcg estrogen) because these tend to have fewer side effects (such as blood clots, breast tenderness, bloating, and nausea).

The newest and most popular oral contraceptive used in acne treatment is Yaz (ethinyloestradiol and drospirenone), which blocks testosterone significantly and has added benefits over other oral contraceptives in that it tends not to cause weight gain and has less potential to decrease your mood. Worldwide, the combination of ethinyloestradiol and cyproterone acetate is very effective.

Antibiotics Your doctor may prescribe a short course (three to six months) of antibiotics for your acne. The most common antibiotics are doxycycline, tetracycline, and minocycline, which are usually used while the gels, wash, or creams are taking effect. Once they have, then the antibiotics are gradually reduced.

Isotretinoin This powerful drug is derived from vitamin A and reduces inflammation, loosens the keratin, reduces sebum production, and diminishes the number of *P. acnes* bacteria on the skin. It has received a lot of media attention because of its potential side effects. You cannot take it during pregnancy since it can cause serious birth defects in the fetus. As a result, any woman of childbearing age who is prescribed isotretinoin must be monitored closely with blood tests to ensure that she is not pregnant and she must use the appropriate contraception.

Isotretinoin is given twice daily for 20 weeks, with the dosage

"Acne is a common problem, especially in the teenage years, but there are many effective treatments available."

based on your body weight. The results are both dramatic and long-lasting: over 85 percent of people are clear of acne after the treatment period.

However, such success comes with a downside, because there are a number of potential side effects. During treatment with isotretinoin you will probably experience a measure of dryness—of your skin, eyes, and lips, among others. The drug can also raise the cholesterol levels in the blood and this is another reason why blood tests need to be done and monitored.

This drug is usually reserved for the worst cases of acne vulgaris or for those who have not benefited from other treatment options. One of the main concerns is that isotretinoin can worsen depression and that there have been some suicides of patients while on the drug. So for women who have a tendency toward depression, it is important to get medical clearance from a psychiatrist.

HOW CAN I HELP MYSELF?

In addition to following your pre-scribed medical treatment, try one or more of the following self-help measures.

Keep your skin clean Wash your skin with warm water and a gentle cleanser no more than twice a day (especially after exercising) on the problem areas.

Avoid irritating the skin Facial scrubs, astringents, face masks, and overwashing irritate the skin and can worsen acne.

Don't pick or squeeze pimples Tempting though it may be, resist the urge to either pick or squeeze your acne pimples. This can lead to infection or scarring.

Wear your hair off your face If you have long hair, tie it back; if it is short, ensure it doesn't sit on your face, otherwise any oil from your hair can sit on your skin.

Don't block the pores Choose skin-care products that are either water-based or non-comedogenic (non-pore-clogging) and always remove your makeup before going to bed. Keeping makeup on all night long will clog pores.

Use lightweight makeup Opt for powder cosmetics rather than cream versions because they're less irritating to the skin.

Rosacea

WHAT IS IT?

This is a chronic skin condition affecting the face that starts with flushing on the cheeks, nose, and forehead then develops into more persistent redness of the face. The small blood vessels in the skin become broken, and there may be outbreaks of inflamed pimples and pus-filled spots. Rosacea is more common in women than men, often runs in families, and typically first appears after 30.

WHAT NEXT?

Your doctor will usually be able to make a firm diagnosis after thoroughly examining your skin.

Sometimes a tiny skin biopsy (a small sample of skin) may be taken for tests to exclude other rare types of facial rash.

MY TREATMENT OPTIONS

Your doctor may recommend any of a number of treatments to help your combat rosacea:

Oral antibiotics The mainstay of treatment is tetracycline, but your doctor may also prescribe doxycycline or minocycline.

Antibiotic creams Creams with metronidazole reduce inflammation and improve the complexion.

Sunscreen Sunscreen containing zinc, which has anti-inflammatory properties, can reduce the inflammation of rosacea.

DO I HAVE THE SYMPTOMS?

Rosacea affects more women than men and often runs in families. It first appears as red flushing on the cheeks, nose, and forehead. Other symptoms may include:

- Red, puffy skin
- Small red bumps
- Small pimples with white or yellow heads
- Tiny broken blood vessels
- If the rosacea affects the nose, the skin may thicken and turn a purplish red color.

See your doctor if you have any of these symptoms.

Laser treatment After the rosacea has cleared up, laser treatment can reduce any underlying redness and broken blood vessels on the nose and cheeks. The laser heat seals the blood vessels back together so that any red wiggly lines at the corners of the nose vanish. Laser treatment may also be helpful in reducing any thickening of the skin on the nose.

HOW CAN I HELP MYSELF?

There are a number of measures you can take to avoid making your rosacea worse:

Avoid trigger foods See below for a list of food that may trigger rosacea or make it worse.

Mild cleansers Only use gentle, non-irritating skin-care products to avoid stripping your face of its essential oils.

Avoid excess heat Sessions in a sauna or steam room can aggravate the redness.

Avoid excess cold Exposure to cold temperatures and wind can worsen redness, so use a scarf to protect your face.

Avoid exposure to sun Cover up when you're in the sun because exposure can make your skin condition worse.

Foods that may trigger rosacea

Keep a journal of what you eat and drink, then figure out which are your particular triggers and steer clear of them. Some of the known trigger foods are shown below. Other potential food triggers include dairy products, such as pasteurized milk, yogurt, and cream, as well as chocolate, wheat and wheat products, white flour, sugar, garlic, and eggs.

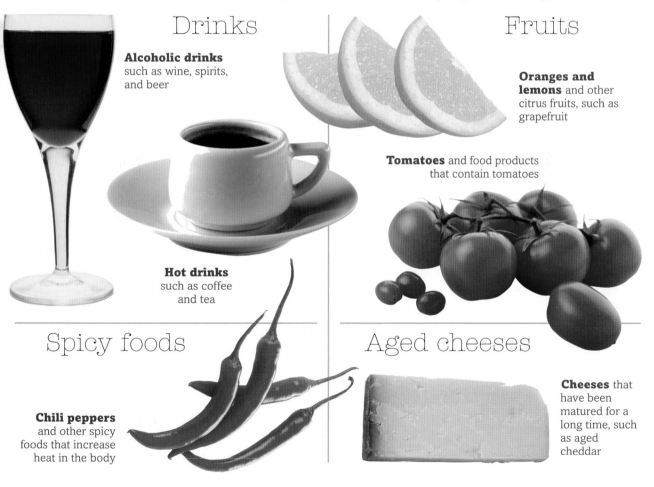

Drinks

Alcoholic drinks such as wine, spirits, and beer

Hot drinks such as coffee and tea

Fruits

Oranges and lemons and other citrus fruits, such as grapefruit

Tomatoes and food products that contain tomatoes

Spicy foods

Chili peppers and other spicy foods that increase heat in the body

Aged cheeses

Cheeses that have been matured for a long time, such as aged cheddar

Skin infections

When the protective barrier of the skin is breached by a microorganism, an infection is the result. Good hygiene routines help you to stay free from infection, and occasional invasions by a virus, bacterium, or fungus can normally be quickly and simply remedied to restore your skin's equilibrium.

Folliculitis

WHAT IS IT?

Infection of a hair follicle is likely to be the result of a cut inflicted while shaving your legs, allowing bacteria to enter. If you have repeated bouts of folliculitis, it may be best to use a different method of hair removal.

WHAT NEXT?

Your doctor will probably be able to diagnose the problem from an examination of the affected area.

MY TREATMENT OPTIONS

Your doctor may prescribe a topical antibiotic to put on the affected area. If a large area is affected, you may also be offered oral antibiotics. Ask your doctor about any side effects.

HOW CAN I HELP MYSELF?

Razor safety Soak reusable razors in an antiseptic solution for five minutes before use, and never share razors.
Get wet first Shaving after showering, when your hair is softer, makes it less likely that you will cut yourself while shaving.

DO I HAVE THE SYMPTOMS?

In folliculitis you may have:
● Small, yellow, pussy pimples
● Itching.
See your doctor if you have the above symptoms and are at all worried.

Warts

WHAT ARE THEY?

These skin growths come and go, and it can be difficult to eliminate them forever. They are caused by human papilloma viruses and can occur anywhere. Verrucas are warts on the soles of the feet.

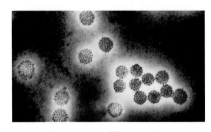

Human papilloma virus
There are over 100 different types of human papilloma virus; the majority are harmless but some lead to cervical cancer.

WHAT NEXT?

Most warts disappear without treatment, but this can take some time. If you have a persistent wart, visit your doctor or buy one of the over-the-counter wart treatments.

MY TREATMENT OPTIONS

Salicylic acid This is the active ingredient in many over-the-counter wart treatments.
Removal Your doctor may freeze off the wart with liquid nitrogen (cryotherapy) or burn it off using acid or electrodesiccation.

DO I HAVE THE SYMPTOMS?

There are three types of wart:
● Common warts on the hands, dotted with black spots
● Plantar warts on the soles of the feet (verrucas); these are dotted with black spots
● Flat warts on the wrists, backs of the hands, and face.
See your doctor if these are bothering you.

HOW CAN I HELP MYSELF?

See your doctor if you want to eliminate them permanently.

Impetigo

WHAT IS IT?

Impetigo is commonly seen on the face as honey-colored crusts. It is the result of a bacterial infection through broken skin, such as a cut, cold sore, or dermatitis (see p354).

WHAT NEXT?

Your doctor will probably be able to diagnose the problem from a close examination of the area. He or she will also take a skin swab and send it for laboratory analysis to identify the offending bacterium. Over 90 percent of cases involve *Staphylococcus* but, rarely, *Streptococcus* may be the culprit. Impetigo is extremely contagious and is spread by direct contact.

MY TREATMENT OPTIONS

Your doctor may prescribe an antibiotic foam, gel, lotion, or pledget (antibiotic-soaked wipe) as well as a ten-day course of oral antibiotics such as cefalexin.

HOW CAN I HELP MYSELF?

To prevent infection, avoid direct contact with others who are infected. If you are infected, see your doctor.

DO I HAVE THE SYMPTOMS?

The symptoms often develop in a typical sequence:
- Red skin and tiny fluid-filled blisters appear
- The blisters burst and release a yellow fluid
- The skin underneath the blisters becomes red and weeping
- The blisters dry out to form an itchy, honey-colored crust.

See your doctor if you experience such symptoms.

Cold sores

WHAT IS IT?

Cold sores have a habit of appearing at the most inopportune of times, often presaged by a telltale tingle. The result of infection with herpes simplex virus type 1, cold sores can come and go throughout life. The virus is very contagious and is passed on by direct skin contact. About six out of ten people have been infected by it by the time they reach adulthood, but only about 25 percent experience symptoms.

WHAT NEXT?

Self-help is sufficient provided you act in time (see below). If not, visit your doctor.

MY TREATMENT OPTIONS

Your doctor will prescribe a course of an antiviral drug such as famiclovir or valacyclovir.

HOW CAN I HELP MYSELF?

When you feel the characteristic tingling on your lip, make sure you have some remedies on hand.
Antiviral medications Apply one of the over-the-counter antiviral medications such as aciclovir. For this cream to be effective, you must apply it as soon as the first symptoms develop.

Trigger factors To prevent cold sores from reccurring, try to steer clear of these well-known trigger factors: stress, fatigue, cold winds, and sunburn.

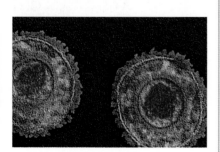

Herpes simplex virus
HSV invades skin cells and travels along nerve paths to the roots of the nerves, where it becomes dormant.

DO I HAVE THE SYMPTOMS?

Cold sores most commonly occur around the lips. Symptoms tend to appear in a certain order:
- The first indication is often a tingling in the affected site
- About six hours later, clusters of tiny, painful blisters begin to develop
- A day or so later, the blisters burst and then become crusty
- The blisters subside after 10–14 days.

See your doctor if you are bothered by these symptoms.

Hair loss

There are few conditions that will reduce a woman to tears but losing her hair is one of them. For many women, having a full head of hair is an integral part of feeling feminine, sexy, and healthy. A bad diet, stress, or overstyling can cause hair to fall out; with temporary hair loss your hair will grow back.

If you're suffering from some form of hair loss, the first thing to do is a hair count—that is, count all the hairs from your hairbrush and the shower drain each day. If after a week of counting you have over 700 hairs, it's time to see your doctor.

POSSIBLE CAUSES

To start with, he or she will want to ask some questions to find out if any new medications (such as lithium, isotretinoin, or heparin) or life events (such as illness requiring surgery, a bereavement, or rapid weight loss) could be the cause.

In addition, your doctor will want to take a blood sample to screen for a variety of other conditions that can cause your hair to fall out, including an underactive thyroid gland (see p327), lupus, (see p269), and iron-deficiency anemia (see pp248–9).

BOOST HAIR GROWTH

Your treatment will depend on what type of hair loss you have. Hair can often regrow, but it just takes time. In the meantime, boost your hair growing power by eating some key foods (see p370).

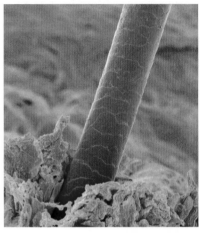

From root to tip
Overlapping scales cover the outside of each hair, the cuticle, to protect its central core of the fibrous protein keratin.

HOW YOUR HAIR GROWS

Each hair grows from a hair follicle within the dermis of the skin. In the hair bulb, or base of the follicle, cells divide rapidly to make each strand of hair. Each follicle follows a cycle of growth and rest, but not all follicles are synchronized, so every day some hairs grow while others fall out.

Your scalp has approximately 100,000 hairs and most are in the growing phase (the anagen phase). Hairs remain in this phase from two to seven years; the exact amount of time depends on your genes.

The anagen phase is followed by an intermediate catagen phase, then a resting, or telogen, phase. At the end of the resting phase, the hair falls out and a new one starts to grow. It's quite normal to lose hair every day (on average, you lose about 100 telogen hairs daily) because hairs are being constantly renewed and replaced.

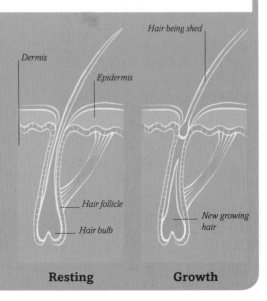

Dermis
Epidermis
Hair being shed
Hair follicle
Hair bulb
New growing hair

Resting　　　**Growth**

Traction alopecia

WHAT IS IT?

Alopecia is the medical term for hair loss, and traction refers to a persistent tug on the hair follicle over time, eventually causing the hair to fall out, This is usually caused by certain severe hairstyles, such as tight buns, chignons, ponytails, and close braiding, tugging too harshly on the hair follicles themselves. This constant strain on the follicles, over time, can lead to scarring of the scalp and permanent damage to the hair root, which can mean that the hair doesn't grow back.

DO I HAVE THE SYMPTOMS?

In traction alopecia, hair loss is associated with:
- Wearing bands in your hair that are too tight
- Always wearing a ponytail
- Wearing braided hair.

See your doctor if self-help measures don't work

WHAT NEXT?

The good news is that hair usually does grow back if the pulling on the follicles ceases.

MY TREATMENT OPTIONS

If you have tried changing your hairstyle and your hair is still not growing back, see your doctor. Bear in mind that African hair is more fragile than Caucasian hair, so if you braid your hair, take time out between braidings to let your follicles recover.

HOW CAN I HELP MYSELF?

Consider cutting your hair; if you always wear it up or back, perhaps it's time to try a different style. If you want to keep it long, avoid wearing it tightly all the time—pinning your hair back while preparing food is fine, but wear it loosely the rest of the time.

Telogen effluvium

WHAT IS IT?

Telogen effluvium is a temporary hair loss that can be alarming since quantities of growing hairs shift into the telogen phase, and your hair starts falling out in clumps.

This type of hair loss is usually due to a change in, or interruption to, your hair's normal cycle. This often occurs after pregnancy—the post-pregnancy "molt"—and is nothing to worry about. At other times, it may be related to a physical or emotional shock, such as an illness in which you had a fever; undergoing surgery that required general anesthesia; sudden weight loss; or a stressful event such as a bereavement.

DO I HAVE THE SYMPTOMS?

In telogen effluvium:
- Handfuls of hair fall out while washing, handling, or brushing your hair
- There is overall hair thinning.

See your doctor if you have the above symptoms.

WHAT NEXT?

If you have persistent hair shedding, your doctor may want to exclude conditions such as hyperthyroidism.

MY TREATMENT OPTIONS

No treatment is required. Typically, the hair follicles become active again in two or three months and your hair soon grows back.

HAIR BREAKAGE

One type of hair loss that is on the rise is from the resurgence in hair straightening. Hairs lost from excessive straightening tend to break off in pieces, so you end up with short strands of hair. Treat your hair kindly and don't choose a hairstyle that involves daily straightening with irons or periodic chemical straightening. Your hair will thank you for it.

HOW CAN I HELP MYSELF?

Avoid breaking your hair through straightening (see above). If your hair loss occurred after pregnancy or is due to illness or stress, your hair will grow back in time. If it doesn't, see your doctor as there may be another cause for the loss.

How to eat to keep your hair healthy

If you don't eat a good balanced diet, say you're trying to lose a few pounds and aren't following your usual good habits, then your hair is the first part of your body to reflect this. For full, lustrous locks, make sure your diet includes the following ingredients.

Zinc

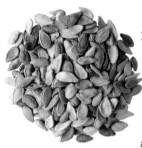

Pumpkin seeds, beef, and chickpeas are all zinc-rich foods, which are vital for hair growth. It helps to oil your scalp and ward off dandruff. In dietary supplement form, you should not take more than 40 mg a day.

B vitamins

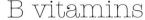

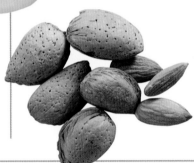

Bananas are rich in B_6, essential for healthy hair, and also contain B_3, B_5, and folic acid (B_9). All the B vitamins contribute to good skin and hair. Avocados are another good source of B vitamins.

Iron

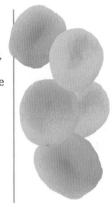

Dried apricots, liver, eggs, and whole-wheat bread are all iron-rich foods that contribute to healthy hair growth. Loss of hair can be a sign of iron-deficiency anemia (see p248–9).

Protein

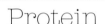

Fish, meat, eggs, tofu, and legumes are all good sources of protein. Eat protein at every meal; healthy hair growth requires a reasonable amount of protein to be able to manufacture the hair protein keratin.

Biotin

Almonds and other nuts contain biotin (100 g/4 oz of almonds = approx. 64 mcg biotin), which helps keep hair and nails thick and healthy. The recommended daily intake is 100–200 mcg.

Alopecia areata

WHAT IS IT?

The cause of alopecia areata is not known, although many doctors believe that it's an autoimmune disease (see p259), in which your body sees your hair as "foreign" and attacks the hair follicles.

WHAT NEXT?

If you are worried, see your doctor.

MY TREATMENT OPTIONS

After examination and testing, your doctor will discuss what treatments are available to you, along with any potential side effects.

Steroids The goal of these drugs is to stop the immune system from attacking your hair. The drugs can be applied as ointments or injected directly into the scalp. Injections are usually done every month for three to six months. Steroid treatment is usually effective and typically yields results within about three months. Early hair regrowth may be with gray hair but don't be alarmed by this since your normal color usually returns eventually.

Other treatments If steroids don't work, your doctor may suggest treatment with topical immunotherapy, topical minoxidil, or phototherapy (see p357).

HOW CAN I HELP MYSELF?

See your doctor and follow the advice and/or treatment.

DO I HAVE THE SYMPTOMS?

In alopecia areata:
- Hair loss usually appears as small, round bald patches all over the scalp.

See your doctor if you have the above symptom.

Female-pattern baldness

It is common for men to lose hair in a certain way as they get older—it gets thin on top and the hairline recedes. Few of us expect women to be similarly affected.

WHAT IS IT?

Female-pattern baldness (also known as androgenetic alopecia) differs from the classic male pattern (although both are related to testosterone levels in the body): women usually have thinning of the hair at the front, sides, or crown, and rarely go completely bald.

As we age, hair thins naturally and this is more apparent in some women: if you have lots of thick hair, you'll fare better than those with less abundant, finer hair.

In female-pattern baldness, the growing phase of the hairs shortens and the hairs become fine and more fragile. With each cycle, the hairs become rooted more superficially and fall out more easily. Female-pattern baldness often runs in families. Heredity will also influence the age at which you start to experience hair loss, as well as the pattern of your baldness, how fast your hairline changes and hair falls out, and how much falls out.

WHAT NEXT?

Because hormones play a part in female-pattern baldness, hair loss may first become apparent during menopause, so if you are worried, make an appointment with your doctor.

MY TREATMENT OPTIONS

When discussing treatments, ask your doctor about any potential side effects.

Hormone replacement therapy Such treatment can help stall the hair loss but is always given on a case by case basis.

Minoxidil lotion This comes in two strengths (2 and 5 percent) used twice daily (2 percent) or once daily (5 percent). This treatment is beneficial in up to half of affected women. To continue the success, you must use it each and every day or within a few months the new hairs that have grown will all fall out.

Spironolactone This drug blocks the actions of testosterone and can be taken in pill form.

Oral contraceptives serve to iron out hormone imbalances and can be used with good success.

Hair transplants If the hair loss can be stabilized, then hair transplanting can be effective. Transplanting single follicular units works best rather than multiple follicles. The hair takes three months to grow in.

HOW CAN I HELP MYSELF?

There's nothing you can do to stop the hair loss, but many women find that changing their hairstyle, hair extensions, or wigs help improve their appearance.

HAIR-LOSS PATTERNS

Female-pattern baldness can be inherited from either side of your family. Women's hair loss tends to follow a different pattern from men's: it becomes thinner overall, especially at the front, sides, and crown. Doctors assign a category to the amount of hair left from grade 1 (mild loss) to grade 3 (marked loss).

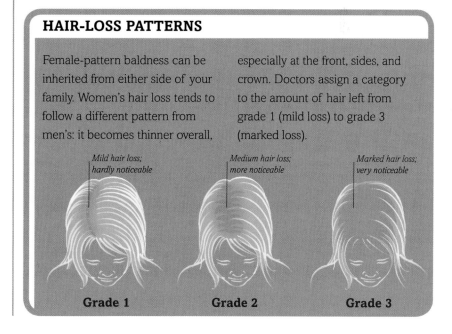

Mild hair loss; hardly noticeable

Medium hair loss; more noticeable

Marked hair loss; very noticeable

Grade 1   **Grade 2**   **Grade 3**

Cosmetic dermatology

As we get older we tend to become more critical of our skin—noticing every new wrinkle or blemish. Many women want to improve their complexion and retain a more youthful appearance. Whether it's achieving a more even skin tone or plumping up some laugh lines, there are plenty of options available.

DO I HAVE THE SYMPTOMS?

Cosmetic dermatology can help hide the effects of a wide range of skin symptoms, including:

- Lines and wrinkles
- Uneven pigmentation
- Noncancerous moles
- Sun-related aging
- Acne scars.

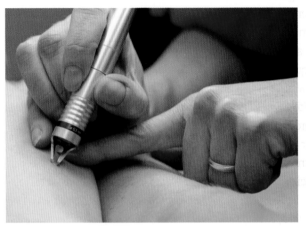

Laser treatment
A targeted laser beam can be positioned over your skin to treat just the right area. Dermatologists use laser treatments both for removing brown spots and melasma and for fading blood vessels.

WHAT IS IT?

Cosmetic dermatology is treatment of the skin, for example laser treatment or chemical peeling. These techniques help improve the physical appearance of the skin, such as acne scarring or skin discoloration. The treatment may or may not include healing a medical condition.

WHAT NEXT?

When assessing what procedures to use to improve your overall complexion, your dermatologist will consider:

- The texture of your skin
- The tone (firmness) of your skin
- The evenness of color
- How much laxity there is (that is, how your skin drapes and sags)
- The size of the pores
- Any lumps and bumps
- Any clogged pores or cysts.

Many studies show that when people evaluate age, they think that someone is older than they really are if they have brown spots. It seems that anything that mars the surface makes us appear older.

MY TREATMENT OPTIONS

Your cosmetic dermatologist will talk you through the most common procedures and advise you on which is best for your skin problem. Each treatment is usually delivered over several sessions. Be sure to ask about any potential side effects. You may feel that your skin needs time to settle before you go out in public.

Bleaching If you have brown spots or melasma (see p361), your doctor may suggest bleaching.

Chemical peels Your doctor will apply an acid to the area. It can target brown spots or fade blood vessels. The depth of skin removed by a peel can be varied. Superficial peels remove only a portion of the epidermis, whereas a medium-depth peel removes the whole epidermis and a tiny part of the underlying dermal tissue too. Peels stimulate the fibroblasts in the skin, and new skin forms to replace what has been peeled off. Your skin will have some redness, which can last a while. After a series of peels, your skin will look smoother and less wrinkled, and your complexion more even.

> "Between ages 25 and 30, collagen-making slows, yet collagen breakdown continues."

Microdermabrasion This removes surface skin but uses tiny crystals instead of acid. It is a more refined technique, removing only a fine layer of skin. A targeted stream of aluminium oxide crystals "sandblasts" your skin. You may notice a slight redness to the treated areas, but this fades quickly; several sessions two to four weeks apart result in younger-looking skin. This procedure is not appropriate for those with eczema or acne rosacea since it can cause flare-ups.

Laser skin resurfacing Your dermatologist uses a laser beam to destroy the epidermal layer and heat the underlying dermis. This stimulates the fibroblasts to produce new collagen fibers, to make skin appear smoother. The laser destroys tissue, which then repairs itself with new cells. This treatment is harsher than others, so can take a few months to heal fully.

There are less intense lasers available, called non-ablative lasers and radiofrequency devices. These treatments heat up the dermis, but without any damage to the epidermis. Recovery time is shorter; but you'll need more treatments to make your skin appear younger.

Laser skin resurfacing can remove brown spots and melasma (see p361), and fade prominent or broken blood vessels. About six sessions are necessary.

Botox is short for botulinum toxin type A. When injected into specific muscles, this neurotoxin blocks nerve impulses and paralyzes and relaxes muscles. The skin flattens and smooths. Each treatment last three to six months, so repeat injections are needed. Botox works well on deep, upper face lines, especially frown lines, horizontal forehead lines, and crow's feet.

Injectable dermal fillers can plump up and smooth out lines. Such fillers can be based on fat, collagen, hyaluronic acid, or calcium hydroxyapatite. These plumping agents give only temporary effects and the procedure will need to be repeated every few months. You may experience temporary redness, swelling, and bruising. The week before treatment you should not take aspirin or vitamin E, or drink any alcohol, to reduce your chances of bruising. You may have needle marks or swelling afterward.

There is some research to suggest that products based on

COSMECEUTICALS— THE FUTURE?

Products once restricted to the use of qualified medical practitioners are making their way into moisturizers and over-the-counter products. The dermal filler Restylane™, for example, can now be applied to the surface of your skin in a cream that promises great results. It will be interesting to see how many dermatological techniques covered will soon be available to buy yourself to do in the comfort of your own home.

hyaluronic acid may stimulate your body to make its own collagen, so long after treatment your skin may still look younger.

HOW CAN I HELP MYSELF?

Reduce the need for cosmetic dermatology by protecting yourself against potential sun damage. Use a high-factor sunscreen and avoid excessive sunbathing. This will reduce the build-up of lines and wrinkles and the possibility of unsightly skin discoloration.

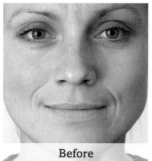
Before

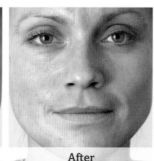
After

Disappearing wrinkles
Injectable dermal fillers can smooth out deep frown lines and wrinkles. After treatment, the wrinkles between nose and mouth and under the eyes are less prominent.

Resources

CHAPTER 2: UNDERSTANDING THE CHANGES

Dr.Donnica.com
www.drdonnica.com
A women's health information website that provides easily accessible, up-to-date, accurate information on specific areas of women's health.

Society for Women's Health Research
1025 Connecticut Avenue, NW
Suite 701
Washington, DC 20036
Tel: 202-223-8224
www.womenshealthresearch.org
E-mail: info@womenshealthresearch.org
A nonprofit organization whose mission is to improve the health of all women through research, education, and advocacy. Through its website, the society shares information on various conditions, and women's health research and policy issues.

The National Women's Health Information Center
US Department of Health & Human Services
Office on Women's Health
8270 Willow Oaks Corporate Drive
Fairfax, VA 22031
Tel: 800-994-9662
www.4woman.gov
The Office on Women's Health seeks to educate health professionals and motivate behavior change in consumers through health information. Its website offers free information on over 800 topics concerning women.

Women's Health Matters
Women's College Hospital
790 Bay Street
Suites 902-908
Toronto, ON M5G 1N8
www.womenshealthmatters.ca
Email: info@womenshealthmatters.ca

Women's Health Matters is a website dedicated to providing reliable, up-to-date information and research specifically for Canadian women.

CHAPTER 3: STAYING WELL

American Heart Association
National Center
7272 Greenville Avenue
Dallas, TX 75231
Tel: 800-242-8721
www.hearthub.org
Find out about healthy lifestyle changes and beneficial diets, such as the Mediterranean diet, on the American Heart Association website. It also provides information about heart conditions, tools such as a BMI calculator, and resources in an interactive format.

Centers for Disease Control and Prevention (CDC)
1600 Clifton Road
Atlanta, GA 30333
Information line: 800-232-4636
24-hour help line: 888-232-6348
www.cdc.gov/nccdphp/dnpa/nutrition.htm
Email: cdcinfo@cdc.gov
This public health agency aims to protect everyone's health through promotion, prevention, and preparedness. In addition to information on nutritional health, its website includes health protection goals and a Healthiest Nation Initiative (www.healthiestnation.org).

Celiac Disease Foundation
13251 Ventura Blvd. No 1
Studio City, CA 91604
Tel: 818-990-2354
www.celiac.org
Email: cdf@celiac.org
This organization gives information on common allergies to gluten and wheat.

The Dash Diet
www.nhyoko.med.navy.mil/pdf/DASH%20Program.pdf
Information on a healthy eating plan to lower blood pressure.

Fruit and Veggies Matter
www.fruitandveggiesmatter.gov
This website (developed by the CDC) gives specific information on your personal daily requirement of fruit and vegetables. It also provides recipes and a calendar showing which produce is in season when.

Health Canada
www.hc-sc.gc.ca/index-eng/php
Email: info@hc-sc.gc.ca
Health Canada is the federal department responsible for helping people maintain and improve their health. This website includes a useful feature on Canada's food guide.

Medline Plus
www.nlm.nih.gov/medlineplus/womenshealth.html
The National Institutes of Health and National Library of Medicine website provides extensive information, overviews, and news on a wide variety of women's health issues.

MyPyramid.gov
www.mypyramid.gov
This website by the Department of Agriculture Center for Nutrition Policy and Promotion offers dietary guidelines, personalized eating plans, and advice on how to assess your food choices.

National Sleep Foundation
1522 K Street, NW, Suite 500
Washington, DC 20005
Tel: 202-347-3471
www.sleepfoundation.org
Email: nsf@sleepfoundation.org
Learn more about sleep on this website's A-Z of topics and conditions.

CHAPTER 5: HORMONES, FERILITY, AND MENOPAUSE

The American College of Obstetricians and Gynecologists
409 12th Street, SW
PO Box 96920
Washington, DC 20090-6920
Tel: 202-638-5577
www.acog.org
A nonprofit organization of women's physicians that promotes patient education and understanding of obstetric and gynecologic issues.

Association of Reproductive Health Care Professionals
1901 L Street, NW, Suite 300
Washington, DC 20036
Tel: 202-466-3825
www.arhp.org
Although this is a membership association for physicians, nurses, and public health professionals, it includes news and information that patients can use on all aspects of reproductive health, such as contraception and sexuality.

The North American Menopause Society
PO Box 94527
Cleveland, Ohio 44101-4527
Tel: 440-442-2660
www.menopause.org
Email: info@menopause.org
Information is provided on all aspects of menopause and long-term health effects, symptoms, and therapies.

Women's Health Matters
See entry under Chapter 2

CHAPTER 6: BREAST HEALTH

American Cancer Society
24-hour helpline for immediate information: 1-866-228-4327
www.americancancersociety.org
www.cancer.org
Provides information about the disease for patients, family, and friends, and facilitates support programs, message boards, and discussion groups.

Breastcancer.org
www.breastcancer.org
Through its website, this organization seeks to provide reliable, comprehensive, and up-to-date information on breast cancer and treatments. All information on the site is reviewed by members of a professional advisory board.

Comprehensive Breast Care Associates
3300 Tillman Drive
Bensalem, PA 19020
Tel: 215-633-3456
www.comprehensivebreastcare.com
Supportive website offering advice on how to come to terms with the diagnosis, clinical trials, and treatment options.

Health Canada
See entry under Chapter 3

CHAPTER 7: HEART AND CIRCULATION

American Heart Association
See entry under Chapter 3

American Stroke Association
National Center
7272 Greenville Avenue
Dallas, TX 75231
Tel: 800-787-8984
www.strokeassociation.org
The American Stroke Association offers patient education materials, scientific statements, information on stroke support groups, and practical advice for caregivers on its website.

Heart and Stroke Foundation of Canada
222 Queen Street, Suite 1402
Ottawa, ON K1P 5V9
Tel: 613-569-4361
www.heartandstroke.ca
This website provides information on risk assessment, blood pressure, and cholesterol among other issues, and includes features on healthy living and recipes for life.

CHAPTER 8: BRAIN AND NERVES

Alzheimer's Association
225 North Michigan Avenue, Fl 17
Chicago, IL 60601-7633
Tel: 312-335-8700
24/7 helpline for information, referral and support: 800-272-3900
www.alz.org
This website explains what Alzheimer's is and how to live with it, and includes information on the latest research and treatments. It also has an interactive tour of the brain and links to other websites with additional information.

MAGNUM The National Migraine Association
100 North Union Street, Suite B,
Alexandra, VA 22314
www.migraines.org
This association was created to raise awareness of the condition and assist migraine sufferers and their families. The website includes medical news, myths and realities about migraines, and suggested reading materials.

Mayo Clinic
www.mayoclinic.com/health/tension-headache
A website with lots of sensible advice for people suffering from tension-type headaches, including drug therapies, lifestyle and home remedies, and advice on coping and support.

Multiple Sclerosis Society of Canada
National office tel: 416-922-6065
To contact the division office in your area, tel: 800-268-7582
www.mssociety.ca
Email: info@mssociety.ca
This website provides information on the disease, treatments, and support in your community.

National Institute of Neurological Disorders and Stroke (NINDS)
National Institutes of Health
9000 Rockville Pike
Bethesda, Maryland 20892
www.ninds.nih.gov
This is a very comprehensive website of the section of the US National Institutes of Health that deals with neurological disorders and strokes. If you know your diagnosis, this site will give you good information about your condition.

National Multiple Sclerosis Society
www.nationalmssociety.org
A comprehensive website for anyone living with MS. There's information on what MS is, how to manage the condition, and the latest research, and there's an online community, which includes personal stories and online chat and message boards.

National Parkinson Foundation
1501 NW 9th Avenue/Bob Hope Road
Miami, Florida 33136-1494
Tel: 305-243-6666/800-327-4545
www.parkinson.org
Email: contact@parkinson.org
This website gives clear information and advice on Parkinson's and how to maintain optimum health. It includes a useful glossary of terms, and has an online community.

CHAPTER 9: MENTAL HEALTH

Canadian Mental Health Association
Phoenix Professional Building
595 Montreal Road, Suite 303
Ottawa ON K1K 4L2
Tel: 613-745-7750
www.cmha.ca
Email: info@cmha.ca
A really practical and informative website, with advice on emotional wellness; how to keep a good work/life balance and cope with stress; the family, and mental health; and understanding different mental illnesses. There's also an online

discussion group and information on various support centers.

National Institute of Mental Health
www.nimh.nih.gov
This organization seeks to transform the understanding and treatment of mental illness through research. The website's health and outreach section provides clear, precise information on various conditions, their treatment, what kind of help is available and how to get it, and links to articles and other websites on related information.

National Mental Health America
2000 North Beauregard Street
6th Floor
Alexandria, VA 22311
Tel: 703-684-7722/800-969-6642
Crisis line: 800-273-TALK
www.nmha.org
This organization was formerly known as the National Mental Health Association. Its website contains fact sheets on mental health topics, treatments and medications, frequently asked questions, and how to find help.

CHAPTER 10: BREATHING AND RESPIRATION

American Lung Association
61 Broadway, 6th Floor
New York, NY 10006
Tel: 212-315-8700
To contact your nearest American Lung association call: 800-LUNGUSA
To speak to a lung professional, call the helpline: 800-548-8252
www.lungusa.org
This website has detailed information on the most common lung disease issues and risk factors, and provides fact sheets, special reports, and information on support services. There's also a section on air quality and related stories.

Canadian Lung Association
1750 Courtwood Crescent, Suite 300
Ottawa, ON K2C 2B5

Tel: 613-569-6411
Toll-free: 888-566-LUNG (5864)
www.lung.ca
Email: info@lung.ca
This website covers all aspects of breathing problems, and provides valuable advice on how to protect your lungs and hot topics by season.

Medline Plus
See entry in Chapter 3

CHAPTER 11: BLOOD DISORDERS

National Heart, Lung, and Blood Institute (NHLBI)
PO Box 30105
Bethesda, MD 20824-0105
Tel: 301-592-8573
www.nhlbi.nih.gov
The website for this organization provides information for health professionals, researchers, patients, and the public.

CHAPTER 12: BONES AND JOINTS

American Academy of Orthopaedic Surgeons
www.aaos.org
Although this website is geared toward health professionals, there is a useful patient information section for the public on orthopedic conditions and treatments, wellness advice, and so on.

Arthritis Foundation
PO Box 7669
Atlanta, GA 30357-0669
Tel: 800-283-7800
www.arthritis.org
Provides support and information about arthritis and living with the disease, and publishes *Arthritis Today,* the consumer health magazine.

Canadian Orthopaedic Association
www.coa-aco.org
This website provides patient information and resources, and links to other websites.

National Institute of Arthritis and Musculoskeletal and Skin Diseases (NIAMS)
1 AMS Circle
Besthesda, MA 20892-3675
Tel: 301-495-4484
Toll free: 877-22-NIAMS (226-4267)
www.niams.nih.gov
Email: NIAMSinfo@mail.nih.gov
Provides a health information index for easily accessible details on a wide range of conditions.

CHAPTER 13: DIGESTIVE SYSTEM

American College of Gastroenterology
PO BOX 342260
Bethesda, MD 20827-2260
Tel: 301-263-9000
www.acg.gi.org
A website for professionals that includes a GI patient center providing information on GI diseases, and answers to frequently asked questions.

American Gastroenterological Association (AGA)
4930 Del Ray Avenue
Bethesda, MD 20814
Tel: 301-654-2055
www.gastro.com
Includes information on digestive disorders and support programs.

CHAPTER 14: ENDOCRINOLOGY AND METABOLISM

American Diabetes Association
ATTN: National Call Center
1701 North Beauregard Street
Alexandria, VA 22311
Email: AskADA@diabetes.org
www.diabetes.org
A comprehensive website detailing all types of diabetes and treatments with sections on nutrition and lifestyle and prevention.

Canadian Diabetes Association
1400-522 University Avenue
Toronto ON M5G 2R5
Tel: 800 BANTING (226-8464)
www.diabetes.ca
Email; info@diabetes.ca
User-friendly website on all aspects of diabetes with nutritional advice and literature to order online.

The Hormone Foundation
8401 Connecticut Avenue, Suite 900
Chevy Chase, MD 20815-5817
Tel: 800-HORMONE
www.hormone.org
Email: hormone@endo-society.org
The Hormone Foundation is a source of hormone-related health information for the public and professionals alike. Learn more about glands and hormones and a wide range of endocrine conditions and topics on its website.

UpToDate Inc
95 Sawyer Road
Waltham, MA 02453
Tel: 800-998-6374
www.uptodate.com/patients
Email: customerservice@uptodate.com
Uptodate is an information resource for clinicians and patients on a huge variety of conditions. The information is regularly updated by a group of expert clinicians. It also has a section on patient stories.

CHAPTER 15: BLADDER AND URINARY TRACT

National Institute of Diabetes and Digestive and Kidney Diseases
Building 31, Rm 9A06
31 Center Drive, MSC 2560
Bethesda, MD 20892-2560
Tel: 301-496-3583
www2.niddk.nih.gov
Various health and disease topics and treatments are included, as well as information on clinical trials for patients.

Women's Health Matters
See entry in Chapter 2

CHAPTER 16: SKIN AND HAIR

American Academy of Dermatology
930 East Woodfield Road
Schaumberg, IL 60173
Tel: 866-503-SKIN (7546)
www.aad.org
Email: MRC@aad.org
The Academy is committed to promoting healthier skin, and its website gives relevant details on sun safety and various skin conditions and diseases, including skin cancer.

American Society for Dermatologic Surgery (ASDS)
24154 Network Place
Chicago, IL 60673
Tel: 847-956-0900
www.asds.net
This website has a section on consumer information that gives advice on skin health and safety through the year and throughout your life, advice on what causes skin problems, and various dermatologic procedures.

The Skin Cancer Foundation
149 Madison Avenue
Suite 901
New York, NY 10016
Tel: 212-725-5176
www.skincancer.org
This website offers information on skin cancer and advice on prevention of the disease. There are sections on preventing and treating sunburn, anti-aging, and sun-protective clothing.

Canadian Dermatology Association (CDA)
www.dermatology.ca
This website includes sun safety information for outdoor workers, a sun awareness program, general information on various skin conditions, and access to related organizations that run support groups for those with skin conditions.

Index

intrauterine devices (IUDs) 132–3, 135
intravenous urogram (IVU) 346
IQ 19
irritable bowel syndrome (IBS) 63, 276, 302, 304–5
itching, vaginal 108–9

J

joints 72, 84, 258–83

K

Kegel exercises
ketoacidosis 320
kidneys 334–5
   cancer 348–9
   kidney stones 330, 335, 338, 346–7
   pyelonephritis 338
knees, osteoarthritis 263

L

labyrinthitis 193
laparoscopy 98, 112–13
laryngitis 236
leg pain 85
leukemia 248, 250, 254–5
leukoplakia 289
libido 34–5, 44
life expectancy 16, 23, 26–7, 89
lifting, preventing back pain 275
lip disorders 74
liver 78, 334
   disorders 72, 118, 254, 296–9, 306
lobular carcinoma in-situ (LCIS) 155
lobular neoplasia (LN) 155
lumbar puncture 179
lungs 230–1
   asthma 76, 238–9
   cancer of 231, 242–3
   chronic obstructive pulmonary disease 240–1
   pneumonia 76, 234
   pulmonary embolism 252–3
lupus 259, 269–70, 368
luteinizing hormone (LH) 89, 112
lymph system 72, 156–7
lymphedema 157
lymphocytes 254
lymphomas 254–5

M

macromastia 150
macular degeneration 68, 191
magnetic resonance imaging scans (MRI) 179
major depressive disorder (MDD) 211, 215, 218
malnutrition 216
mammography 144–5, 151, 152–3, 154
mania 211, 212
manic depression 212
mastalgia 146–9
mastectomy 156, 157
mastitis 146, 148, 153
medication, for mental health 226–7
meditation 62
melanoma 358, 360
melasma 361, 372, 373
memory loss 16, 40, 47, 184–5
Ménière's disease 188, 192
meningitis 72, 181
menopause 30, 34, 41, 136–41
   adenomyosis in 102
   atrophic vaginitis in 108
   breasts 145
   depression 17
   hair loss 371
   heart disease 16, 163
   hysterectomy 103
   insomnia 61
   migraines 182
   osteoporosis 260–1
   "postmenopausal zest" 38, 137
   sexual disorders 222, 223
   uterine cancer 104
menorrhagia 35, 91, 101
menstruation 13, 15, 35, 88, 89
   anemia 247, 248
   breasts 144–5, 146–7
   diabetes 324
   disorders 90–3, 102, 250–1, 276
   epilepsy 195
   migraines 182
   PMDD 211
mental health 16, 202–27
   at different life stages 28, 36, 40, 42, 44
   treatment 224–7
mesothelioma 243
metabolic syndrome 36, 324
metabolism 15, 318–31
micromastia 151
micturating cystourethrogram (MCUG) 338

migraines 17, 63, 182–3, 192, 194
miscarriage 124, 125, 126
moles 360
mononucleosis 296
moods
   changes 74, 212
   stabilizers 227
mouth
   care 68–9
   disorders 75, 271, 288–9
multiple births 131
multiple sclerosis (MS) 192, 198
muscles 15, 57, 259
myeloma 254–5
myocardial infarction 166
myocardial perfusion scan 169

N

nails 72, 84, 85
nature versus nurture 20–1, 26
neck
   pain 67, 83, 272–5, 282
   swelling 75
nerve cells 179
nervous system 178–81
neuroleptics 226
neurological disorders 178–99
nipples 77
nodes, swollen 81
nodules 236
nose disorders 75, 250, 251, 254
nutrition see diet; food

O

obesity 32, 58–9
   abdominal 322–4
   and diabetes 322–4
   and heart disease 163
obsessive compulsive disorder (OCD) 207
oligomenorrhea 90, 101
oral health 26, 45, 68–9, 162
orgasms 223
osteoarthritis 16, 263–5, 272–3, 282
osteoporosis 16, 38, 45–6, 258–62
   and HRT 138
   and obesity 59
   prevention 140
   and smoking 64
otitis externa 186
otitis media 187, 188

Acknowledgments

Publisher's Acknowledgments

Dorling Kindersely would like to thank the following: Hilary Mandleberg for her unfailing professionalism throughout this project; John Freeman for photography; model Holly Newbury; Dawn Bates and Emma Forge; Dr. Naomi Craft; Jane de Burgh; Dr. Laszlo Tabar for the information in the graph on p153; Fiona Hunter, Bsc (Hons) Nutrition, Dip Dietetics; Yvonne Bishop-Weston, Foods for Life nutrition clinics, www.optimumnutritionists.com, email: clinic@ foodsforlife.co.uk, tel: 0871 288 4642; Elma Aquino, Will Hicks, and Adam Walker for design assistance; Stephanie Schwartz for proofreading; Vanessa Bird for the index.

All illustrations by Juliet Percival

Picture Credits
The publisher would like to thank the following for their kind permission to reproduce their photographs:

(Key: a-above; b-below/bottom; c-center; f-far; l-left; r-right; t-top)

Alamy Images: amana images inc. 7tc; Daniel Dempster Photography 172; FogStock 41c; Guy Croft SciTech 197l; Bubbles Photolibrary 305b; Phototake Inc 162, 243; botonics Limited (www.botonics.co.uk): 373; Corbis: Heide Benser 37c; Bettmann 17; Envision 93l; Howard Sochurek 166; DK Images: Stephen Oliver 141cla; Courtesy of the Royal Botanic Gardens, Edinburgh 93r; Getty Images: Alterndo Images 20r; altrendo images 7tr; Cornelia Doerr 62; Michael Goldman 50; Hulton Archive 22; William McCoy-Rainbow 205; Benn Mitchell 47r; Thomas Northcut 140; Marc Romanelli/The Image Bank 47l; Terry Vine 37r; Health and Safety Executive: poster Skin Checks for Dermatitis (c) Crown copyright material is reproduced with the permission of the Controller of HMSO and Queen's Printer for Scotland 354t; iStockphoto.com: Carmen Martínez Banús 20l; Jill Chen 141cl; Martina Ebel 353b; Quavondo Nguygen 353t; Anthony Rosenberg 23; Thomas Stange 32c; Valeria Titova 139; Mediscan: 153; Owen Mumford Ltd: 110; Photolibrary: 133ca; BananaStock 40c; Big Cheese 46l; Blend Images 32l, 33r, 41l, 353ca; Brand X Pictures 237; Corbis 7bc, 353cb; Digital Vision 2, 41r, 46r, 202; image100 168; Juice Images 33l; moodboard 40r, 353c; Photoalto 226; Photodisc 37l, 46c; Photographer's Choice 145; Purestock 36c; Phototake: PDSN 171; PunchStock: Mixa 32r; Rex Features: Garo/ Phanie 138, 195r; RESO 40l; Voisin / Phanie 204; Science Photo Library: 106r, 114, 174, 260l, 260r, 295, 296b, 299, 309; AJ Photo 271; Samuel Ashfield 155; Biophoto Associates 12; Dee Breger 319; BSIP / Laurent / Laetitia 217; BSIP, Cavallini James 255; BSIP, Ducloux 197r; CDC 296t; Centre for infections/ Health protection agency 366; CNRI 338, 349b, 360fbl; Custom Medical Stock Photo 133cb, 195l, 360r; Michael Donne 372; Du Cane Medical Imaging Ltd 253, 313; Eye of Science 120, 367; Simon Fraser 273, 298; Dr. Robert Friedland 185; Chris Gallagher 169; Adam Gault 161, 344; GJLP 331; Steve Gschmeissner 251, 251cr, 254, 289, 297, 343, 349t; Gusto Images 95, 347; Institut Pasteur/ Unite Des Virus OncongenesF 278; ISM 94, 97, 328; Kwangshin Kim 336; James King-Holmes 123, 252; Mehau Kulyk 148, 264; Dr. Najeeb Layyous 131; Living Art Enterprises 282; Dr. Karl Lounatmaa 115; Dr. P. Marazzi 260c, 265, 272, 360c, 360l; BSIP 291b; David M. Martin, M.D. 291t; Moredun Animal Health Ltd 119; Don Fawcett 122, 305t; Professors P.M. Motta & F.M. Magliocca 301; Dr. Gopal Murti 232; Susumu Nishinaga 368; D. Phillips 300; Dr. Linda Stannard, UCT 116; James Stevenson 360fbr; Saturn Stills 135b, 355b; Andrew Syred 246; Dr. E. Walker 106l, 249, 288; Dr. Keith Wheeler 89; Zephyr 267l; Shutterstock: J.T. Lewis 268; William Stuart: 139r; SuperStock: 47c; age fotostock 135c

All other images © Dorling Kindersley
For further information see: www.dkimages.com